Clinical Dilemmas in
Diabetes

Clinical Dilemmas in

Diabetes

EDITED BY

Adrian Vella, MD

Associate Professor of Medicine
Department of Endocrinology
Mayo Clinic
Rochester, MN, USA

Robert A. Rizza, MD

Professor of Medicine
Department of Endocrinology
Mayo Clinic
Rochester, MN, USA

⊛WILEY-BLACKWELL

A John Wiley & Sons, Ltd., Publication

This edition first published 2011, © 2011 by Blackwell Publishing Ltd

Blackwell Publishing was acquired by John Wiley & Sons in February 2007. Blackwell's publishing program has been merged with Wiley's global Scientific, Technical and Medical business to form Wiley-Blackwell.

Registered office: John Wiley & Sons Ltd, The Atrium, Southern Gate, Chichester, West Sussex, PO19 8SQ, UK

Editorial offices: 9600 Garsington Road, Oxford, OX4 2DQ, UK
The Atrium, Southern Gate, Chichester, West Sussex, PO19 8SQ, UK
111 River Street, Hoboken, NJ 07030-5774, USA

For details of our global editorial offices, for customer services and for information about how to apply for permission to reuse the copyright material in this book please see our website at www.wiley.com/wiley-blackwell

Library of Congress Cataloging-in-Publication Data

Clinical dilemmas in diabetes / Edited by Adrian Vella, MD, Associate Professor of Medicine, Department of Endocrinology, Mayo Clinic, Rochester, MN, USA, Robert A. Rizza, MD, Professor of Medicine, Department of Endocrinology, Mayo Clinic, Rochester, MN, USA.
      p. ; cm.
   Includes bibliographical references and index.
   ISBN 978-1-4051-6928-8 (pbk. : alk. paper)
   1. Diabetes.   2. Evidence-based medicine.   I. Vella, Adrian, editor.   II. Rizza, Robert A., editor.
   [DNLM: 1. Diabetes Mellitus–therapy.   2. Diabetes Mellitus–diagnosis.   3. Evidence-Based Medicine–methods. WK 810]
   RC660.C4635 2011
   616.4′62–dc22
                                                                                      2010052327

A catalogue record for this book is available from the British Library.

This book is published in the following electronic formats: ePDF 9781444340266; Wiley Online Library 9781444340280; ePub 9781444340273

Set in 8.75/12pt Minion by Aptara® Inc., New Delhi, India
Printed and bound in Singapore by Fabulous Printers Pte Ltd

1   2011

Contents

Contributors

Rami Almokayyad, MD
Endocrine Fellow
Division of Endocrinology, Department of
    Medicine, University of Minnesota
    Medical School
University of Minnesota
Minneapolis, MN, USA

Morgan L. Brown, MD, PhD
Resident
University of Alberta
Edmonton, AB, Canada

William T. Cefalu, MD
Douglas L. Manship, Sr. Professor of
    Diabetes
Chief, Joint Program on Diabetes,
    Endocrinology and Metabolism
Pennington Biomedical Research Center &
    LSUHSC School of Medicine
New Orleans, LA and Baton Rouge, LA,
    USA

Maria L. Collazo-Clavell, MD
Associate Professor of Medicine
Division of Endocrinology, Diabetes,
    Metabolism & Nutrition
Mayo Clinic
Rochester, MN, USA

Robert M. Cuddihy, MD
Medical Director
International Diabetes Center
World Health Organization Collaborating
    Center for Diabetes Education,
    Translation and Computer Technology
Minneapolis, MN, USA

Sean F. Dinneen, MD, FRCPI
Senior Lecturer in Medicine
Department of Medicine
Clinical Science Institute
NUI Galway
Galway, Ireland

Vivian Fonseca, MD
Professor of Medicine and Pharmacology
Tullis Tulane Alumni Chair in Diabetes
Chief, Section of Endocrinology
Tulane University Health Sciences Center
New Orleans, LA, USA

Robert L. Frye, MD
Professor of Medicine
Division of Cardiovascular Diseases
Mayo Clinic
Rochester, MN, USA

Praveena Gandikota, MD
Endocrine Fellow
Endocrine, Diabetes and Nutrition Division
Department of Medicine
St Luke's Roosevelt Hospital
New York, NY, USA

Chiara Guglielmi, MD, PhD
PostDoc Fellow
Department of Endocrinology & Diabetes
University Campus Bio-Medico
Rome, Italy

Michael D. Jensen, MD
Tomas J. Watson, Jr. Professor in Honor of
    Dr. Robert L. Frye
Mayo Foundation
Rochester, MN, USA

Blandine Laferrère, MD
Assistant Professor of Medicine
Division of Endocrinology
Diabetes and Nutrition Obesity Research
    Center Department of Medicine
St Luke's Roosevelt Hospital Center
Columbia University College of Physicians
    and Surgeons
New York, NY, USA

Stephen H. McKellar, MD, MSc
Resident
Division of Cardiovascular Surgery
Mayo Clinic
Rochester, MN, USA

L. Yvonne Melendez-Ramirez, MD
Assistant Professor of Medicine
Joint Program on Diabetes, Endocrinology
    and Metabolism
Pennington Biomedical Research Center &
    LSUHSC School of Medicine
New Orleans, LA & Baton Rouge, LA, USA

John M. Miles, MD
Professor of Medicine
Endocrine Research Unit
Mayo Clinic
Rochester, MN, USA

Manpreet S. Mundi, MD
Senior Associate Consultant
Division of Endocrinology
Mayo Clinic
Rochester, MN, USA

Kalpana Muthusamy, MD
Clinical Fellow
Division of Endocrinology
Mayo Clinic
Rochester, MN, USA

Timothy O'Brien, MD, PhD
Professor of Medicine,
Consultant Endocrinologist/Director of
  REMEDI
Department of Medicine and
  Endocrinology/Diabetes Mellitus
University College Hospital/National
  University of Ireland Galway
Galway, Ireland

Aonghus O'Loughlin, MB, MRCPI
Specialist Registrar in
  Endocrinology/Diabetes Mellitus
Department of Medicine and
  Endocrinology/Diabetes Mellitus
University College Hospital/National
  University of Ireland
Galway, Ireland

Michael O'Reilly, MB, BCh, BAO, MRCPI
Specialist Registrar in
  Endocrinology/Diabetes Mellitus
Department of Medicine and
  Endocrinology/Diabetes Mellitus
University College Hospital/National
  University of Ireland
Galway, Ireland

Paolo Pozzilli, MD
Professor of Endocrinology
Head of Department of Endocrinology &
  Diabetes
University Campus Bio-Medico, Rome,
  Italy;
Professor of Diabetes Research
Barts & the London School of Medicine &
  Dentistry
London, UK

Philip Raskin, MD
Professor of Medicine
Clifton and Betsy Robinson Chair in
  Biomedical Research
University of Texas Southwestern Medical
  Center at Dallas
Dallas, TX, USA

Deepika S. Reddy, MD
Assistant Professor
Department of Endocrinology
Scott & White Clinic
Temple, TX, USA

John W. Richard III, MD
Endocrinology Fellow
Division of Endocrinology, Diabetes,
  Nutrition and Metabolism
University of Texas Southwestern Medical
  Center at Dallas
Dallas, TX, USA

Robert J. Richards MD
Associate Professor of Medicine
Joint Program on Diabetes, Endocrinology
  and Metabolism
Pennington Biomedical Research Center &
  LSUHSC School of Medicine
New Orleans, LA and Baton Rouge, LA,
  USA

Matheni Sathananthan, MD
Endocrinology Fellow
Division of Endocrinology, Diabetes,
  Nutrition and Metabolism
Mayo Clinic
Rochester, MN, USA

F. John Service MD, PhD
Professor of Medicine
Mayo Clinic College of Medicine
Rochester, MN, USA

Steven A. Smith, MD
Associate Professor of Medicine
Medical Director, Mayo Patient Education
Consultant in Endocrinology, Diabetes
  Nutrition and Metabolism
Health Care Policy & Research
Mayo Clinic
Rochester, MN, USA

Galina Smushkin, MD
Fellow
Mayo Clinic
Division of Endocrinology
Rochester, MN, USA

Preface

Clinical Dilemmas in Diabetes is a book that arose out of several different motivations. The primary motivator may have been a desire to shed some light onto how to translate results of clinical trials to individual patient care. Indeed, the passage of time continues to demonstrate that "common sense" is still (unfortunately) an uncommon commodity, but one which is necessary for the optimal management of Diabetes.

Another potential motivator is the realization that blind adherence to algorithm-based approaches to clinical care is a poor substitute for informed decision making in the clinic. With this in mind, we chose several subjects of relevance to diabetes that deserve discussion and debate. We hope this will be the first iteration of a book that will develop and grow over time – assimilating new chapters and topics for debate – in much the same way that diabetes care continues to develop.

Adrian Vella
Robert A. Rizza
February 2011

PART I
Prediabetes and the Diagnosis of Diabetes

1 Is prediabetes a risk factor or is it a disease?

Kalpana Muthusamy[1] and Adrian Vella[2]

[1] Clinical Fellow, Division of Endocrinology, Mayo Clinic Rochester, MN, USA
[2] Associate Professor of Medicine, Department of Endocrinology, Mayo Clinic, Rochester, MN, USA

LEARNING POINTS

- The diagnostic criteria for prediabetes and diabetes are based on the relationship of hyperglycemia with microvascular disease.
- Defects in insulin secretion and action occur in people with impaired fasting glucose and impaired glucose tolerance.
- An oral glucose tolerance test may help to better characterize patients at higher risk of progression to type 2 diabetes.
- Intervention may delay the progression to diabetes.

Prediabetes, as previously defined by the American Diabetes Association (ADA), includes subjects with fasting plasma glucose (FPG) >100 mg/dl and <126 mg/dl and/or 2-hour plasma glucose following a 75-g oral glucose load >140 mg/dl and <200 mg/dl. The rate of progression to diabetes without any intervention is about 28.9% over a 3-year period as seen in the placebo arm of the Diabetes Prevention Program [1]. A 9-year longitudinal study from Olmsted County, Minnesota, reported a similar rate of diabetes progression of 34% [2]. The prevalence rate of prediabetes in the American adult population, as reported by CDC from 2003 to 2006, was 25.9% [3]. This represents 57 million American adults, a significant number of whom are predisposed to developing diabetes if adequate intervention is not undertaken. Therefore, understanding the definition of prediabetes, its implications, pathogenesis, and appropriate management becomes critical to any clinician.

Prediabetes includes two categories, impaired fasting glucose (IFG) and impaired glucose tolerance (IGT). Examining the evolution of these criteria will help us understand not only the basis of the current definitions, but also provide us guidance for the necessary evaluation and management.

Prediabetes, diabetes, micro- and macrovascular disease

Impaired glucose tolerance (IGT) is defined by a plasma glucose 2 hours after a 75-g oral glucose load >140 mg/dl and <200 mg/dl, while impaired fasting glucose (IFG) is defined by a fasting plasma glucose >100 mg/dl and <126 mg/dl.

IGT is a terminology that has been long known and has been a part of the ADA classification since 1979 [4]. IFG as a separate entity was established in an ADA report published in 1997 [5] and was later adopted by an expert WHO panel in 1999 [6]. These categories were intended to be seen as risk factors for future diabetes and cardiovascular disease rather than distinct clinical groups. The definition for IGT has undergone little change since its inception. IFG was initially defined as fasting plasma glucose >110 mg/dl and <126 mg/dl. This classification was rather arbitrary and reflected the then available evidence suggesting an insulin secretory defect and an increased risk of cardiovascular disease.

Brunzell et al. performed intravenous glucose tolerance tests in 66 subjects with a wide range of fasting glycemia [7]. Acute insulin response and glucose disappearance rate were markedly lower in subjects with fasting plasma glucose above 115 mg/dl in comparison to those with a fasting glucose below 115mg/dl. The main limitation of this data was

Clinical Dilemmas in Diabetes, First Edition. Edited by Adrian Vella and Robert A. Rizza
© 2011 Blackwell Publishing Ltd. Published 2011 by Blackwell Publishing Ltd.

the relatively small number of patients in the fasting plasma glucose group 115–149 mg/dl ($n = 3$). The Paris Prospective Study noted an increasing risk of diabetes with incremental fasting plasma glucose, despite normal glucose tolerance (2-hour-value after a 75-g oral glucose tolerance test <140 mg/dl). The relative risk of developing subsequent diabetes in the IGT and IFG (fasting plasma glucose >109 mg/dl) groups was 9.6 and 5.6, respectively [8]. The impact of hyperglycemia on cardiovascular mortality was also examined in this study, with the age-adjusted relative risk for coronary heart disease death noted to be 1.32 (1.04–1.67) in subjects in the fasting plasma glucose category of 104–124 mg/dl in comparison to the group <104 mg/dl [9]. A similar increase in risk was observed with increased post-challenge glucose in the Whitehall study that followed 18,403 male civil servants for a total of 7.5 years [10].

The microvascular effects of prediabetes were investigated in a few studies with mostly uniform results. Subjects with a capillary blood glucose between 120 and 200 mg/dl, following a 50-g oral glucose load did not have any discernible difference from controls in the prevalence of retinal abnormalities over a 10-year follow-up period [11]. Klein et al. evaluated the effect of impaired glucose tolerance, with plasma glucose between 140 and 200 mg/dl after a standard 75-g oral glucose load [12]. Age-adjusted frequency of visual impairment as measured by visual acuity of ≤ 20/40 was higher in the IGT group when compared to men with diabetes and normoglycemic women. However, the rates of retinopathy were uniformly low across all groups with no significant intergroup differences. In another report from two different groups of patients, including Pima Indians and male civil servants, development of retinopathy was mostly confined to subjects with 2-hour plasma glucose exceeding 200 mg/dl, without any marked change in the intermediate groups [13].

Following these earlier studies, one of the important debates that ensued was the comparability between IGT and IFG with regard to outcomes. Data from a longitudinal study of Pima Indians showed greater prevalence of IGT over IFG among nondiabetic subjects [14]. However, the 5-year cumulative incidence of diabetes was much higher for IFG at 31% in comparison to 19.9% for subjects with IGT. The combination of these two risk factors was better than either alone with an incidence of 41.2%. A receiver operating characteristic (ROC) curve analysis showed that, by defining IFG using a fasting glucose ≥ 102 mg/dl, the prevalence in the two groups was mirrored. This might not have necessarily led to identifying the same set of sub-jects, as these two cohorts might have included subjects who were mutually exclusive. However, the sensitivity and specificity of diabetes prediction was equaled in the IFG and IGT groups when using a definition of IFG >103 mg/dl as opposed to 110 mg/dl. In a Mauritian [15] cohort of 3,229 nondiabetic subjects, 148 had IFG alone in comparison to 489 with isolated impaired post-challenge glucose. A combination of IFG and IGT was present in 118 subjects. The sensitivity, specificity, and positive predictive value for prediction of progression to diabetes were 50, 84, and 24%, respectively, for IGT. Although IFG was less sensitive, it had a better specificity and positive predictive value at 26, 94, and 29%, respectively. These data would suggest that IFG defines a smaller, yet a more extreme category of glycemia that progresses to diabetes more predictably. However, from a population perspective, IFG identifies a lesser percentage of people progressing to diabetes, making it difficult to successfully implement diabetes prevention measures based on fasting plasma glucose alone. In this study, the optimal definition of IFG that gave the best combination of sensitivity and specificity for diabetes prediction was a fasting glucose >99 mg/dl [16]. These data formed the basis for the revised IFG criteria of plasma glucose >100 mg/dl and less than 125 mg/dl, in a follow-up report in 2003 [17].

It is important to remember that in clinical practice, the risk of progression to diabetes follows a gradient across a seamless continuum of glucose levels [16]. While scrutinizing the evidence to decide the optimal definitions of IGT and IFG and their individual value, it is critical to understand if IGT and IFG act as risk factors for micro- and macrovascular disease independently of diabetes.

It is generally accepted that microvascular disease, such as retinopathy, neuropathy, and nephropathy, is a function of the degree and duration of hyperglycemia. Contrary to the earlier studies that did not reveal an increased frequency of retinopathy among people with prediabetes, some recent studies demonstrated an elevated risk of microvascular disease even in subjects with hyperglycemia less than the diabetic range. A subset of the Diabetes Prevention Program cohort was investigated with fundus photographs at a mean 5.6 years of follow-up [18]. Changes of diabetic retinopathy were reported in 7.9% of the impaired glucose group and in 12.6% of the group that developed diabetes on follow-up. Although the subjects who developed retinal changes were not significantly different from those without these changes in the impaired glucose group, they tend to have a higher baseline prevalence of hypertension, lower HDL, higher triglycerides, and a history of gestational diabetes.

The rates of retinopathy and nephropathy were higher in individuals with impaired fasting glucose in comparison to those with impaired glucose tolerance on 10 years of follow-up of a group of Pima Indians, also supporting the previous evidence that IFG might denote a metabolically advanced state [19]. As opposed to these results, the incidence of diabetic retinopathy was reported to be very low at 28–31/10,000 person-years of follow-up in a large Japanese cohort of atomic bomb survivors with impaired glycemia [20]. A steep rise in the incidence and prevalence of fundus changes were noted only when the fasting plasma glucose was >125 mg/dl and the 2–hour post-challenge glucose >198 mg/dl. A similar threshold for retinopathy also evolved in the AusDiab study [21]. A clear threshold effect was not evident for microalbuminuria and the relation to rise in glucose was more gradual. Subjects with neuropathy were more likely to have retinopathy and microalbuminuria in the AusDiab cohort with impaired glucose metabolism [22]. Collectively, although there is evidence for increased prevalence and incidence of microvascular changes before the onset of diabetes, these changes predominantly occur with higher levels of glycemia.

In summary, the recently proposed definitions of prediabetes are dependent on their ability to identify individuals with a high risk of progression to diabetes. Defining IFG using a fasting glucose >100mg/dl increased the prevalence of prediabetes from 19.3% to 36.3% on evaluation of the NHANES III data [23]. Whether this definition portends true benefit or places a higher societal burden for preventive measures has been questioned [24]. We also have to factor in the behavioral impact of this labeling on individuals [25]. Strong antagonistic opinions to the new cutoff cite the lack of net proven benefit based on a detailed decision analysis [26].

Most recently in 2010, the title "Prediabetes" was renamed as "Categories of increased risk for diabetes" to reflect the risk of progression to diabetes rather than the subsequent micro- and macrovascular outcomes. An equivalent intermediate category for A1C was also identified, with values between 5.7% and 6.4% indicating a heightened risk for diabetes development [27–29].

Prediabetes and atherosclerosis: Why do they associate and how to best predict the risk?

A progressive increase in cardiovascular risk has been shown with rising blood sugars, across a spectrum ranging from normal to significant hyperglycemia. The DECODE study group showed a J-shaped relationship between all-cause mortality and plasma glucose, whether fasting or post-challenge [30]. A plausible and intuitive explanation for the increased cardiovascular risk is the clustering of other well-known traditional risk factors in patients who develop prediabetes [31]. The San Antonio Heart Study followed 614 nondiabetic Mexican American individuals and demonstrated that subjects who developed diabetes had a more atherogenic profile at baseline, including higher triglycerides, LDL and total cholesterol, BMI, blood pressure, insulin, and lower HDL than the group that did not develop diabetes [32]. The clustering of risk variables explained all the observed metabolic features rather than a single underlying etiology [33]. Low cardiorespiratory fitness had a significant impact on all-cause mortality in women with IFG in the 16-year follow-up in the Aerobic Center Longitudinal Study (ACLS) [34].

Studies that examined the ability of IGT and IFG to predict cardiovascular risk and mortality suggest that IGT is a better predictor of all-cause mortality [35, 36] and cardiovascular disease [37–39]. In contrast, data from Norwegians followed over 22 years showed that fasting plasma glucose was an important predictor of cardiovascular death [40]. Adding to these already varied results, a Chinese study showed equivalent performance of IGT and IFG in predicting cardiovascular disease risk [41]. The Atherosclerosis Risk in Communities Study (ARIC) also showed that both IGT and IFG were associated with an increased prevalence of cardiovascular risk factors with none being worse than the other [42]. It is also important to remember the important role of other cardiovascular risk factors in the development of atherogenesis. In agreement, the Framingham Offspring and San Antonio Heart Studies have shown that the knowledge we gain from post-challenge hyperglycemia might add little to what we might already know from traditional cardiovascular risk factors [43, 44].

Is there a role for OGTT in clinical practice?

This has been a topic of considerable debate, which was fueled by the 1997 ADA recommendation to favor the use of fasting plasma glucose over OGTT. The huge influx of data that followed in favor and disfavor of this recommendation has helped shape the definition of prediabetes as reviewed earlier. Prevalent use of OGTT has been limited by its inconvenience, cost, and poor reproducibility. Marked intra- and interindividual variation in postload glucose has been demonstrated in multiple studies [45–48]. McDonald et al. showed that the standard deviation for fasting glucose was about 5 mg/dl, whereas it was substantially higher for 1- and 2-hour postload glucose where the deviation around the mean was 20–30 mg/dl [46]. This degree of fluctuation leads to misclassification, with nearly 39% of people diagnosed with IGT found to be normal on a repeat OGTT within 2–6 weeks [49].

Given that individuals spend at least 6–9 hours on a given day in the postprandial state, knowledge gained from a standardized glucose load cannot be ignored [50]. As discussed earlier, IGT is a better predictor of diabetes and macrovascular risk than fasting glucose. Although in practice clinicians almost never use the OGTT except in special situations such as pregnancy, it continues to remain a valuable epidemiological tool.

What is the underlying pathogenesis and natural history of IGT and IFG?

Hyperglycemia develops when, in response to impaired insulin sensitivity, the secretion of insulin declines. As we would expect, the spectrum of disorders with disturbed glucose metabolism en route from normoglycemia to development of diabetes would encompass defects of insulin action and β-cell secretion. Butler et al., using pancreatic tissue obtained from autopsy, showed that β-cell volume is decreased by 40% in IFG compared to normoglycemic individuals [51]. It has also been shown that the usual 0.7% per year rate of β-cell deterioration is doubled in IGT with accelerated progression to diabetes [52]. There have been attempts to dissect IGT and IFG to denote specific defects in glucose homeostasis, but these have yielded contrasting results. Most studies reported increased insulin resistance in IGT [53–55] and decreased β-cell function in IFG [53, 54, 56] as the predominant metabolic derangements, using data from insulin clamps and glucose tolerance tests. In contrast, the Botnia study concluded that IFG is more characterized by insulin resistance and IGT by impaired insulin secretion with decreased I/G ratio (Insulin/glucose ratio) [57]. The amplitude of insulin secretion and its response to oscillations in glucose were blunted in IGT [58]. Bock et al. reported both defective insulin secretion and action with meal ingestion in IGT, whereas in individuals with isolated IFG the postprandial glucose metabolism was completely normal but they had an inappropriately elevated fasting

endogenous glucose production [59]. Understandably, a combination of IGT and IFG presents a morphologically advanced group with more severe metabolic impairments than isolated presentation of either [56].

In the progression from normoglycemia, it is not imperative that both IGT and IFG develop before transition to diabetes, as we have learnt from the Baltimore Longitudinal Study of Aging [60]. During a 10-year follow-up, only 37% with IFG went on to develop IGT and only 15% with IGT developed IFG. The progression from baseline IGT/IFG to diabetes happened at an accelerated rate of 39.3%. This has also been confirmed in a cohort of Pima Indians, where one-fourth of the subjects with IGT developed diabetes in 5 years and two-thirds in 10 years [61]. The best predictors of this progression were age, male gender, BMI, and central obesity [60, 61]. The progression from normoglycemia to diabetes is more slow and gradual with a 10-year cumulative incidence of 7.01% by 2-hour glucose and 1.48% by fasting glucose.

Management of prediabetes

Relatively few studies have addressed the role of intervention in people with prediabetes. In the Diabetes Prevention Program (DPP) [1], lifestyle intervention in affected individuals decreased the incidence of diabetes by 58% and by 31% when treated with metformin in comparison to the control group. The average weight loss achieved was 0.1, 2.1, and 5.6 kg in the placebo, metformin, and lifestyle groups, respectively. Similar studies have been replicated in different populations, with the Finnish Diabetes Prevention Study demonstrating a comparable weight loss of 4.2 kg with lifestyle modification and a 58% reduction in diabetes incidence over 3.2 years [62]. In the Indian Diabetes Prevention Programme and the Da Qing IGT and Diabetes Study, in accordance with the impression that the South Asians represent a metabolically disadvantaged group for a given weight, the BMI of the subjects with prediabetes was lower in comparison to Caucasians; 25–26 kg/m^2 [63, 64]. They experienced a more rapid rate of progression to diabetes of 55% and 67% in their control groups, respectively, over 3–6 years. Despite minimal or no weight loss with lifestyle intervention, they still had a 28% and a 46% reduction in diabetes progression.

Apart from metformin, the pharmacologic agents that have been utilized in this setting include troglitazone in several studies, and acarbose in STOP-NIDDM. Troglitazone, during its short span of use in DPP before the drug discontinuation in 1998 due to concerns of liver toxicity, lowered the diabetes incidence rate more significantly in comparison to the other groups [65]. Two short-term studies concluded that the ability of this drug to prevent progressive secretory dysfunction and improve insulin action contributed to its effect on slowing diabetes progression [66, 67]. The increased glycemic durability of rosiglitazone in the ADOPT trial and the decreased incidence of diabetes in the rosiglitazone subgroup in the DREAM trial suggests that this is a class effect for the thiazolidinediones [68, 69]. On the other hand, there are potential risks associated with thiazolidinedione use that must be considered—including an increased risk of hospitalization for heart failure, edema, and fracture.

Acarbose, although successful in decreasing the incidence of diabetes in the STOP-NIDDM study, had a 31% discontinuation rate due to gastrointestinal side effects [70]. Blockade of the renin angiotensin system did not offer any significant advantage, as noted in the DREAM trial, but a modest 3.7% absolute risk reduction in the incidence of diabetes by valsartan was reported in the recently published NAVIGATOR trial [71]. The nateglinide arm in the NAVIGATOR trial did not show any benefit, despite the association of postprandial hyperglycemia with diabetes and cardiovascular risk [72]. Collectively, despite variable glycemic effects, none of the therapeutic agents have been shown to have micro- or macrovascular benefit in the prediabetes population.

One of the commonly cited criticisms of DPP is the replicability of the aggressive lifestyle intervention in their protocol, in common practice. The support and the education offered to the subjects were individualized and included a total of 22 visits in the first year. This is in sharp contrast to current practice, even in the diabetic population. Despite these challenges, we should note that the moderate weight loss achieved in these trials had significant beneficial effects on blood pressure and cholesterol [1, 73]. Risk factor reduction in this population is highly desirable given the high incidence of cardiovascular disease and mortality with diabetes development. Lifestyle modification also resulted in an overall change to healthier habits in this cohort with reduction in smoking. The 10-year follow-up of the DPP cohort confirms that the glycemic benefits of lifestyle intervention are long lasting [74]. One of the key points to be addressed is, if successful intervention at this stage, apart from lowering glycemia, would also lower the risk of future macrovascular disease. The emergent macrovascular and mortality benefits noted from early glycemic intervention in the 10-year follow-up of the UKPDS cohort, in comparison to the ADVANCE and ACCORD trials that included subjects with advanced diabetes, mandate further investigation in the prediabetic population. The beneficial effect in the UKPDS cohort was most pronounced in the metformin arm. The strongest intervention trial in individuals with prediabetes, DPP, has established the superior efficacy of lifestyle intervention over metformin in the short term. This further strengthens our argument to favor behavior and lifestyle modification over early initiation of drugs. The cost–benefit analysis of this approach in people with prediabetes is sparse [75]. Further research into the long-term cost-effectiveness of early lifestyle intervention is needed.

In conclusion, prediabetes identifies a group of individuals at high risk of progression to diabetes and who have increased cardiovascular mortality compared to the normoglycemic population. Clustering of other cardiovascular risk factors might explain the increased macrovascular events in this group. Early lifestyle intervention is needed to decrease the risk of progression to diabetes and potentially offer protection against accelerated atherogenesis.

Reference

1. Knowler WC, Barrett-Connor E, Fowler SE, et al. Reduction in the incidence of type 2 diabetes with lifestyle intervention or metformin. *N Engl J Med.* **346**(6):393–403, 2002.

2. Dinneen SF, Maldonado D, IIIrd, Leibson CL, et al. Effects of changing diagnostic criteria on the risk of developing diabetes. *Diabetes Care.* **21**(9):1408–1413, 1998.

3. National Diabetes Fact Sheet 2007 [cited 2010 February 17th]; Available from: http://www.searchfordiabetes.org/public/documents/CDCFact2008.pdf

4. National Diabetes Data Group. Classification and diagnosis of diabetes mellitus and other categories of glucose intolerance. *Diabetes.* **28**(12):1039–1057, 1979.

5. Report of the Expert Committee on the Diagnosis and Classification of Diabetes Mellitus. *Diabetes Care.* **20**(7):1183–1197, 1997.

6. Alberti KG, Zimmet PZ. Definition, diagnosis and classification of diabetes mellitus and its complications. Part 1: diagnosis and classification of diabetes mellitus provisional report of a WHO consultation. *Diabet Med.* **15**(7):539–553, 1998.

7. Brunzell JD, Robertson RP, Lerner RL, et al. Relationships between fasting plasma glucose levels and insulin secretion

during intravenous glucose tolerance tests. *J Clin Endocrinol Metab.* **42**(2):222–229, 1976.

8. Charles MA, Fontbonne A, Thibult N, Warnet JM, Rosselin GE, Eschwege E. Risk factors for NIDDM in white population. Paris prospective study. *Diabetes.* **40**(7):796–799, 1991.

9. Charles MA, Balkau B, Vauzelle-Kervroedan F, Thibult N, Eschwege E. Revision of diagnostic criteria for diabetes. *Lancet.* **348**(9042):1657–1658, 1996.

10. Fuller JH, Shipley MJ, Rose G, Jarrett RJ, Keen H. Coronary-heart-disease risk and impaired glucose tolerance. The Whitehall study. *Lancet.* **1**(8183):1373–1376, 1980.

11. McCartney P, Keen H, Jarrett RJ. The Bedford Survey: observations on retina and lens of subjects with impaired glucose tolerance and in controls with normal glucose tolerance. *Diabete Metab.* **9**(4):303–305, 1983.

12. Klein R, Barrett-Connor EL, Blunt BA, Wingard DL. Visual impairment and retinopathy in people with normal glucose tolerance, impaired glucose tolerance, and newly diagnosed NIDDM. *Diabetes Care.* **14**(10):914–918, 1991.

13. Jarrett RJ, Keen H. Hyperglycaemia and diabetes mellitus. *Lancet.* **2**(7993):1009–1012, 1976.

14. Gabir MM, Hanson RL, Dabelea D, et al. The 1997 American Diabetes Association and 1999 World Health Organization criteria for hyperglycemia in the diagnosis and prediction of diabetes. *Diabetes Care.* **23**(8):1108–1112, 2000.

15. Shaw JE, Zimmet PZ, de Courten M, et al. Impaired fasting glucose or impaired glucose tolerance. What best predicts future diabetes in Mauritius? *Diabetes Care.* **22**(3):399–402, 1999.

16. Shaw JE, Zimmet PZ, Hodge AM, et al. Impaired fasting glucose: how low should it go? *Diabetes Care.* **23**(1):34–39, 2000.

17. Genuth S, Alberti KG, Bennett P, et al. Follow-up report on the diagnosis of diabetes mellitus. *Diabetes Care.* **26**(11): 3160–3167, 2003.

18. Diabetes Prevention Program Research Group. The prevalence of retinopathy in impaired glucose tolerance and recent-onset diabetes in the Diabetes Prevention Program. *Diabet Med.* **24**(2):137–144, 2007.

19. Gabir MM, Hanson RL, Dabelea D, et al. Plasma glucose and prediction of microvascular disease and mortality: evaluation of 1997 American Diabetes Association and 1999 World Health Organization criteria for diagnosis of diabetes. *Diabetes Care.* **23**(8):1113–1118, 2000.

20. Ito C, Maeda R, Ishida S, Harada H, Inoue N, Sasaki H. Importance of OGTT for diagnosing diabetes mellitus based on prevalence and incidence of retinopathy. *Diabetes Res Clin Pract.* **49**(2–3):181–186, 2000.

21. Tapp RJ, Zimmet PZ, Harper CA, et al. Diagnostic thresholds for diabetes: the association of retinopathy and albumin-

uria with glycaemia. *Diabetes Res Clin Pract.* **73**(3):315–321, 2006.

22. Barr EL, Wong TY, Tapp RJ, et al. Is peripheral neuropathy associated with retinopathy and albuminuria in individuals with impaired glucose metabolism? The 1999–2000 AusDiab. *Diabetes Care.* **29**(5):1114–1116, 2006.

23. Benjamin SM, Cadwell BL, Geiss LS, Engelgau MM, Vinicor F. A change in definition results in an increased number of adults with prediabetes in the United States. *Arch Intern Med.* **164**(21):2386, 2004.

24. Davidson MB, Landsman PB, Alexander CM. Lowering the criterion for impaired fasting glucose will not provide clinical benefit. *Diabetes Care.* **26**(12):3329–3330, 2003.

25. Lara C, Ponce de Leon S, Foncerrada H, Vega M. Diabetes or impaired glucose tolerance: does the label matter? *Diabetes Care.* **30**(12):3029–3030, 2007.

26. Schriger DL, Lorber B. Lowering the cut point for impaired fasting glucose: where is the evidence? Where is the logic? *Diabetes Care.* **27**(2):592–601, 2004.

27. American Diabetes Association. Diagnosis and classification of diabetes mellitus. *Diabetes Care.* **33**(Suppl 1):S62–S69.

28. Edelman D, Olsen MK, Dudley TK, Harris AC, Oddone EZ. Utility of hemoglobin A1c in predicting diabetes risk. *J Gen Intern Med.* **19**(12):1175–1180, 2004.

29. Pradhan AD, Rifai N, Buring JE, Ridker PM. Hemoglobin A1c predicts diabetes but not cardiovascular disease in non-diabetic women. *Am J Med.* **120**(8):720–727, 2007.

30. The DECODE Study Group and on behalf of the European Diabetes Epidemiology Group. Is the current definition for diabetes relevant to mortality risk from all causes and cardiovascular and noncardiovascular diseases? *Diabetes Care.* **26**(3):688–696, 2003.

31. Douaihy K. Prediabetes & atherosclerosis: what's the connection? *Nurse Pract.* **30**(6):24–35 quiz 6–7, 2005.

32. Haffner SM, Stern MP, Hazuda HP, Mitchell BD, Patterson JK. Cardiovascular risk factors in confirmed prediabetic individuals. Does the clock for coronary heart disease start ticking before the onset of clinical diabetes? *JAMA.* **263**(21): 2893–2898, 1990.

33. Meigs JB, D'Agostino RB, Sr., Wilson PW, Cupples LA, Nathan DM, Singer DE. Risk variable clustering in the insulin resistance syndrome. The Framingham Offspring Study. *Diabetes.* **46**(10):1594–1600, 1997.

34. Lyerly GW, Sui X, Lavie CJ, Church TS, Hand GA, Blair SN. The association between cardiorespiratory fitness and risk of all-cause mortality among women with impaired fasting glucose or undiagnosed diabetes mellitus. *Mayo Clin Proc.* **84**(9):780–786, 2009.

35. Sorkin JD, Muller DC, Fleg JL, Andres R. The relation of fasting and 2-h postchallenge plasma glucose concentrations to mortality: data from the Baltimore Longitudinal Study of

Aging with a critical review of the literature. *Diabetes Care.* **28**(11):2626–2632, 2005.

36. Shaw JE, Hodge AM, de Courten M, Chitson P, Zimmet PZ. Isolated post-challenge hyperglycaemia confirmed as a risk factor for mortality. *Diabetologia.* **42**(9):1050–1054, 1999.

37. The DECODE Study Group and on behalf of the European Diabetes Epidemiology Group. Glucose tolerance and cardiovascular mortality: comparison of fasting and 2-hour diagnostic criteria. *Arch Intern Med.* **161**(3):397–405, 2001.

38. Tominaga M, Eguchi H, Manaka H, Igarashi K, Kato T, Sekikawa A. Impaired glucose tolerance is a risk factor for cardiovascular disease, but not impaired fasting glucose. The Funagata Diabetes Study. *Diabetes Care.* **22**(6):920–924, 1999.

39. Smith NL, Barzilay JI, Shaffer D, et al. Fasting and 2-hour postchallenge serum glucose measures and risk of incident cardiovascular events in the elderly: the Cardiovascular Health Study. *Arch Intern Med.* **162**(2):209–216, 2002.

40. Bjornholt JV, Erikssen G, Aaser E, et al. Fasting blood glucose: an underestimated risk factor for cardiovascular death. Results from a 22-year follow-up of healthy nondiabetic men. *Diabetes Care.* **22**(1):45–49, 1999.

41. Chien KL, Hsu HC, Su TC, Chen MF, Lee YT, Hu FB. Fasting and postchallenge hyperglycemia and risk of cardiovascular disease in Chinese: the Chin-Shan Community Cardiovascular Cohort study. *Am Heart J.* **156**(5):996–1002, 2008.

42. Pankow JS, Kwan DK, Duncan BB, et al. Cardiometabolic risk in impaired fasting glucose and impaired glucose tolerance: the Atherosclerosis Risk in Communities Study. *Diabetes Care.* **30**(2):325–331, 2007.

43. Meigs JB, Nathan DM, D'Agostino RB, Sr., Wilson PW. Fasting and postchallenge glycemia and cardiovascular disease risk: the Framingham Offspring Study. *Diabetes Care.* **25**(10):1845–1850, 2002.

44. Stern MP, Fatehi P, Williams K, Haffner SM. Predicting future cardiovascular disease: do we need the oral glucose tolerance test? *Diabetes Care.* **25**(10):1851–1856, 2002.

45. Feskens EJ, Bowles CH, Kromhout D. Intra- and interindividual variability of glucose tolerance in an elderly population. *J Clin Epidemiol.* **44**(9):947–953, 1991.

46. McDonald GW, Fisher GF, Burnham C. Reproducibility of the Oral Glucose Tolerance Test. *Diabetes.* **14**:473–480, 1965.

47. Riccardi G, Vaccaro O, Rivellese A, Pignalosa S, Tutino L, Mancini M. Reproducibility of the new diagnostic criteria for impaired glucose tolerance. *Am J Epidemiol.* **121**(3): 422–429, 1985.

48. Eschwege E, Charles MA, Simon D, Thibult N, Balkau B. Reproducibility of the diagnosis of diabetes over a 30-month follow-up: the Paris Prospective Study. *Diabetes Care.* **24**(11):1941–1944, 2001.

49. Mooy JM, Grootenhuis PA, de Vries H, et al. Intra-individual variation of glucose, specific insulin and proinsulin concentrations measured by two oral glucose tolerance tests in a general Caucasian population: the Hoorn Study. *Diabetologia.* **39**(3):298–305, 1996.

50. Tuomilehto J. Point: a glucose tolerance test is important for clinical practice. *Diabetes Care.* **25**(10):1880–1882, 2002.

51. Butler AE, Janson J, Bonner-Weir S, Ritzel R, Rizza RA, Butler PC. Beta-cell deficit and increased beta-cell apoptosis in humans with type 2 diabetes. *Diabetes.* **52**(1):102–110, 2003.

52. Szoke E, Shrayyef MZ, Messing S, et al. Effect of aging on glucose homeostasis: accelerated deterioration of beta-cell function in individuals with impaired glucose tolerance. *Diabetes Care.* **31**(3):539–543, 2008.

53. Wasada T, Kuroki H, Katsumori K, Arii H, Sato A, Aoki K. Who are more insulin resistant, people with IFG or people with IGT? *Diabetologia.* **47**(4):758–759, 2004.

54. Davies MJ, Raymond NT, Day JL, Hales CN, Burden AC. Impaired glucose tolerance and fasting hyperglycaemia have different characteristics. *Diabet Med.* **17**(6):433–440, 2000.

55. van Haeften TW, Pimenta W, Mitrakou A, et al. Relative conributions of beta-cell function and tissue insulin sensitivity to fasting and postglucose-load glycemia. *Metab: Clin Exp.* **49**(10):1318–1325, 2000.

56. Weyer C, Bogardus C, Pratley RE. Metabolic characteristics of individuals with impaired fasting glucose and/or impaired glucose tolerance. *Diabetes.* **48**(11):2197–2203, 1999.

57. Tripathy D, Carlsson M, Almgren P, et al. Insulin secretion and insulin sensitivity in relation to glucose tolerance: lessons from the Botnia Study. *Diabetes.* **49**(6):975–980, 2000.

58. Polonsky KS. Evolution of beta-cell dysfunction in impaired glucose tolerance and diabetes. *Exp Clin Endocrinol Diabetes.* **107**(Suppl 4):S124–S127, 1999.

59. Bock G, Dalla Man C, Campioni M, et al. Pathogenesis of prediabetes: mechanisms of fasting and postprandial hyperglycemia in people with impaired fasting glucose and/or impaired glucose tolerance. *Diabetes.* **55**(12):3536–3549, 2006.

60. Meigs JB, Muller DC, Nathan DM, Blake DR, Andres R. The natural history of progression from normal glucose tolerance to type 2 diabetes in the Baltimore Longitudinal Study of Aging. *Diabetes.* **52**(6):1475–1484, 2003.

61. Saad MF, Knowler WC, Pettitt DJ, Nelson RG, Mott DM, Bennett PH. The natural history of impaired glucose tolerance in the Pima Indians. *N Engl J Med.* **319**(23):1500-1506, 1988.

62. Tuomilehto J, Lindstrom J, Eriksson JG, et al. Prevention of type 2 diabetes mellitus by changes in lifestyle among

subjects with impaired glucose tolerance. *N Engl J Med.* **344**(18): 1343–1350, 2001.

63. Ramachandran A, Snehalatha C, Mary S, Mukesh B, Bhaskar AD, Vijay V. The Indian Diabetes Prevention Programme shows that lifestyle modification and metformin prevent type 2 diabetes in Asian Indian subjects with impaired glucose tolerance (IDPP-1). *Diabetologia.* **49**(2):289–297, 2006.

64. Pan XR, Li GW, Hu YH, et al. Effects of diet and exercise in preventing NIDDM in people with impaired glucose tolerance. The Da Qing IGT and Diabetes Study. *Diabetes Care.* **20**(4):537–544, 1997.

65. Knowler WC, Hamman RF, Edelstein SL, et al. Prevention of type 2 diabetes with troglitazone in the Diabetes Prevention Program. *Diabetes.* **54**(4):1150–1156, 2005.

66. Buchanan TA, Xiang AH, Peters RK, et al. Preservation of pancreatic beta-cell function and prevention of type 2 diabetes by pharmacological treatment of insulin resistance in high-risk hispanic women. *Diabetes.* **51**(9):2796–2803, 2002.

67. Nolan JJ, Ludvik B, Beerdsen P, Joyce M, Olefsky J. Improvement in glucose tolerance and insulin resistance in obese subjects treated with troglitazone. *N Engl J Med.* **331**(18): 1188–1193, 1994.

68. Kahn SE, Haffner SM, Heise MA, et al. Glycemic durability of rosiglitazone, metformin, or glyburide monotherapy. *N Engl J Med.* **355**(23):2427–2443, 2006.

69. Bosch J, Yusuf S, Gerstein HC, et al. Effect of ramipril on the incidence of diabetes. *N Engl J Med.* **355**(15):1551–1562, 2006.

70. Chiasson JL, Josse RG, Gomis R, Hanefeld M, Karasik A, Laakso M. Acarbose for prevention of type 2 diabetes mellitus: the STOP-NIDDM randomised trial. *Lancet.* **359**(9323): 2072–2077, 2002.

71. The NAVIGATOR Study Group. Effect of valsartan on the incidence of diabetes and cardiovascular events. *N Engl J Med.* **362**:1477–1490, 2010.

72. The NAVIGATOR Study Group. Effect of nateglinide on the incidence of diabetes and cardiovascular events. *New Engl J Med.* 362: 1463–1476, 2010.

73. Eriksson KF, Lindgarde F. Prevention of type 2 (non-insulin-dependent) diabetes mellitus by diet and physical exercise. The 6-year Malmo feasibility study. *Diabetologia.* **34**(12): 891–898, 1991.

74. Knowler WC, Fowler SE, Hamman RF, et al. 10-year follow-up of diabetes incidence and weight loss in the Diabetes Prevention Program Outcomes Study. *Lancet.* **374**(9702): 1677–1686, 2009.

75. Ramachandran A, Snehalatha C, Yamuna A, Mary S, Ping Z. Cost-effectiveness of the interventions in the primary prevention of diabetes among Asian Indians: within-trial results of the Indian Diabetes Prevention Programme (IDPP). *Diabetes Care.* **30**(10):2548–2552, 2007.

2 Early diagnosis of type 1 diabetes: Useful or a phyrrhic victory?

Chiara Guglielmi[1] and Paolo Pozzilli[2]

[1] PostDoc Fellow, Department of Endocrinology & Diabetes, University Campus Bio-Medico, Rome, Italy
[2] Professor of Endocrinology, Head of Department of Endocrinology & Diabetes, University Campus Bio-Medico, Rome, Italy; Professor of Diabetes Research, Barts & the London School of Medicine & Dentistry, London, UK

LEARNING POINTS

- Type 1 diabetes (T1D) is one of the most widespread chronic diseases in the world affecting children, adolescents, and young adults.
- Early diagnosis of T1D is crucial because it is a condition leading to early complications.
- Genetic, immunological, and environmental factors are involved in the pathogenesis of T1D.
- The importance of understanding the natural history of immune-mediated prediabetes lies in the development of prevention strategies.
- Many clinical trials are attempting to modify the course of disease progress at many points along the presumed pathogenic pathway.

Introduction

Type 1 diabetes (T1D) is one of the most widespread chronic diseases of childhood, affecting children, adolescents, and young adults. In 1985, 30 million people worldwide were reported with diabetes (all types included), in 1995 135 million, in 2001 approximately 177 million, and it is predicted that some 285 million people worldwide will live with diabetes in 2010 [1].

As the prevalence of diabetes continues to grow worldwide, disease-related morbidity and mortality are emerging as major health care problems. Epidemiologic evidence suggests the relationship between diabetes and complications begins early in the progression from normal glucose tolerance to impaired fasting glucose (IFG) and impaired glucose tolerance (IGT) to diabetes than previously thought. These observations indicate that early identification and management of individuals with diabetes and prediabetes have the potential to reduce both the incidence of diabetes and its related complications.

The global incidence of T1D in children and adolescents is rising with an estimated overall annual increase of approximately 3%. The increase in incidence of T1D has been shown in countries having both high and low prevalence figures, with an indication of a steeper increase in some of the low-prevalence countries. Several European studies have suggested that, in relative terms, the increase is more pronounced in young children. Although T1D usually accounts for only a minority of the total burden of diabetes in a population, it is the predominant form of the disease in younger age groups in most developed countries.

T1D accounts for about 10% of all cases of diabetes, occurs most commonly in people of European descent and affects 2 million people in Europe and North America. The lowest incidence has been found in Asia and Oceania, the highest in Europe.

T1D results from the autoimmune destruction of insulin-producing beta cells in the pancreas. Genetic, metabolic, and environmental factors act together to precipitate the onset of the disease. The excess mortality associated with complications of T1D and the increasing incidence of childhood T1D emphasize the importance of therapeutic strategies to prevent this chronic metabolic disorder. Increasingly, efforts need to be directed toward early diagnosis of T1D because it is a condition leading to early complications, and the potential availability of disease-modifying interventions underscore the need for early diagnosis.

Clinical Dilemmas in Diabetes, First Edition. Edited by Adrian Vella and Robert A. Rizza
© 2011 Blackwell Publishing Ltd. Published 2011 by Blackwell Publishing Ltd.

Pathogenesis of T1D: an update in view of defining preventive tools

There are three main categories of factors involved in the pathogenesis of T1D. These are genetic, immunological, and environmental factors (Figure 2.1).

Like other organ-specific autoimmune diseases, T1D has human leukocyte antigen (HLA) associations. The HLA complex on chromosome 6 comprises the first gene shown to be associated with the disease, which is considered to contribute about half of the familial basis of T1D. Two combinations of HLA haplotypes are of particular importance. They are DR4-DQ8 and DR3-DQ2, which are present in 90% of children with T1D [2]. A third haplotype, DR15-DQ6, is found in less than 1% of children with T1D, compared with more than 20% of the general population and is considered to be protective. The genotype combining the two susceptibility haplotypes (DR4-DQ8/DR3-DQ2) contributes the greatest risk of disease and is most common in children in whom the disease develops very early in life. First-degree relatives of these children are themselves at greater risk of T1D than are the relatives of children in whom the disease develops later.

Candidate gene studies also identified the insulin gene on chromosome 11 as the second most important genetic susceptibility factor, contributing 10% of the genetic susceptibility to T1D [3]. An allele of the gene acting as a negative regulator of T-cell activation, cytotoxic T lymphocyte antigen 4 (CTLA-4), found on chromosome 2q33, is considered to be another susceptibility gene for T1D and has been associated with increased levels of soluble CTLA-4 and the frequency of regulatory T cells [4]. A variant of

PTPN22, the gene encoding lymphoid phosphatase (LYP), also a suppressor of T-cell activation, has been deemed as another susceptibility gene [5]. The observation that these four most important susceptibility genes for T1D can all be represented on a single diagram of antigen presentation to T cells, emphasizes the potential importance of current therapeutic strategies targeting this interaction.

Genetic studies have highlighted the importance of large, well-characterized populations in the identification of susceptibility genes for T1D. Recruitment of increasingly large populations of patients with T1D and their families is required to provide statistically powerful cohorts in which to identify other disease-associated genes. Some genes have a relatively minor individual impact on susceptibility to disease but identify important pathways in the pathogenesis of T1D, which could be targets for drug development.

The presence of autoantibodies to beta cells is the hallmark of T1D. Abnormal activation of the T-cell-mediated immune system in susceptible individuals leads to an inflammatory response within the islets as well as to a humoral response with production of antibodies to beta-cell antigens. Islet cell antibodies (ICA) were the first described, followed by more specific autoantibodies to insulin (IAA), glutamic acid decarboxylase (GAD), and the protein tyrosine phosphatase (IA-2), all of which can be easily detected by sensitive radioimmunoassay to identify subjects at risk of developing T1D [6]. These autoantibodies are common in both childhood and adult onset T1D, with many subjects being positive for multiple autoantibodies. The type of immune response is age-dependent, but seroconversion to multiple autoantibody positivity usually

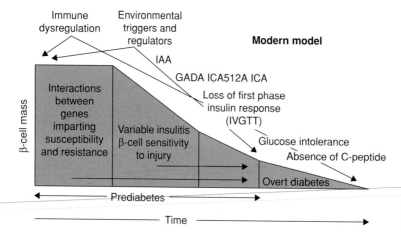

FIG 2.1 Pathogenesis and natural history of type 1 diabetes. (Atkinson MA, Eisenbarth GS. *Lancet* 2001).

occurs in close temporal relationship and is associated with higher genetic risk.

The presence of one or more types of antibody can precede the clinical onset of T1D by years or even decades. These autoantibodies are usually persistent, although a small group of individuals may revert back to being seronegative without progressing to clinical diabetes. The presence and persistence of positivity to multiple antibodies increases the likelihood of progression to clinical disease.

Continuing destruction of beta cells leads to a progressive reduction of insulin-secretory reserve and loss of first-phase insulin secretion in response to an intravenous glucose tolerance test, followed by clinical diabetes when insulin secretion falls below a critical amount, and finally, to a state of absolute insulin deficiency.

What are the environmental factors?

As regards the role of environmental factors, it should be underlined that the increase in incidence of T1D is too rapid to be caused by alterations in the genetic background and is likely to be the result of environmental changes.

Certain viral infections may play a role in the pathogenesis of human T1D. *Congenital rubella* is the classical example of virus-induced diabetes in human beings, but effective immunization programs have eliminated congenital rubella in most Western countries. Currently, the main candidates for a viral trigger of human diabetes are members of the group of *Enterovirus* [7]. They are small nonenveloped RNA viruses, which belong to the Picornavirus family. They consist of more than 60 different serotypes, with the Polioviruses being their best-known representatives. Enterovirus infections are frequent among children and adolescents causing aseptic meningitis, myocarditis, rash, hand-food-and-mouth disease, paralysis, respiratory infections and severe systemic infections in newborn infants. Most infections, however, are subclinical or manifest with mild respiratory symptoms. The primary replication of the virus occurs in the lymphoid tissues of the pharynx and small intestine, and during the following viremic phase the virus can spread to various organs including the beta cells.

Theoretically, *Enterovirus* could cause beta-cell damage by two main mechanisms. Enterovirus may infect beta cells and destroy them directly or they may induce an autoimmune response against beta cells. Direct virus-induced damage has been supported by studies showing that *Enteroviruses* are present in beta cells in patients who have died from severe systemic *Enterovirus* infection and

that the islet cells of these patients are damaged. *Enterovirus* can also infect and damage beta cells in vitro and induce the expression of interferon-alpha and HLA-class I molecules in beta cells, thus mimicking the situation observed in the pancreas of patients affected by T1D. The first reports connecting *Enterovirus* infections to T1D were published more than 30 years ago, showing that the seasonal variation in the onset of T1D follows that of *Enterovirus* infections. At the same time antibodies against *Coxsackievirus B* serotypes were found to be more frequent in patients with newly diagnosed T1D than in control subjects [8]. *Enteroviruses* have also been isolated from patients with newly diagnosed T1D. In one case report *Coxsackievirus B4* was isolated from the pancreas of a child who had died from diabetic ketoacidosis, and this virus caused diabetes when transferred to a susceptible mouse strain. The beta cells of diabetic patients also express interferon-alpha, a cytokine that is induced during viral infections, suggesting the presence of some virus in the beta cells. Prospective studies are particularly valuable in the evaluation of viral triggers because they cover all stages of the beta-cell damaging process.

Enteroviruses are not the only viruses that have been connected to the pathogenesis of T1D. *Mumps, measles, cytomegalovirus* and *retroviruses* also have been found to be associated with T1D but the evidence is less convincing than that for *Enterovirus*.

The role of cow's milk

There is evidence that cow's milk proteins can act as triggers for the autoimmune process of beta-cell destruction based on studies indicating bottle feeding as a triggering factor for an autoimmune response to beta cells.

There are several arguments for the milk hypothesis in T1D, including the following (reviewed in ref. 9):

- Epidemiological studies show increased risk for T1D if the breastfeeding period is short and cow's milk is introduced before 3–4 months of age.
- Skim milk powder can be "diabetogenic" in diabetes-prone BB rats.
- Patients with T1D have increased levels of antibodies against cow's milk constituents.
- Milk albumin and beta casein have some structural similarity to the islet autoantigen ICA69 and GLUT2, respectively.

A number of hypotheses have been postulated to explain the pathogenic role of cow's milk. One of the most convincing ones is that immature gut mucosa allows the passage of high molecular weight, potentially antigenic proteins which share some molecular mimicry with pancreatic beta cells. Among diabetogenic proteins in cow's milk, beta casein, beta lactoglobulin, and albumin have been implicated as sources of potential antigens.

Casein represents the major protein in cow's milk. Human and bovine beta casein are approximately 70% homologous and 30% identical. There are several reasons why it is thought that beta casein is a good candidate to explain the observed association between cow's milk consumption and T1D: (a) it has several structural differences from the homologous human protein; (b) casein is probably the milk fraction promoting diabetes in the NOD mouse, since a protein-free diet prevents the disease while a diet containing casein as the sole source of protein produces diabetes in the same animals; (c) several sequence homologies exist between bovine beta casein and beta-cell autoantigens; (d) specific cellular and humoral immune responses toward bovine beta casein are detectable in most T1D patients at the time of diagnosis, highly suggestive that this protein may participate in the immune events triggering the disease; (e) casein hydrolysate was shown to be nondiabetogenic in the BB rat and NOD mouse models, therefore it was thought that this dietary intervention might be beneficial in humans as well for disease prevention.

The rationale behind the use of cow's milk hydrolysate for primary prevention of T1D is based on several epidemiological and in vitro studies indicating that intact cow's milk, if given before three months of age, may induce an immune response toward beta cells.

The role of vitamin D deficiency

Several epidemiological studies have described an intriguing correlation between geographical latitude and the incidence of T1D and an inverse correlation between monthly hours of sunshine and the incidence of diabetes. A seasonal pattern of disease onset has also been described for T1D, once again suggesting an inverse correlation between sunlight and the disease [10]. Vitamin D is an obvious candidate as a mediator of this effect.

Dietary vitamin D supplementation is often recommended in pregnant women and in children to prevent vitamin D deficiency. Cod liver oil taken during the first year of life reportedly reduced the risk of childhood-onset T1D and a multicentre case-control study also showed an association between vitamin D supplementation in infancy

and a decreased risk of T1D. A further study found that an intake of 2000 IU of vitamin D during the first year of life diminished the risk of developing T1D and showed that the incidence of childhood diabetes was three times higher in subjects with suspected rickets [11]. It remains to be determined whether these observations are the result of supplementation of vitamin D to supraphysiological levels, or are simply the result of the prevention of vitamin D deficiency. Observations in animal models suggest the latter, since regular supplements of vitamin D in neonatal and early life offered no protection against T1D in non-obese diabetic (NOD) mice or in BB rats, whereas the prevalence of diabetes is doubled in NOD mice rendered vitamin D-deficient in early life [12]. The results of genetic studies investigating a possible relationship between VDR polymorphisms and T1D are inconsistent: a clear correlation exists in some populations, whereas no correlation is observed in others.

Prediction of T1D as the basis for disease prevention

There are different approaches for the identification of individuals at risk for T1D. These approaches are based on family history of T1D, genetic disease markers, autoimmune markers, or metabolic markers of T1D. These alternatives may also be combined in various ways to improve the predictive characteristics of the screening strategy. The importance of understanding the natural history of immune-mediated prediabetes lies in the development of prevention strategies. Several randomized clinical intervention trials have been concluded and the next generation of such trials will rely upon improved and simplified identification of individuals who are at high risk of progression to T1D. This is essential to ensure that trials have sufficient statistical power to detect a given effect of the intervention within the time available for the study. Such understanding is also needed to avoid exposing those who will not develop T1D to the risk of adverse effects of the intervention.

Prevention of T1D: current status

Although the process by which pancreatic beta cells are destroyed is not well understood, several risk factors and immune-related markers are known to accurately identify first-degree relatives of patients with T1D who may develop the disease. Since we now have the ability to predict the development T1D, investigators have begun to explore the

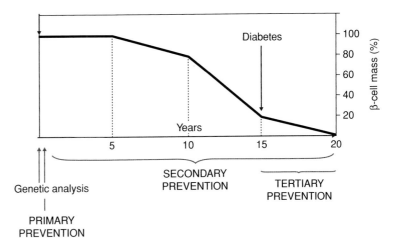

FIG 2.2 Strategies to preserve beta-cell mass in T1D. (Modified from Reimann M et al. *Pharmacology & Therapeutics* 2009).

use of intervention therapy to halt or even prevent beta-cell destruction in such individuals. The autoimmune pathogenesis of T1D determines the efforts to prevent it (Figure 2.2). Susceptible individuals are identified by searching for evidence of autoimmune activity directed against beta cells. While direct evaluation of T-cell activity might be preferable, antibody determinations are generally used for screening because these assays are more robust. Antibody titers are often used in combination with an assessment of the genetic susceptibility, primarily evaluated by HLA typing.

Interventions are generally designed to delay or prevent T1D by impacting some phases of the immune pathogenesis of the disease. As discussed below, current trials are attempting to modify the course of disease progress at many points along the presumed pathogenic pathway. Most prevention trials include only relatives of T1D patients, a group in which risk prediction strategies are most established. Trials in genetically at-risk infants evaluate whether avoiding one of the putative environmental triggers for T1D can delay or prevent its onset (Table 2.1).

TABLE 2.1 Prevention in T1D

	Study
Primary prevention	
	TRIGR: Casein hydrolysate vs. cow's milk formula
	PREVEFIN: Vitamin D supplementation and beta-casein-free diet
	BABYDIET: Delayed introduction of dietary gluten
	DIPP: Intranasal insulin
Secondary prevention	
	ENDIT: Nicotinamide
	DPT-1: Insulin/oral insulin
Tertiary prevention	
	Cyclosporine
	Nicotinamide
	Vitamin D (Calcitriol)
	Anti-CD3 Monoclonal antibody
	GAD
	DIAPEP277
	Anti-IL-1

Primary prevention

Primary prevention identifies and attempts to protect individuals at risk from developing T1D. It can therefore reduce both the need for diabetes care and the need to treat diabetes-related complications.

T1D is relatively easy to prevent in animal models of the disease and an array of therapies is effective. However, the mechanism of prevention is usually poorly defined, and

there is a lack of surrogate assays of the immune response to define which therapies are likely to prevent diabetes in humans. Inability to define surrogate assays probably results from a fine balance of the immune system, so that even with inbred strains of animals, only a subset progress to diabetes, and thus, relatively small changes in immune function may prevent disease. These observations have led to the hypothesis that identifying children at a very high genetic risk for diabetes, prior to development of measurable beta-cell autoimmunity, and treating them at that point may be a more effective means of diabetes prevention. Studies for the primary prevention of T1D, i.e., prior to the expression of islet autoantibodies, are currently being designed and implemented. These studies target young children at a very high genetic risk for T1D and propose treatments that are very safe. These studies require large-scale screening to identify high-risk subjects and follow-up over a long period of time to observe the outcome of anti-islet autoimmunity as a surrogate marker for the disease and onset of hyperglycemia as the final end point.

A large worldwide trial called TRIGR (Trial to Reduce IDDM in the Genetically at Risk) *and a small one in Italy called* PREVEFIN aim to answer the question of whether cow's milk administered in early life is diabetogenic and whether the use of a cow's milk hydrolysate can protect from the disease. The rationale behind the use of cow's milk hydrolysate for primary prevention of T1D is based on several epidemiological and in vitro studies indicating that intact cow's milk, if given before 3 months of age, may induce an immune response toward beta cells.

TRIGR is a randomized double-blind intervention study with the intention to treat as well as statistically analyze the incidence of predictive islet cell autoantibodies vs. the actual occurrence of clinical diabetes in two treatment groups [13]. This trial, which investigates cow's milk as an environmental factor, has several key features. First, it is designed to intervene specifically in first-degree relatives of T1D patients. The newborns enrolled must have a genotype with diabetogenic HLA alleles without protective alleles and a mother, father, or a sibling who suffers from T1D. Second, the sample size is highly significant, since previous trials were used to estimate the number of newborns necessary to participate. This is an international trial and recruitment has been carried out during a 2-year period in nine European countries, six major centers in the USA, 12 centers in Canada, and three centers in Australia. Due to statistical considerations, the frequency of the high-risk HLA genotype, consent and dropout rates, the trial required initial access to 8000 pregnancies that ultimately yielded 5156 infants necessary for randomization. Each formula milk used in the two treatment groups is a nutritionally complete infant formula. The study formula contains extensively hydrolyzed casein as the protein source, vegetable oils as fat source, and glucose polymers and modified starch as carbohydrate source.

The control formula is a mixture of a standard commercial cow's milk-based formula powder made by the same company plus casein hydrolysate powder in a 4:1 ratio designed to mask the flavor and smell distinctions between the two study formulas. The major outcome for the first phase is the frequency of T1D-associated islet cell autoantibodies and/or the development of clinical diabetes by the age of 6 years. The outcome of the second phase will be the manifestation of T1D by the age of 10 years. The manifest diabetes outcome will be assessed as the proportion of subjects in each group who develop T1D, as well as age at diagnosis.

In *PREVEFIN*, the first national preventive trial of T1D in Italy, newborns from the general population (approximately 12,000 at birth) were screened for the presence of the high-risk genotype HLA-DR/ DQ for T1D (DRB1*-DQB1*0201/DRB1*04- DQB1*0302) [14]. This high-risk genotype has been found to have a frequency of only 0.9% in the general Italian population, lower than in other Caucasian populations, thus explaining the low incidence of T1D in continental Italy. Many centers participated in the project that will yield information concerning acceptability of and compliance with early childhood intervention to prevent T1D. The HLA screening was performed within the first 2 weeks of life, so that randomization occurs before 1 month of age. High risk newborns were recruited into two treatment arms from the time mothers have stopped breastfeeding or if they did not breast-feed. Treatment consists of (i) normal cow's milk formula with vitamin D supplementation (500 IU/day) or (ii) cow's milk hydrolysate with vitamin D supplementation (500 IU/day) continued for up to 1 year. Vitamin D supplementation was included following recent evidence that administration of this vitamin to newborns can reduce T1D incidence later in life.

Detection of islet cell autoantibodies and later development of diabetes are used as end points. Subjects who participate in a similar project called *DIABFIN* [15] form the control group, where newborns with the same high-risk HLA genotype as in the *PREVEFIN* trial are being followed for the appearance of islet cell autoantibodies and diabetes. While the proposed trial may not allow all questions to be fully answered, this national collaborative network provides safety, efficacy, and logistic data necessary to design a Phase III trial. Results will be available in 2015.

Another pilot study called *BABYDIET* is currently underway to determine whether primary intervention through delayed introduction of dietary gluten is feasible and may reduce the incidence of islet autoimmunity in high-risk first-degree relatives of patients with T1D [16]. The study is based on the premise that introduction of foods containing gluten or cereal before the age of 3 months is associated with an increased risk of islet autoimmunity in childhood. Newborn children are eligible if they are younger than 3 months, are offspring or siblings of patients with T1D, and have HLA genotypes that confer a high T1D risk.

Finally, the Diabetes Prediction and Prevention Project (*DIPP Study*) [17] is a longitudinal study on T1D prediction and prevention carried out in the university hospitals of Turku, Tampere, and Oulu (Finland). The aim of the study is to investigate longitudinally the dietary factors in relation to the development of diabetic autoantibodies and clinical T1D. The diet of children is followed up by a structured questionnaire and by 3-day dietary records at various ages. A food frequency questionnaire is applied for studying the dietary intake of pregnant and lactating mothers.

The aims of this project are: (1) to identify infants at increased genetic risk for T1D from the general population at birth, (2) to monitor such children for the appearance of diabetes-associated autoantibodies, so as to identify those at high risk of developing clinical disease and characterize the natural course of T1D, (3) to identify the environmental factors inducing the seroconversion to autoantibody-positivity in children at increased genetic risk; and (4) to evaluate whether it is possible to delay or prevent progression to clinical T1D by daily administration of intranasal insulin. Whereas the aims given in points 1–4 have been fulfilled and useful information has been obtained, the trial with intranasal insulin did not show any beneficial effect of this treatment in preventing the disease.

In conclusion, since the failure of *ENDIT* and *DPT1* trials (see secondary prevention) in preventing the onset of T1D in subjects who are beta-cell autoantibody positive, interest has switched to prevention trials starting *before* islet cell autoimmunity has developed. These primary prevention trials of T1D offer an exciting view of how our knowledge of the pathogenesis of this disease can lead to the possibility of intervening at birth. There is still a long way to go, however, the rationale is sound and the prospects seem good.

Secondary prevention

Secondary prevention of T1D aims to reduce the incidence of the disease by stopping progression of beta-cell destruction in individuals with signs of such a process. A number of early studies of secondary prevention were carried out,

in some cases interesting results were obtained (as in the case of the gluten-free diet study), but the majority of these studies suffered from the limitation of inadequate power or an insufficient follow-up time.

To this end consortia of investigators have been created, extended to numerous centers, with the objective to generate the required critical mass for the development of studies with sufficient numbers of subjects at risk for T1D.

European Nicotinamide Diabetes Intervention Trial (ENDIT)

The **ENDIT** study, conducted predominantly in Europe, examined whether nicotinamide could lead to a reduction in the rate of progression to T1D in at-risk relatives of T1D probands. Over 40,000 first-degree relatives aged 5–40 years, were screened in centers in Europe and North America. The study was designed to recruit at least 422 subjects with ICA titers $\geq$ 20 JDF units to be randomized to either a nicotinamide- or a placebo-treated group. With an expected rate of progression to diabetes of 40% in the placebo arm, the proposed 5-year observation period should have allowed a 90% power to observe a 35% reduction in the incidence of disease [18].

Nicotinamide treatment at the doses used did not show any significant effect on the primary outcome—progression to T1D. A total of 159 participants developed the disease within 5 years of randomization to treatment, 82 (30%) in the active treatment group and 77 (28%) in the placebo group. The unadjusted Cox proportional hazard estimate showed no difference between the placebo and nicotinamide groups on an intention-to-treat basis. Nor any difference was found between groups after adjustment for age at baseline, glucose concentrations at 2-h glucose in the OGTT, and number of islet autoantibodies. The proportion of relatives who developed diabetes within 5 years was almost identical in those treated with nicotinamide and those treated with placebo, and there was no suggestion of a treatment effect in any of the subgroups defined by well-established markers of additional risk.

DPT-1 trials

The Diabetes Prevention Trial—Type 1 (*DPT*-1) consisted of two clinical trials that sought to delay or prevent T1D. Nine medical centers and more than 350 clinics in the United States and Canada took part in the two trials of the *DPT-1* [19, 20].

Individuals who were eligible for testing were identified as follows: age 3 to 45 years, with a brother or sister, child or parent with T1D; age 3 to 20 years, with a cousin, uncle or aunt, nephew or niece, grandparent, or half-sibling with T1D. Those who met these criteria had ICA antibodies measured. To be eligible, a subject had to be positive for ICAs.

Animal research and small studies indicated that small, regular doses of insulin could prevent or delay T1D in subjects at risk. One *DPT-1* trial tested whether low-dose insulin injections could prevent or delay the development of T1D in people at high risk for developing T1D within 5 years.

First-degree relatives, 3 to 45 years of age, and second-degree relatives, 3 to 20 years of age, of patients with T1D were screened for islet-cell antibodies. Those with an islet-cell antibody titer of 10 JDF units or higher were offered staging evaluations.

Subjects identified as having a high risk of T1D were eligible for random assignment to the experimental intervention (parenteral insulin therapy) or to a control group that underwent close observation.

The results demonstrated that insulin, in small doses, can indeed be administered safely to persons who are at risk for T1D. The increase in presumed and definite hypoglycemia among the subjects in the intervention group did not adversely affect cognitive function.

In high-risk relatives of patients with diabetes, the insulin regimen did not delay or prevent the development of T1D [19]. Long-term follow-up, to detect any effects on the course of diabetes, has begun. There are several potential explanations for the lack of effect observed so far. One is that the intervention took place too late in the disease process to slow down the progression of disease. Studies conducted earlier in the disease process, such as the ongoing DPT-1 oral-insulin trial in relatives of patients with T1D who have a projected five-year risk of 26 to 50%, may be more successful. Moreover, oral insulin may have a greater immunologic effect, although it does not provide for beta-cell rest. In fact, the low-dose insulin used in the trial may have failed to achieve such an effect on beta cells, but the dose was limited by the risk of hypoglycemia. With a different dosing scheme or a different regimen, insulin or insulin-like peptides might alter the course of development of diabetes.

The other study was an oral insulin trial that sought to prevent T1D in subjects with a moderate risk for developing diabetes.

First-degree (ages 3–45 years) and second-degree (ages 3–20 years) relatives of patients with T1D were screened for ICAs. Those with ICA titer ≥ 10 JDF units were invited to undergo staging evaluations.

Staging confirmed ICA positivity, measured insulin autoantibody (IAA) status, assessed first-phase insulin response (FPIR) to intravenous glucose, assessed oral glucose tolerance (OGT), and determined the presence or absence of HLADQA1*0102/DQB1*0602 (a protective haplotype that excluded subjects from participation).

The study was a double-masked, placebo-controlled, randomized clinical trial, in which participants were assigned to receive capsules of either oral insulin, 7.5 mg of recombinant human insulin crystals (Eli Lilly, Indianapolis, IN), or matched placebo. Subjects consumed the capsule (insulin or placebo) as a single daily dose before breakfast each day, either by taking the capsule or, if the subject could not swallow capsules, sprinkling its contents in juice or on food.

In the primary analysis of relatives selected and randomized in DPT-1, oral insulin did not delay or prevent development of diabetes. There was greater variability in the IAA assay for values 39–79 nU/ml than for values ≥ 80 nU/ml, particularly in confirmation of a positive result (98.7% overall confirmation for values ≥ 80 nU/ml compared with 70.6% for values 39–79 nU/ml). This prompted comparison of the rate of evolution of diabetes by entry IAA level. The cohort with confirmed IAA ≥ 80 nU/ml (the original entry IAA criterion) progressed to diabetes at a faster rate than those subjects who did not have confirmed IAA ≥ 80 nU/ml. In addition, those with confirmed IAA ≥ 80 nU/ml had other risk characteristics that suggested more rapid evolution to diabetes, including younger age, greater likelihood of having other antibodies, and greater loss of beta-cell function [20].

The effect of intervention in each of these two subgroups was further evaluated.

The group with confirmed IAA ≥ 80 nU/ml showed a beneficial effect of oral insulin, whereas the group who did not have confirmed IAA ≥ 80 nU/ml showed a trend suggesting a detrimental effect of oral insulin [20]. This group also had a much lower overall rate of development of diabetes.

In conclusion, neither low-dose insulin injections in subjects at high risk for developing T1D nor insulin capsules taken orally by those at moderate risk for T1D were successful at preventing or delaying the disease.

Tertiary prevention

Tertiary prevention is aimed at delaying or preventing the development of complications in subjects who already have T1D. A landmark trial investigating patients with T1D showed that good glycemic control can reduce the likelihood of microvascular complications leading to blindness or kidney disease, but the trend toward a decrease in macrovascular disease was not statistically significant. Diabetes education of health care professionals and those affected by diabetes plays a key role in the tertiary prevention of the disease. Tertiary prevention is identified by the maintenance of the residual beta-cell function present at disease onset and can be realized by immune suppression or immune modulation since the time of clinical diagnosis of T1D.

The best results in this field were obtained 20 years ago with the use of *cyclosporine* [21], subsequently abandoned because of transient benefits and undesired adverse effects.

In the following years none of the several treatments that have been proposed has obtained appreciable results but for *nicotinamide* [22].

Recently, there has been growing interest in *vitamin D* and its active metabolites in relation to T1D and its immune pathogenesis. Vitamin D metabolites have been shown to exert several immunomodulatory effects and 1,25-dihydroxyvitamin D3 [1,25-(OH)2D3] can either prevent or suppress autoimmune encephalomyelitis, inflammatory bowel disease, and T1D.

Recent data in humans demonstrated that reduction in vitamin D supplementation is associated with a higher risk of the disease, whereas its supplementation is associated with a decreased frequency of T1D [23].

Based on this rationale, an open-label randomized trial was designed to determine whether supplementation with the active form of vitamin D (*calcitriol*) at diagnosis of T1D could improve parameters of glycemic control (24). The secretion of C-peptide as an index of residual pancreatic β-cell function was the primary end point, with HbA1c and insulin requirement as secondary end points. The aim of this study was to investigate whether supplementation with the active form of vitamin D (calcitriol), in subjects with recent-onset T1D, protects residual pancreatic beta-cell function and improves glycemic control (HbA1c and insulin requirement). In this open-label randomized trial, 70 subjects with recent-onset T1D, mean age 13.6 ± 7.6 years, were randomized to calcitriol (0.25 mg on alternate days) or nicotinamide (25 mg/kg daily) and

were followed up for 1 year. Intensive insulin therapy was implemented with three daily injections of regular insulin + NPH insulin at bedtime. No significant differences were observed between calcitriol and nicotinamide groups in respect of baseline/stimulated C-peptide or HbA1c 1 year after diagnosis, but the insulin dose at 3 and 6 months was significantly reduced in the calcitriol group. In conclusion, at the dosage used, calcitriol had a modest effect on residual pancreatic beta-cell function and only temporarily reduced the insulin dose [24].

Other strategies for prevention of beta-cell damage with immune intervention at onset of the disease are based on immune tolerance (Anti CD3 monoclonal antibody, GAD65, Diapep277, Anti-Interleukin1).

Only recently, experience obtained with the use of the *antiCD3 monoclonal antibody* in two studies (one in the United States and the other in Europe) has revitalized the interest in this type of interventions [25, 26]. The drug, a modified form of anti-CD3 antibody that minimizes first-dose side effects, was studied by comparing 12 subjects, aged 7 to 30, who were treated with the antibody to an equal number of patients in a control group who did not receive the drug. One year after treatment with anti-CD3, the treated patients produced more insulin and needed less insulin therapy than the untreated patients. Those who received the antibody treatment also had better HbA1c levels. The anti-CD3 was designed to act on the immune system's T cells in a more specific manner than previous attempts at immune intervention in early diabetes.

GAD65 (the 65 kDa isoform of glutamic acid decarboxylase) is a human enzyme that has an important role in the nervous system and in several nervous system diseases, e.g. Parkinson's disease and chronic pain.

GAD65 is also found in the insulin-producing beta cells of the pancreas, although its function at this site is not yet fully established. It is however clear that GAD65 is one of the most important targets when the immune system attacks the insulin-producing beta cells in autoimmune diabetes.

Ongoing studies aim to investigate whether rhGAD65 can preserve beta-cell function in recently diagnosed children and young adults (10–20 years) with T1D.

This treatment is thought to induce tolerance to GAD65, thereby intervening in the autoimmune attack and preserving the capacity to produce insulin in patients with autoimmune diabetes [27].

Another study is based on the administration of *Heat Shock Protein 60 peptide 277 (Diapep 277)*. This is a 24 amino acids synthetic peptide derived from human heat shock protein (Hsp60) and it modulates the immune response by inducing tolerance to a specific peptide present in inflamed beta cells [28]. The purpose of the ongoing studies is to determine if DiaPep277 can effectively protect the internal production of insulin in patients newly diagnosed with T1D, by stopping the immune destruction of insulin-producing beta-cells in the pancreas. DiaPep277 acts on the immune system and is expected to prevent further destruction of the beta cells by stimulating regulatory responses, without causing immunological suppression [29].

The aim of using the *Anti-interleukin-1 (Kineret)* in newly diagnosed T1D subjects is to test the feasibility, safety/tolerability, and potential efficacy of anti-IL-1 therapy in maintaining or enhancing beta-cell function in people with new onset T1D. Kineret is already being used in the treatment of patients suffering from rheumatoid arthritis and preclinical studies are now suggesting that it may also be useful for patients with T1D. The active substance is interleukin-1 receptor antagonist, a blocker of an immune-signal molecule named interleukin-1 [30].

A randomized, placebo-controlled, double-masked, parallel group, multicentre trial of IL-1 antagonism in subjects with newly diagnosed T1D is ongoing. Patients are instructed to inject 100 mg of Kineret or placebo s.c. once daily for 9 months.

Conclusions

Today, one of the therapeutic goals in T1D is the preservation of the residual C-peptide secretion that is detected in a significant percentage of patients at diagnosis and which potentially may influence the clinical course of the disease.

Several studies have demonstrated that residual C-peptide secretion, after T1D diagnosis, depends on genetic factors, the patient's age at diagnosis, the number of anti-islet antibodies, and residual C-peptide secretion. Intensive insulin therapy and immunomodulatory drugs may be useful in this regard.

The ultimate goal of any therapeutic intervention is to prevent or reverse T1D by abrogation of pathogenic autoreactivity and by preservation or restoration of the beta-cell mass and function to physiologically sufficient levels to maintain stable glucose control. Early diagnosis of T1D is crucial if we want to restore and to save beta-cell mass. Different trials using antigen-specific or nonspecific interventions have shown some benefit in modulation of the autoimmune process and in preventing the loss of insulin secretion in the short term after early diagnosis of T1D.

Unfortunately, there are many limitations to current strategies, including a lack of suitable markers to predict and monitor the success of interventions, uncertainty about the long-term adverse effects, or the duration of treatment effect and the feasibility of restoration of beta-cell mass. Moreover, we should remember that T1D is a heterogeneous disease with an age at onset spanning from childhood to adult age.

Ideally, the interventions would be specific for T1D, free of adverse effects and effective prior to disease onset, with long-term and clinically meaningful improvements over standard therapies. The success of these approaches will eventually be evaluated by their impact on glycemic control, as this is the definitive determinant of long-term outcome of the disease.

In conclusion, we can affirm that early diagnosis of T1D is very valuable and is not a *phyrrhic victory*. Early diagnosis of T1D is more akin to David and Goliath: T1D (Goliath) could be vanquished with a simple intervention made possible by early diagnosis of the disease

Acknowledgments

We would like to thank Juvenile Diabetes Research Foundation (JDRF), National Institute of Health (NIH) Consortia, Centro Internazionale Studi Diabete (CISD), Diabete e Metabolismo (DEM) Foundation and University Campus Bio-Medico that support clinical research on T1D in our University Hospital.

References

1. International Diabetes Federation (IDF) Atlas data. http://www.diabetesatlas.org/.
2. Park Y, Eisenbarth GS. Genetic susceptibility factors of type 1 diabetes in Asians. *Diabetes Metab Res Rev.* **17**(1):2–11, 2001.
3. Bennett ST, Wilson AJ, Cucca F, et al. IDDM2-VNTR-encoded susceptibility to type 1 diabetes: dominant protection and parental transmission of alleles of the insulin gene-linked minisatellite locus. *J Autoimmun.* **9**:415–421, 1996
4. Ueda H, Howson JM, Esposito L, et al. Association of the T-cell regulatory gene CTLA4 with susceptibility to autoimmune disease. *Nature.* **423**(6939):506–511, 2003.

5. Ladner MB, Bottini N, Valdes AM, Noble JA. Association of the single nucleotide polymorphism C1858T of the PTPN22 gene with type 1 diabetes. *Hum Immunol*. **66**:60–64, 2005.

6. Wasserfall CH, Atkinson MA. Autoantibody markers for the diagnosis and prediction of type 1 diabetes. *Autoimmun Rev*. **5**:424–428, 2006.

7. Peng H, Hagopian W. Environmental factors in the development of type 1 diabetes. *Rev Endocr Metab Disord*. **7**:149–162, 2006.

8. Gamble DR, Taylor KW, Cumming H. Coxsackie viruses and diabetes mellitus. *Br Med J*. **4**:260–262, 1973.

9. Vaarala O. Is type 1 diabetes a disease of the gut immune system triggered by cow's milk insulin? Adv Exp Med Biol. **569**:151–156, 2005.

10. Chatfield SM, Brand C, Ebeling PR, Russell DM. Vitamin D deficiency in general medical inpatients in summer and winter. *Intern Med J*. **37**:377–382, 2007.

11. Hypponen E, Laara E, Reunanen A, Jarvelin MR, Virtanen SM. Intake of vitamin D and risk of type 1 diabetes: a birth-cohort study. *Lancet*. **358**:1500–1503, 2001.

12. Driver JP, Foreman O, Mathieu C, van Etten E, Serreze DV. Comparative therapeutic effects of orally administered 1,25-dihydroxyvitamin D(3) and 1alpha-hydroxyvitamin D(3) on type-1 diabetes in non-obese diabetic mice fed a normal-calcaemic diet. *Clin Exp Immunol*. **151**:76–85, 2008.

13. TRIGR Study Group. Study design of the Trial to Reduce IDDM in the Genetically at Risk (TRIGR). *Pediatr Diabetes*. **8**:117–137, 2007.

14. Lorini R, Minicucci L, Napoli F, et al. Screening for type 1 diabetes genetic risk in newborns of continental Italy. Primary prevention (Prevefin Italy) – preliminary data. *Acta Biomed Ateneo Parmense*. **76**:31–35, 2005.

15. Buzzetti R, Galgani A, Petrone A, et al. Genetic prediction of type 1 diabetes in a population with low frequency of HLA risk genotypes and low incidence of the disease (the DIABFIN study). *Diabetes Metab Res Rev*. **20**:137–143, 2004.

16. Schmid S, Buuck D, Knopff A, Bonifacio E, Ziegler AG. BABYDIET, a feasibility study to prevent the appearance of islet autoantibodies in relatives of patients with type 1 diabetes by delaying exposure to gluten. *Diabetologia*. **47**:1130–1131, 2004.

17. Kupila A, Sipila J, Keskinen P, et al. Intranasally administered insulin intended for prevention of type 1 diabetes–a safety study in healthy adults. *Diabetes Metab Res Rev*. **19**:415–420, 2003.

18. Bingley PJ, Gale EA, European Nicotinamide Diabetes Intervention Trial (ENDIT) Group. Progression to type 1 diabetes in islet cell antibody-positive relatives in the European Nicotinamide Diabetes Intervention Trial: the role of additional immune, genetic and metabolic markers of risk. *Diabetologia*. **49**:881–890, 2006.

19. Diabetes Prevention Trial Type 1 Diabetes Study Group. Effects of insulin in relatives of patients with type 1 diabetes mellitus. *N Engl J Med* **346**:1685–1691, 2002.

20. Skyler JS, Krischer JP, Wolfsdorf J, et al. Effects of oral insulin in relatives of patients with type 1 diabetes: The Diabetes Prevention Trial–Type 1. *Diabetes Care*. **28**:1068–1076, 2005.

21. The Canadian-European randomized control trial group. Cyclosporin-induced remission of IDDM after early intervention: association of 1 year of cyclosporin treatment with enhanced insulin secretion. *Diabetes*. **37**:1574–1582, 1988.

22. Crino A, Schiaffini R, Ciampalini P, et al.; IMDIAB Group. A two year observational study of nicotinamide and intensive insulin therapy in patients with recent onset type 1 diabetes mellitus. *J Pediatr Endocrinol Metab*. **18**:749–754, 2005.

23. Harris SS. Vitamin D in type 1 diabetes prevention. *J Nutr*. **135**:323–325, 2005.

24. Pitocco D, Crinò A, Di Stasio E, et al.; IMDIAB Group. The effects of calcitriol and nicotinamide on residual pancreatic beta-cell function in patients with recent-onset type 1 diabetes (IMDIAB XI). *Diabet Med*. **23**:920–923, 2006.

25. Herold KC, Hagopian W, Auger JA, et al. Anti-CD3 monoclonal antibody in new-onset type 1 diabetes mellitus. *N Engl J Med*. **346**:1692–1698, 2002.

26. Keymeulen B, Vandemeulebroucke E, Ziegler AG, et al. Insulin needs after CD3- antibody therapy in new-onset type 1 diabetes. *N Engl J Med*. **352**:2598–2608, 2005.

27. Ludvigsson J. Therapy with GAD in diabetes. *Diabetes Metab Res Rev*. **25**(4):307–315, 2009.

28. Huurman VA, van der Meide PE, Duinkerken G, et al. Immunological efficacy of heat shock protein 60 peptide DiaPep277 therapy in clinical type I diabetes. *Clin Exp Immunol*. **152**(3):488–497, 2008.

29. Eldor R, Kassem S, Raz I. Immune modulation in type 1 diabetes mellitus using DiaPep277: a short review and update of recent clinical trial results. *Diabetes Metab Res Rev*. **25**(4):316–320, 2009.

30. Pickersgill LM, Mandrup-Poulsen TR. The anti-interleukin-1 in type 1 diabetes action trial–background and rationale. *Diabetes Metab Res Rev*. **25**(4):321–324, 2009.

3 How should secondary causes of diabetes be excluded?

Aonghus O'Loughlin[1] and Sean F. Dinneen[2]

[1]Specialist Registrar in Endocrinology/Diabetes Mellitus, Department of Medicine and Endocrinology/Diabetes Mellitus, University College Hospital/National University of Ireland, Galway, Ireland
[2]Senior Lecturer in Medicine, Department of Medicine, Clinical Science Institute, NUI Galway, Galway, Ireland

LEARNING POINTS

- Diabetes clinical practice guidelines do not currently address the issue of population-wide screening for secondary forms of diabetes.
- Case finding should be undertaken among patients with diabetes and other clinical features of the condition under consideration.
- Both serum ferritin and transferrin saturation should be used to assess iron stores when screening for hereditary hemochromatosis.
- When screening for Cushing's syndrome, the following tests should be considered; a 24-hour urinary-free cortisol, a 1-mg overnight dexamethasone suppression test, a late-night salivary cortisol.
- Annual oral glucose tolerance testing should be considered in adolescents and adults with cystic fibrosis.
- Baseline measurement of height, weight (with calculation of body mass index) and laboratory measurement of fasting plasma glucose and fasting lipid profile should be undertaken before commencement of an atypical antipsychotic drug.

Introduction

In the early 1990s the terminology used to classify diabetes mellitus was based mainly on the approach used to treat the condition; the two main forms of the disease were described as "insulin-dependent" and "non-insulin-dependent" diabetes. The term "other specific types" was used to describe a variety of forms of diabetes for which a cause was clearly identified. Problems arose with this approach because many "non-insulin-dependent" patients ended up being treated with insulin and having the very cumbersome label of "insulin-treated non-insulin-dependent" diabetes. In 1997 an Expert Committee recommended adoption of the terms "type 1" and "type 2 diabetes" to replace "insulin-dependent" and "non-insulin-dependent diabetes" respectively [1]. The category "other specific types" has remained. It is likely that the terms "type 1" and "type 2 diabetes" represent a bridge between a classification based on treatment to a classification based on pathogenesis. We anticipate a time when terms like "autoimmune diabetes" and "non-autoimmune diabetes" will be used and when the number of patients currently assigned the label type 2 diabetes will diminish in favor of an increased number of "other specific types" (including genetic forms) of diabetes. A recent thought-provoking perspective on the classification of diabetes suggests that our current system of classification inhibits scientific progress by "lumping" together diverse groups of patients [2].

In this chapter we will discuss several forms of diabetes that have a specific etiology. In clinical practice the term "secondary diabetes" is usually applied to these forms of diabetes. Their recognition is important because of the potential for improvement in (or cure of) the diabetes through treatment of the underlying cause. The majority of secondary forms of diabetes are rare entities. There is very little mentioned in clinical practice guidelines on when or how to test for secondary diabetes. Even within a group of clinicians it may be difficult to agree on a uniform approach. As well as traditional forms of secondary diabetes we will discuss some of the newer genetic syndromes that have been elucidated in recent years. Although these conditions may

Clinical Dilemmas in Diabetes, First Edition. Edited by Adrian Vella and Robert A. Rizza
© 2011 Blackwell Publishing Ltd. Published 2011 by Blackwell Publishing Ltd.

not be curable their recognition can have a profound effect (therapeutic or otherwise) on an individual patient and/or their family members.

It is worth contrasting the challenge of searching for secondary forms of hypertension with that of searching for secondary forms of diabetes. There are certain "red flags" that most clinicians are alert to in a hypertensive patient that may indicate an underlying secondary cause. These include a young age at onset of hypertension, difficult to control blood pressure (e.g., requiring three or more antihypertensive drugs), and the presence of certain clinical (e.g., paroxysmal symptoms) or biochemical (e.g., hypokalemia) markers at first presentation. Unfortunately these "red flags" do not easily translate into the diabetes setting. Onset of diabetes at a young age is not unusual and is likely to be classified as type 1 diabetes if the patient is lean or as type 2 if the patient is overweight. The latter is increasingly recognized as a feature of the pandemic of obesity and diabetes and is especially common among ethnic minority groups. Similarly, diabetes that is difficult to control with tablets would not typically suggest an underlying cause but rather it would lead to the earlier introduction of insulin. The "failure" of oral antihyperglycemic agents is not unusual and does not represent a red flag for secondary causes. It is in the clinical domain that the similarities between approaches to identifying secondary hypertension and secondary diabetes hold up. Indeed several endocrinopathies such as Cushing's syndrome or Acromegaly are known to lead to both diabetes and hypertension. Because these conditions are so rare, in the majority of cases clinical acumen has been the most important factor in identifying secondary diabetes. In this chapter we will address the question "should we be undertaking more systematic case finding among our patients with diabetes?"

Screening for disease at a population level is an expensive endeavor. Within the National Health Service in the United Kingdom the National Screening Committee (NSC) is charged with providing guidance on conditions for which screening programs should or should not be developed. The criteria by which the NSC adjudicates on the appropriateness of introducing a screening program are rigorous. They include questions relating to *the condition* (e.g., does the natural history of the condition include progression from latent to declared disease?), *the test* (e.g., is it simple, safe, precise, and valid?), *the treatment* (e.g., is there evidence of early treatment leading to better outcomes than later treatment?) and *the screening program* itself (e.g., is there randomized controlled trial evidence that the screening pro-

gram itself is cost effective). Only 7 of the 36 adult conditions that have been considered by the NSC have been recommended for widespread screening. These include breast, bowel, and cervical cancer as well as hypertension, diabetic retinopathy, abdominal aortic aneurysm, and vascular risk status. Conditions that have not been recommended for population-wide screening include type 2 diabetes (although diabetes screening is recommended as part of a vascular risk assessment) and hereditary hemochromatosis. Although the exercise of searching for secondary forms of diabetes is not, strictly speaking, screening (which by definition is searching for disease in a healthy population), it is a very similar process. We will refer to the NSC criteria in our discussion of secondary causes of diabetes and we would recommend that anyone interested in the area of screening take a look at the NSC website. The equivalent resource in the United States is the US Preventive Services Taskforce, which can be accessed through the website of the Agency for Healthcare Research and Quality (www.ahrq.gov.). Table 3.1 summarizes the main secondary forms of diabetes mellitus and screening methods available to detect them.

Hereditary hemochromatosis

Hereditary hemochromatosis is associated with increased and unregulated absorption of iron by enterocytes in the gastrointestinal tract. The disorder is inherited as an autosomal recessive trait and results from one of several mutations in the HFE gene, with the commonest being the C282Y mutation. Affected individuals may develop excessive deposition of iron in the parenchymal cells of certain organs including liver, heart, pancreas, and skin. The clinical manifestations include hepatic fibrosis/cirrhosis, cardiomyopathy, diabetes mellitus, and a bronzed appearance to the skin. Joint pains, fatigue, reduced libido, and erectile dysfunction are other potential problems that can occur. The following vignette illustrates a typical patient who developed diabetes secondary to hemochromatosis.

Natural history of hemochromatosis

In the past hemochromatosis often presented with end-organ damage similar to that described in the case vignette. Although the genetic defect is present from birth the clinical manifestations are not usually seen until the sixth or seventh decade. Certain factors can lead to earlier (e.g., excessive alcohol consumption) or later (female gender with regular menses) presentation. Prior to 1996 confirmation

TABLE 3.1 Overview of secondary diabetes due to pancreatic disease and hormone excess

	Condition	Screening for condition among people with DM	Evidence for benefit from population-wide screening	Screening for DM among individuals with the condition
Pancreatic Disease	Hereditary Hemochromatosis	Serum Ferritin Transferrin Saturation Genotyping	++	OGTT/FG
	CFRD	N/A	+	Annual OGTT
	Pancreatic cancer	Abdominal CT scan +/− EUS	−	OGTT
Hormone Excess	Cushing's syndrome	24-hour UFC 1 mg DST Late night salivary cortisol	+	OGTT
	Acromegaly	IGF-1 and OGTT with growth hormone	+/−	OGTT
	Phaeochromocytoma	Urinary metanephrines, catecholamines and plasma fractionated metanephrines*	+/−	OGTT

Abbreviations: EUS: Endoscopic ultrasound; DST: Dexamethasone suppression test; OGTT: Oral glucose tolerance test; IGF-1: Insulin-like growth factor; FG: Fasting glucose.
*Regional variation.
Evidence for benefit from population screening
++ Very strong evidence and improvement of dysglycemia with treatment
+ Strong evidence
+/− Conflicting evidence
− Little evidence.

of the diagnosis was undertaken by documenting excessive iron stores on biochemistry and measuring hepatic or bone marrow iron levels by quantitative methods. In that year the mutation(s) in the HFE gene, which are known to cause hemochromatosis, were identified. Confirmation of the diagnosis now involves genetic testing of suspected cases for the commonest mutations (C282Y and H63D). The frequency of homozygosity for the C282Y mutation is 4.4 per 1000 in Caucasian populations in the United States. It is less common in Hispanic (0.27 per 1000), African

A 43-year-old Caucasian male was referred with a 3-month history of polydipsia, polyuria, and 4 kg unintentional weight loss. A random blood glucose was 288 mg/dl (16 mmol/L). He was diagnosed with hemochromatosis 12 years before at which time he had a serum ferritin of greater than 4000 ng/mL and hepatic fibrosis on liver biopsy. Regular phlebotomy was instituted but his attendance had become erratic in recent years. His medication included methotrexate and folic acid for hemochromatosis-related arthritis. The patient drank 24 units of alcohol per week. He reported normal libido and erectile function. He had no cardiac symptoms.

On examination he had a bronzed appearance. His body mass index was 26 kg/m^2 and his blood pressure was 135/87 mmHg. He had no stigmata of chronic liver disease. The cardiovascular, respiratory, and gastrointestinal system examinations were normal. His ankles were swollen over the lateral malleoli with scars from previous arthroscopies. He had normal peripheral pulses and no loss of vibration sensation. Biochemical investigations revealed a glycated hemoglobin of 14.3%, normal liver chemistries, a normal level of alphafetoprotein, a serum ferritin of 1340 ng/mL, a transferrin saturation of 97% and a normal serum testosterone and gonadotrophins. He was instructed in self-monitoring of blood glucose and reported home readings that were consistently above 15 mmol/L. A multiple daily injection regimen with insulin glargine and aspart was commenced. He received more intensive phlebotomy to maintain his serum ferritin less than 50 ng/mL. Once this was achieved his glycemic control stabilized and his insulin requirements diminished somewhat.

American (0.14 per 1000) and Asian American (<0.001 per 1000) populations. It has become clear that not everyone homozygous for the C282Y mutation (the commonest genetic defect associated with hemochromatosis) goes on to develop the full-blown clinical syndrome. In fact penetrance of the disease has been reported to be as low as 10% in some cohorts [3]. In the UK homozygosity for C282Y has been reported in as many as 1 in 300 blood donors and studies on first-degree relatives of probands suggest that penetrance is in the region of 50% for men and 30% for women. These data have huge implications for screening (see below).

Among the many organ systems that can become involved in the clinical form of the disease, liver problems are the commonest, occurring in approximately 75% of individuals. Diabetes develops in approximately 50% of cases and results mainly from beta-cell dysfunction (iron deposition in pancreatic islets). Reduced insulin action can also play a part in the etiology of glucose intolerance, particularly in patients with overt liver disease. The major causes of death in patients with hemochromatosis are complications associated with hepatic cirrhosis including hepatocellular carcinoma. Treatment of hemochromatosis involves regular phlebotomy with the goal of achieving a serum ferritin level below 50 ng/ml. This may reverse some of the end-organ damage, particularly if the phlebotomy is instituted early in the course of the disease.

The case for screening

In many ways hemochromatosis would appear to be a perfect condition for screening; it has an insidious onset over many years, there are good biochemical and genetic tests available for detection of cases, and a relatively safe treatment is available that would appear to be associated with benefit. Despite these considerations, both the US Preventive Services Taskforce on Screening [3, 4] and the UK National Screening Committee (http://www.screening.nhs.uk) recommend against population-wide screening for hemochromatosis. In the case of the USPSTF, the rationale for this decision was based on (1) the full-blown clinical disease is rare in the general population, (2) the penetrance of the disease is low among those with a high-risk genotype, (3) evidence that early phlebotomy in the screen-detected patient provides additional benefit over phlebotomy in clinically detected patients is lacking and (4) the potential for harm through labeling of homozygous individuals as "diseased" or "high risk," despite the possibility that they may never develop clinical disease. Harm could arise through anxiety, denial of life insurance, or discrimination through health insurance. The UK NSC acknowledged that, because the benefits of phlebotomy have been demonstrated through case series, it is unlikely that a randomized controlled trial of screening for hemochromatosis will ever be undertaken. It does recommend research to explore these issues further.

The case for screening for hemochromatosis among individuals with preexisting diabetes would appear to be stronger than the case for screening in the general population. This is based on a number of reports of hemochromatosis prevalence of 5 to 6 times that seen in nondiabetic controls [3, 5]. However, these studies did not use a uniform way of screening for iron overload and some were done in the era prior to the availability of genetic testing for the disease. It is the practice in many diabetes clinics to measure iron stores in patients with newly diagnosed diabetes. This does not really amount to a population-wide approach to screening (since not all patients with newly diagnosed diabetes will be referred to the hospital). It is also common for iron stores to be measured in patients with diabetes and another potential manifestation of hemochromatosis (such as abnormal liver function tests or a bronzed appearance to the skin). An important point to remember when measuring iron stores is that serum ferritin may be elevated as an acute phase reactant (particularly in patients with newly diagnosed diabetes) and may not reflect iron overload. A combination of serum ferritin and transferrin saturation is the preferred method of biochemical screening. So where does all of this leave the practicing diabetes clinician? In the absence of guidance from the American Diabetes Association, the 2001 Clinical Practice Guideline of the American Association for the Study of Liver Diseases (AASLD) provides sensible guidance on screening for hemochromatosis in routine clinical practice [6]. It emphasizes the measurement of iron stores as a first step and targets relatives of individuals known to have the genetic disorder as well as patients with symptoms or manifestations linked to the clinical disorder. The AASLD algorithm is reproduced in Figure 3.1.

Cystic fibrosis-related diabetes

Cystic fibrosis is the commonest life-threatening autosomal recessive disorder seen in Caucasian populations affecting approximately 1 in 2500 births. It results from a defect in

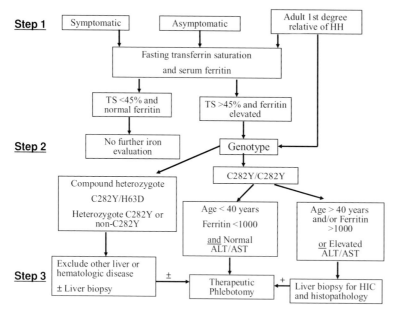

FIG 3.1 Proposed algorithm for screening and treatment of hemochromatosis in diabetic population [6] (TS: transferrin saturation; HIC: hepatic iron concentration) [6].

the cystic fibrosis gene, which encodes a protein called cystic fibrosis transmembrane regulator (CFTR). The genetic defect leads to disordered ion transport, which in turn affects the function of sweat glands, the exocrine pancreas, and the gastrointestinal and respiratory tracts. The classical clinical picture of cystic fibrosis is of recurrent pulmonary infections, exocrine pancreatic insufficiency, malnutrition, and premature death. In the past two to three decades improvements in the pulmonary, antimicrobial, and nutritional management of patients with cystic fibrosis means that patients are now living into their third, fourth, or fifth decades. A major comorbidity that has emerged in older patients is cystic fibrosis-related diabetes (CFRD).

Natural history of CFRD
The primary pathogenetic defect in CFRD is insulin deficiency resulting from pancreatic exocrine damage and pancreatic fibrosis. Glucagon deficiency also occurs and this may explain why ketoacidosis is seldom seen in CFRD. It is uncommon for CFRD to appear in childhood. Various degrees of glucose intolerance become more common as patients get older. A recent North American study from a single center that undertakes annual oral glucose tolerance testing on its patients reported CFRD rates of 2% in children, 19% in adolescents, 40% in individuals in their

20s, and 45–50% in those aged ≥30 years [7]. In the age group of 30–39 years, women with CFRD outnumbered men but typically there is no gender difference in prevalence. The presence of CFRD is associated with reduced survival compared to CF patients without diabetes. This survival difference may be more marked in females.

A comparison with other forms of diabetes
Table 3.2 compares features of CFRD with the two major forms of diabetes seen in the population at large. Although insulin deficiency is the primary defect in patients with CFRD, insulin resistance can also be a factor. This is especially true during periods of intercurrent illness (e.g., respiratory infections). Autoimmunity does not appear to be a factor in the pathogenesis of CFRD. Low body mass index is associated with premature mortality in cystic fibrosis and this can lead to conflict in the dietary management of patients with CFRD. While calorie restriction is usually recommended in the management of patients with type 2 diabetes, this is not the case in CFRD. Instead a liberal diet is recommended and the glucose-lowering therapy (usually insulin) is adjusted to achieve near normal plasma glucose levels. Centers in the United States that have a lot of experience of managing CFRD recommend early use of insulin. As well as achieving and maintaining good glycemic

TABLE 3.2 Clinical features of T1DM, T2DM and CFRD

	T1DM	T2DM	CFRD
BMI	Usually normal	Usually increased	Usually decreased
Presentation	Acute	Sub-clinical	Sub-clinical
Age of onset	Childhood and adolescence	Adulthood	Increasing incidence with age
Autoantibodies	Yes	No	Probably no
β cell function	Severely reduced/absent	Reduced	Severely reduced
Insulin action	Usually normal	Severely impaired	Somewhat impaired*
Treatment	Insulin	Diet, glucose-lowering medication including insulin	Insulin and nutrition
Microvascular complications	Yes	Yes	Reduced
Macrovascular complications	Yes	Yes	No
Cause of death	Cardiovascular disease and nephropathy	Cardiovascular disease	Pulmonary disease

Abbreviations: BMI: body mass index; CFRD: cystic fibrosis-related diabetes; T1DM: type 1 diabetes mellitus; T2DM: type 2 diabetes mellitus.
*Insulin sensitivity reduced during acute illness.
Adapted from O'Riordan *et al.* [9].

control, the anabolic effects of insulin are believed to be advantageous to patients with CFRD. Whereas patients with type 1 and type 2 diabetes require regular surveillance for the microvascular and macrovascular complications of diabetes, this is less of an issue for patients with CFRD. Microvascular complications are infrequent and macrovascular complications virtually never occur. This is likely to be due at least in part to the shortened lifespan. While most patients with diabetes die as a result of macrovascular disease, patients with CFRD most often die from pulmonary complications of their cystic fibrosis.

The case for screening

It is important to reiterate that screening is not a diagnostic exercise but rather it is an exercise in case finding, initiating earlier treatment and (ideally) achieving improved outcomes. It is extremely unlikely that patients with cystic fibrosis would develop diabetes as the first manifestation of their cystic fibrosis. Because of this we will not discuss case finding of cystic fibrosis patients in a general diabetes clinic. Instead, we will discuss the case for screening for diabetes among patients with cystic fibrosis. Glucose tolerance status can vary across individuals with cystic fibrosis and within an individual patient. For example, at times of severe pulmonary infection or during use of corticosteroid therapy, glucose intolerance can develop but may not be permanent. Within the cystic fibrosis literature there was confusion as to how to categorize different states of glucose intolerance. A

Consensus Conference report published in 1999 recognized four glucose tolerance categories based on the results of a 1.75 g/kg (maximum 75 g) oral glucose tolerance test [8]. These are still used today and include (1) normal glucose tolerance, (2) impaired glucose tolerance, (3) CFRD without fasting hyperglycemia and (4) CFRD with fasting hyperglycemia. The literature would suggest that patients with CFRD with fasting hyperglycemia have a worse prognosis than patients with CFRD without fasting hyperglycemia. Because of this, early initiation of insulin therapy is generally recommended for patients with CFRD with fasting hyperglycemia. Insulin may be used for patients with CFRD without fasting hyperglycemia, although some clinicians would consider using oral glucose-lowering agents in this setting. The case for universal screening is not accepted by everyone. However, the most recent guidelines on CFRD management from the International Society for Paediatric and Adolescent Diabetes (ISPAD) recommend universal screening [9]. The guidelines emphasize the importance of undertaking the screening at a time when the patient is at their baseline health status. More intensive monitoring of blood glucose through use of reflectance meters or continuous glucose sensors should be considered if hyperglycemic symptoms develop, or at times of acute pulmonary infection. The oral glucose tolerance test is still the means by which the diagnosis is established. It is unlikely that a clinical trial comparing treatment versus no treatment of screen-detected CFRD will be undertaken. In the absence of such a trial the next best level of evidence comes from well described case series. One such case series was recently reported from the University of Minnesota, a unit that has vast experience in management of CFRD. The report highlights a temporal trend over the past three decades toward improved outcomes and greater longevity in patients with CFRD [7]. The authors attribute this to universal screening (which they undertake from age 6), earlier recognition of CFRD, and more aggressive treatment with insulin and nutritional strategies.

Pancreatic-cancer-associated diabetes

An association between pancreatic cancer and diabetes has been recognized for a long time but whether the pancreatic cancer caused the diabetes or vice versa has been difficult to ascertain. The truth is that the association is bidirectional; long-standing diabetes is a recognized risk factor for pancreatic cancer. At the same time pancreatic cancer can cause new onset diabetes. The latter is likely to be mediated through humoral factors produced by the tumor rather than through destruction of beta cells. Cases have been reported of diabetes disappearing after resection of small, early stage pancreatic cancers. Approximately 50% of cases of sporadic pancreatic cancer have diabetes and in nearly half of these the diabetes is diagnosed shortly before or concomitant with the pancreatic cancer. Because the 5-year survival of pancreatic cancer is so dismal, it has been suggested that new-onset diabetes may be a marker of early stage cancer and could potentially lead to earlier recognition with a greater chance of cure. In the diabetes literature it has been suggested that age over 50 years, a lean body habitus, and lack of a family history of type 2 diabetes are clinical indicators of the potential for underlying pancreatic cancer. However, this clinical impression has not been borne out by careful comparison of the characteristics of patients with pancreatic-cancer-associated diabetes and type 2 diabetes. A group at the Mayo Clinic has shown that a similar percentage of patients in both of these groups are overweight and obese and have a positive family history for diabetes [10]. In fact, as these authors point out, obesity itself is a risk factor for pancreatic cancer.

In order for new onset diabetes mellitus to be useful as a potential indicator of the presence of underlying pancreatic cancer it needs to be combined with some tumor biomarker. No such biomarker has yet been identified. The presence of symptoms such as jaundice, abdominal pain, anorexia, and weight loss is problematic because by the time the patient develops symptoms the tumor is almost always unresectable. It is hoped that studies into the pathogenesis of pancreatic-cancer-associated diabetes will lead to the identification of a measurable biomarker which, among patients with recent onset diabetes, may be used as a screening tool. In the meantime widespread use of abdominal imaging among older patients with new onset diabetes cannot be recommended as a method of searching for occult pancreatic cancer.

Diabetes due to hormone excess

Several disorders resulting in hormone excess can cause diabetes. These include Cushing's syndrome (due to glucocorticoid excess), acromegaly (due to growth hormone excess), pheochromocytoma (due to catecholamine excess), glucagonoma, somatostatinoma, and Conn's syndrome (due to aldosterone excess). The latter two conditions cause glucose intolerance by interfering with insulin secretion, while the others predominantly affect insulin action. The benefit of identifying one of these conditions in a patient with concomitant diabetes is that cure of the endocrinopathy may lead to cure or amelioration of the glucose intolerance. In the case of acromegaly and pheochromocytoma, routine screening among individuals with diabetes is not justified, since both conditions are extremely rare and routine screening would very likely be associated with high rates of false positive test results with resultant increased distress and cost from unnecessary testing. Instead, case finding should be undertaken when additional clinical features consistent with the endocrinopathy are present. In the case of acromegaly these would include enlargement of the hands and feet, characteristic changes in facial appearance, headache, and increased perspiration. Because these changes are often subtle and take many years to appear, they may not be apparent to the patient or even to family members. A comparison of the patient's current appearance with that obtained from old photographs is often very informative. The classical features of pheochromocytoma include paroxysmal hypertension, palpitations, pallor, perspiration, and pain. Table 3.2 includes initial testing that can be undertaken if the clinical suspicion of growth hormone or catecholamine excess is sufficiently high to justify a case-finding exercise. One caveat with acromegaly screening is that poorly controlled diabetes is associated with elevated levels of growth hormone.

Cushing's syndrome merits particular mention because it is by far the commonest endocrine disorder associated with diabetes. This is because of the widespread use of exogenous glucocorticoids in the treatment of a host of inflammatory and malignant diseases. A careful medication history should highlight the use of exogenous steroids in a patient with diabetes. Sometimes glucocorticoids may be contained in over-the-counter or herbal preparations or may be taken surreptitiously. In addition, use of some steroids (such as medroxyprogesterone acetate) that are not primarily glucocorticoids has been associated with Cushing's syndrome. The mechanism whereby glucocorticoid excess causes diabetes is through increased insulin resistance and a failure of the beta cells to respond appropriately to this challenge. If Cushing's syndrome from exogenous glucocorticoid use is excluded, then (endogenous) Cushing's syndrome is rare. In population studies its incidence has been reported to be as low as two to three cases per million persons per year. However, among populations of patients with diabetes who have undergone screening for Cushing's syndrome, prevalence as high as 3–5% has been reported [11, 12]. Some authors have advocated screening all patients with newly diagnosed diabetes (in a hospital setting), while others have suggested that screening for Cushing's syndrome should be limited to patients with poorly controlled diabetes. Recent guidelines from the Endocrine Society support testing for Cushing's syndrome among groups of patients with certain "overlap disorders," i.e., conditions which, although common in the community, can also be a feature of occult Cushing's syndrome [13]. These include osteoporosis, hypertension, and diabetes mellitus. The guidelines state that Cushing's syndrome is more likely when these conditions occur at a young age. Another way of increasing the pre-test probability of Cushing's syndrome is to limit screening to those patients with diabetes and one or more of the clinical features associated with tissue glucocorticoid excess. These include (but are not limited to) facial plethora, easy bruising, proximal myopathy, and striae. The tests recommended by the Endocrine Society are listed in Table 3.2. The choice of which test(s) to use depends on several factors including concomitant medication use, local laboratory expertise, as well as the index of clinical suspicion for severe Cushing's syndrome. Diagnostic criteria that suggest Cushing's syndrome are a 24-hour urinary-free cortisol above the upper limit of normal for the assay, an 08:00 cortisol above 50 nmol/L after administration of dexamethasone 1 mg at midnight, and a late-night salivary cortisol above 4 nmol/L.

Some authors have advocated using higher cutoff levels as a way of reducing the number of false positives. There is a need for better evidence to support a screening/treatment strategy for Cushing's syndrome among patients with diabetes. Whether an opportunistic approach to screening (which is likely to be what most clinicians currently practice) or whether a more systematic approach (at a population level) should be adopted could be addressed in a randomised controlled trial.

Post-transplant diabetes mellitus

The term "post-transplant diabetes mellitus" (PTDM) refers to the recognition of diabetes in recipients of solid organ transplants. Recently the terms "new-onset diabetes mellitus after transplantation" (NODAT) and "transplant associated hyperglycemia" have been recommended to differentiate new-onset hyperglycemia from that present prior to transplantation. There is wide variation in the reported incidence of PTDM ranging from as low as 2% to as high as 50%. This variation relates in part to varying definitions of hyperglycemia between studies. Risk factors for PTDM include increasing age, non-Caucasian ethnicity, increasing body weight, a family history of diabetes, and a history of cytomegalovirus or hepatitis C infection. Hepatitis C leads to increased risk of PTDM with either liver or kidney transplantation. Treatment with interferon for hepatitis C results in increased insulin resistance. Many immunosuppressant drugs including tacrolimus and cyclosporin (calcineurin inhibitors), as well as corticosteroids, are diabetogenic. The latter cause diabetes predominantly through increasing insulin resistance in patients whose beta-cell response is compromised. The mechanism whereby the calcineurin inhibitors cause diabetes is less clear but appears to involve toxicity to the beta cell as well as effects on insulin action.

Clinical features

Weight gain is a common occurrence after transplantation and the risk of developing PTDM increases by a factor of 1.4 for every 10 kg increase in weight over 60 kg [14]. Taken with the increasing insulin resistance associated with the immunosuppressant medication, the clinical features of PTDM resemble those of type 2 diabetes. The diagnosis of PTDM can be problematic following pancreas transplantation for type 1 diabetes, as a persistence of autoimmune beta-cell destruction has been reported.

The case for screening

Hyperglycemia in the post-transplant period can result in an increased risk of infection, graft failure, and death from cardiovascular causes. Myocardial infarction was commoner in the 3 years following transplantation in a group with PTDM compared to nondiabetic transplant recipients. Early recognition of PTDM with the potential to prevent the associated morbidity and mortality has been advocated. The screening tests used are fasting plasma glucose or the oral glucose tolerance test. Management of PTDM involves use of oral antihyperglycemic medication and insulin. The biguanides are contraindicated in the presence of impaired renal function. Modification of the immunosuppressant regimen must be balanced with the risk of graft rejection. Furthermore, the benefits of reducing corticosteroid dosage and reducing or substituting calcineurin inhibitors have not been proven fully in clinical trials. A screening program should involve pre- and post-transplant testing of glucose tolerance. A knowledge of pre-transplant risk factors is essential to characterize the subsequent risk of PTDM. The recommended intervals for post-transplant screening (initially with a fasting plasma glucose) are 4 weeks, 3, 5, and 12 months and annually thereafter [15].

Diabetes associated with atypical antipsychotic drug use

Antipsychotic drugs are licensed for use in schizophrenia and related psychotic disorders. The first-generation antipsychotics were useful for alleviating the positive symptoms of psychosis such as hallucinations and delusions. They are less efficacious at managing the negative symptoms of psychosis that include withdrawal, poverty of speech, and cognitive problems. The introduction of the second-generation (or atypical) antipsychotics in the early 1990s was greeted with enthusiasm, as they were efficacious against both positive and negative psychotic symptoms. In addition, they were not associated with the (often very debilitating) extrapyramidal side effects of the first-generation agents. These drugs, which include clozapine, olanzapine, quetiapine and respiridone, have transformed the lives of many patients with schizophrenia and have enabled many individuals to live in the community as opposed to being managed as inpatients in psychiatric institutions. The drugs have become very popular among psychiatrists and general practitioners and are now prescribed for many psychiatric conditions other than those for which

they are licensed. One report published in 2001 estimated that as much as 70% of prescriptions for atypical antipsychotics were for off-label use [16]. Their side effect profile includes the very rare agranulocytosis associated with clozapine (and for which regular monitoring of the patient's full blood count is mandatory) to the much commoner metabolic disorders that we will discuss in detail.

Natural history

The underlying disorders for which the atypical antipsychotic drugs are used (schizophrenia, other psychotic disorders, major depression, etc.) are often associated with a sedentary lifestyle and poor dietary habits. Although high-quality cohort studies have been difficult to undertake, it is generally accepted that these disorders are associated with an increased risk of obesity, dyslipidemia, diabetes, and resultant increased cardiovascular morbidity. Because of the effect of the underlying disease it has been difficult to tease out the exact contribution of an additional drug effect on top of this. Clinical experience does suggest that many of the atypical antipsychotics are associated with weight gain and metabolic abnormalities. Occasionally, use of these agents has been associated with profound metabolic disturbance including diabetic ketoacidosis (DKA). In some case reports the presentation with DKA is followed by subsequent recovery of beta-cell function akin to the so-called "Flatbush" or "ketosis-prone type 2 diabetes." More commonly the metabolic derangement is less profound and associated with weight gain and dyslipidemia. As well as causing new diabetes among individuals not previously recognized as having the disease, these drugs can also lead to worsening of preexisting diabetes and a need for intensification of antihyperglycemic therapy.

The case for screening

On a background of increasing concern about the metabolic consequences of these drugs, a Consensus Conference was convened in late 2003 involving a number of professional organizations, including the American Diabetes Association and the American Psychiatric Association. The report from this conference highlighted a gradation of metabolic risk across drugs in the class with clozapine and olanzapine carrying a higher risk of metabolic side effects than quetiapine and risperidone [17]. The conference participants felt that insufficient experience was available with newer members of the class, such as aripiprazole and ziprasidone, to classify their risk. The conference called for research into the potential mechanisms whereby these drugs cause diabetes. The suspicion that the mechanism may not be as simple as weight gain leading to increased central adiposity and insulin resistance was borne out by subsequent studies in which the metabolic effects of the drugs were studied in an animal model. In a series of elegant experiments Dr. Ader and her colleagues showed that the beta-cell response to increasing insulin resistance on exposure to olanzapine was less than that seen with simple diet-induced weight gain of a similar degree [18]. This inability of the beta cell to respond to (mainly hepatic) insulin resistance could be centrally mediated, although the mechanism remains speculative. Further work in this area is keenly anticipated and may shed light on some of the complex interplay between the beta cell and insulin action in commoner forms of diabetes.

An important message that came from the Consensus Conference report was the need for baseline monitoring of metabolic parameters prior to (or as early as possible after) commencing long-term prescribing of atypical antipsychotic drugs. At a minimum this should include clinical recording of height and weight (and calculation of body mass index), waist circumference, and blood pressure, as well as biochemical measurement of fasting glucose and lipid levels. Although these are measured routinely in diabetes clinics around the world, they are not undertaken routinely in departments of psychiatry. However, if we are to have any chance of stemming the rise in metabolic disorders that would appear to be happening with increasing use of these drugs, then this is an important first step. The consensus group went on to suggest that repeat measurement of fasting glucose and lipids at 12 weeks and then annually thereafter should be undertaken. Several variations on how to screen patients at risk have been published since the report. A recent summary of the various recommendations and a pragmatic approach to screening has been published from a group in the UK [19].

Diabetes associated with HIV infection and its treatment

Over the past 20 years patients living with human immunodeficiency virus (HIV) infection in the developed world have seen a transformation in the disease from one associated with opportunistic infection and premature death to a chronic disease associated with good long-term survival. A consequence of this success story has been the develop-

ment in this group of patients of metabolic abnormalities including diabetes, dyslipidemia, and increased cardiovascular event rates [20]. Much of the metabolic derangement that occurs in HIV patients is due to the drugs that are used to treat the disease. The use of highly active antiretroviral therapy (HAART) has been responsible for much of the benefit but also much of the side effects. Similar to the story with the atypical antipsychotics, clinicians prescribing these drugs need to be aware of the risk of metabolic derangement that varies between the different agents [21]. Clinicians also need to be aware of the importance of screening their patients for the metabolic consequences of drug use. One aspect of the diabetes that occurs with use of HAART is its frequent association with partial lipodystrophy. This acquired abnormality in body fat distribution is associated with insulin resistance and has been amenable to treatment with agents from the thiazolidinedione class of antihyperglycemic drugs.

A 23-year-old Caucasian male was admitted to hospital with acute urinary retention and renal failure. He had been experiencing progressive thirst, polyuria, and nocturia over the last eighteen months. He had a past history of diabetes mellitus diagnosed 10 years previously and was managing this with insulin aspart and insulin glargine. He had poor eyesight since childhood and this was attributed to Leber's optic atrophy. His mother had type 2 diabetes mellitus and was on insulin. She had a history of gestational diabetes. His father had hypercholesterolemia and was otherwise well. His grandmother had diabetes mellitus and died aged 73 years. His other grandparents died in old age. He had three sisters who were alive and well.

On examination he was noted to be very hard of hearing. His blood pressure was 170/95 mmHg and his body mass index was 29.8 kg/m^2. He had markedly decreased visual acuity. Dilated fundoscopy revealed pale optic disks and scattered retinal hemorrhages. He had no evidence of peripheral neuropathy. Remainder of physical examination was normal. An ultrasound revealed bilateral hydronephrosis. His renal failure resolved with insertion of a suprapubic catheter. An audiogram revealed bilateral sensorineural deafness. A water deprivation test confirmed cranial diabetes insipidus.

Genetic testing revealed a complex heterozygote state with c.506G and c.1611_1624del14 mutations in the WFS1 gene on chromosome 4 confirming the clinical impression of Wolfram's or DIDMOAD (Diabetes Insipidus, Diabetes Mellitus, Optic Atrophy and Deafness) syndrome. Both parents were confirmed to be carriers and the family received genetic counselling on the inheritance of this autosomal recessive disorder.

Genetic forms of diabetes

If secondary forms of diabetes are rare, then genetic forms of diabetes are rarer again. The main justification for identifying secondary forms of diabetes is the potential for cure through treatment of the underlying condition. This does not apply to genetic forms of diabetes (although advances in gene therapy may make this a reality in the future). Instead the justification comes from (1) the ability to provide an individual patient and their family with a more accurate prognosis; (2) the potential to better match the treatment regimen to the form of diabetes resulting from the genetic defect and (3) the potential to advance science and our understanding of diabetes in general through elucidation of rare molecular and cellular defects causing diabetes [22]. In the case described above, the family was not aware of the progressive nature of Wolfram syndrome with almost inevitable death before age 50; most families appreciate the additional knowledge gained through genetic testing and genetic counselling. Examples of the recognition of a genetic form of diabetes resulting in a better fit between the diabetes syndrome and the treatment regimen come from the maturity onset diabetes of the young (MODY) syndromes. Several different gene defects have been recognized as causing MODY [23]. The commonest form of MODY results from a defect in the hepatocyte nuclear factor 1-alpha (HNF1A) gene and leads to a form of diabetes that can be managed adequately with oral sulfonylurea therapy. Because the diabetes is often diagnosed in childhood or adolescence, many of these patients are started on insulin on the assumption that they have type 1 diabetes. The ability to recognize previously undiagnosed HNF1A diabetes and potentially remove the need for lifelong insulin is a huge benefit to the patient. This phenomenon (of stopping insulin after many years of use) has also been reported in patients with permanent neonatal diabetes due to mutations in the Kir6.2 subunit of the ATP-sensitive potassium channels in the beta cell [24]. The cellular mechanism relates to the mutated channels remaining open and resulting in the beta-cell membrane remaining in a hyperpolarized state thereby preventing insulin from being secreted. The sulfonylurea drug leads to closure of the channel, thus enabling insulin secretion.

Other monogenic forms of diabetes that can be misdiagnosed as type 1 diabetes (if childhood onset) or type 2 diabetes (if adult onset) include that associated with the m.3243A>G mutation in mitochondrial DNA as well as lipodystrophic forms of diabetes due to mutations in the LMNA gene causing familial partial lipodystrophy. The phenotypic characteristics that should alert the clinician to the possibility of a monogenic form of diabetes include (1) young age of onset, (2) family history demonstrating either a pattern of autosomal dominant inheritance (e.g., in MODY kindreds) or of maternal transmission (e.g., in mitochondrial diabetes), (3) association with deafness (e.g., mitochondrial diabetes) or (4) neurological or neuromuscular disorders.

References

1. Report of the Expert Committee on the Diagnosis and Classification of Diabetes Mellitus. *Diabetes Care.* **20**(7):1183–1197, 1997.
2. Gale EA. Declassifying diabetes. *Diabetologia.* **49**(9):1989–1995, 2006.
3. Whitlock EP, Garlitz BA, Harris EL, Beil TL, Smith PR. Screening for hereditary hemochromatosis: a systematic review for the U.S. Preventive Services Task Force. *Ann Intern Med.* **145**(3):209–223, 2006.
4. U.S. Preventive Service Task Force. Screening for hemochromatosis: recommendation statement. *Ann Intern Med.* **145**(3):204–208, 2006.
5. O'Brien T, Barrett B, Murray DM, Dinneen S, O'Sullivan DJ. Usefulness of biochemical screening of diabetic patients for hemochromatosis. *Diabetes Care.* **13**(5):532–534, 1990.
6. Tavill AS. Diagnosis and management of hemochromatosis. *Hepatology.* **33**(5):1321–1328, 2001.
7. Moran A, Dunitz J, Nathan B, Saeed A, Holme B, Thomas W. Cystic fibrosis-related diabetes: current trends in prevalence, incidence, and mortality. *Diabetes Care.* **32**(9):1626–1631, 2009.
8. Moran A, Hardin D, Rodman D, et al. Diagnosis, screening and management of cystic fibrosis related diabetes mellitus: a consensus conference report. *Diabetes Res Clin Pract.* **45**(1): 61–73, 1999.
9. O'Riordan SM, Robinson PD, Donaghue KC, Moran A. Management of cystic fibrosis-related diabetes. *Pediatr Diabetes.* **9**(4 Pt 1):338–344, 2008.
10. Pannala R, Basu A, Petersen GM, Chari ST. New-onset diabetes: a potential clue to the early diagnosis of pancreatic cancer. *Lancet Oncol.* **10**(1):88–95, 2009.
11. Reimondo G, Pia A, Allasino B, et al. Screening of Cushing's syndrome in adult patients with newly diagnosed diabetes mellitus. *Clin Endocrinol (Oxf)* **67**(2):225–229, 2007.

12. Boscaro M, Arnaldi G. Approach to the patient with possible Cushing's syndrome. *J Clin Endocrinol Metab.* **94**(9): 3121–3131, 2009.

13. Nieman L, Biller B, Findling J, et al. The diagnosis of Cushing's syndrome: an endocrine society clinical practice guideline. *J Clin Endocrinol Metab.* **93**:1526–1540, 2008.

14. Cosio FG, Pesavento TE, Kim S, Osei K, Henry M, Ferguson RM. Patient survival after renal transplantation: IV. Impact of post-transplant diabetes. *Kidney Int.* **62**(4):1440–1446, 2002.

15. Bodziak KA, Hricik DE. New-onset diabetes mellitus after solid organ transplantation. *Transpl Int.* **22**(5):519–530, 2009.

16. Glick ID, Murray SR, Vasudevan P, et al. Treatment with atypical antipsychotics: new indications and new populations. *J Psychiatr Res.* **35**(3):187–191, 2001.

17. Consensus development conference on antipsychotic drugs and obesity and diabetes. *Diabetes Care.* **27**(2):596–601, 2004.

18. Ader M, Kim SP, Catalano KJ, et al. Metabolic dysregulation with atypical antipsychotics occurs in the absence of underlying disease: a placebo-controlled study of olanzapine and risperidone in dogs. *Diabetes.* **54**(3):862–871, 2005.

19. Churchward S, Oxborrow SM, Olotu VO, Thalitaya MD. Setting standards for physical health monitoring in patients on antipsychotics. *Psychiatr Bull.* **33**: 451–454, 2009.

20. Morse CG, Kovacs JA. Metabolic and skeletal complications of HIV infection: the price of success. *JAMA.* **296**(7): 844–854, 2006.

21. De Wit S, Sabin CA, Weber R, et al. Incidence and risk factors for new-onset diabetes in HIV-infected patients: the Data Collection on Adverse Events of Anti-HIV Drugs (D:A:D) study. *Diabetes Care.* **31**(6):1224–1229, 2008.

22. O'Rahilly S. Human genetics illuminates the paths to metabolic disease. *Nature.* **462**(7271):307–314, 2009.

23. Fajans SS, Bell GI, Polonsky KS. Molecular mechanisms and clinical pathophysiology of maturity-onset diabetes of the young. *N Engl J Med.* **345**(13):971–980, 2001.

24. Hattersley A, Bruining J, Shield J, Njolstad P, Donaghue KC. The diagnosis and management of monogenic diabetes in children and adolescents. *Pediatr Diabetes.* **10**(Suppl 12): 33–42, 2009.

4 Screening patients with prediabetes and diabetes for cardiovascular disease

Deepika S. Reddy[1] and Vivian Fonseca[2]

[1] Assistant Professor, Department of Endocrinology, Scott & White Clinic, Temple, TX, USA
[2] Professor of Medicine and Pharmacology, Tullis Tulane Alumni Chair in Diabetes, Chief, Section of Endocrinology, Tulane University Health Sciences Center, New Orleans, LA, USA

LEARNING POINTS

- Patients with dysglycemia are at risk for developing cardiovascular disease before and after they develop frank diabetes.

- Current guidelines for screening with cardiac imaging have limitations.

- Assessment of risk factors to stratify a patient's risk may be helpful.

- Treating traditional risk factors (such as blood pressure, elevated LDL cholesterol, etc.) for cardiovascular disease help reduce the patient's risk.

- When traditional risk factors have been treated, normalization of nontraditional risk factors such as highly sensitive C-reactive protein may prove to be useful.

- The optimal "screening tool" therefore may not be a single imaging study, instead it may be a multistep process of assessment and treatment of risk factors to improve cardiovascular outcomes in patients with prediabetes and diabetes.

Introduction

Patients with diabetes are at increased risk for developing and dying from cardiovascular disease (CVD). People with diabetes have been shown to have twice the risk of CVD as the general population [1]. Patients with prediabetes in the San Antonio Heart Study had atherogenic risk factors suggesting that risk for CVD may start before the diagnosis of diabetes [2]. In a study of Finnish patients with and without diabetes followed for seven years, the risk of a recurrent event was greatest in diabetic patients with a known history of CVD [3]. The risk was similar in patients with diabetes and no history of CVD and patients without diabetes who had a history of known CVD. This gave rise to the notion of "cardiac risk equivalent" and the need to evaluate and treat patients with diabetes in the same way as those with preexisting heart disease. With the worldwide incidence of diabetes rising steadily, CVD in patients with diabetes will continue to be a major public health concern requiring a concerted effort to detect those at risk and to intervene early to reduce this risk.

The aim of this review is to discuss optimal identification of patients at risk, current recommendations for such identification, recent developments, and possible future directions in such efforts.

Current screening guidelines in asymptomatic patients with diabetes

In guidelines published in 1998 by the American Diabetes Association [4] (ADA), a risk factor guided approach was suggested. In the asymptomatic patient, presence of two or more risk factors, EKG abnormalities, or evidence of vascular disease were described as reasons to perform specialized screening for inducible ischemia. In 2004, ADA guidelines [5] recommended cardiac stress testing before initiation of an exercise regimen in all patients with diabetes who were over the age of 40. In those between 35 and 40 years of age, pre-exercise stress testing was recommended if other risk factors for cardiovascular disease were present. In 2007 [6], an ADA consensus panel recognized that the "risk

Clinical Dilemmas in Diabetes, First Edition. Edited by Adrian Vella and Robert A. Rizza
© 2011 Blackwell Publishing Ltd. Published 2011 by Blackwell Publishing Ltd.

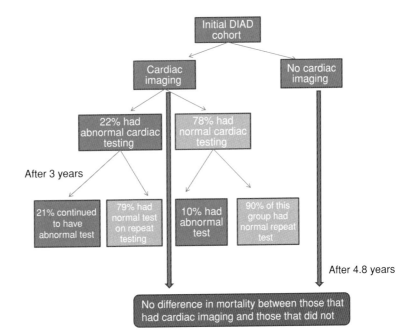

FIG 4.1 Composite of data from the three DIAD studies.

factor approach" to screening for CVD in the asymptomatic patient had some shortcomings that are listed below.

First, in the Detection of Ischemia in Asymptomatic Diabetics (DIAD) study [7], patients with type 2 diabetes with no symptoms of CVD were randomized to "no imaging" or "cardiac perfusion imaging" groups. Of all the patients who underwent perfusion imaging, 22% had abnormal testing. Of these, 40% had less than two risk factors for CVD. Three years later when the testing was repeated, of those that had a negative test, 10% now had a positive test [8]. A more striking finding was the resolution of inducible ischemia in 79% of those that had ischemia initially and no intervening revascularization procedure. On follow up, 4.8 years after the original study, the incidence of CV events was low. There was a significant increase in primary prevention efforts in both groups and there was no difference in mortality between those that had myocardial perfusion testing and those that did not [9] (see Figure 4.1). Thus, screening by the guidelines may lead to both false positives and negatives and high-risk patients may be better served by aggressive risk factor modification as suggested by a number of guidelines such as NCEP/ATPIII.

Second, there is increasing awareness that in patients with stable CVD, medical management and percutaneous coronary intervention (PCI) were equally effective. In the

COURAGE study [10], patients with CAD were randomized to just medical care or medical care plus PCI. There was no difference in death or major cardiovascular events between the groups, although there was a greater incidence of repeat catheterizations and PCI in those initially assigned to medical management alone. The results were the same in the subset of patients with diabetes.

In asymptomatic patients, therefore, the value of screening with cardiac stress testing is unclear, as aggressive risk factor identification and medical management appears to be equally efficacious in reducing the risk of future CV events.

Hyperglycemia and the risk of cardiovascular disease

Glucose is a continuous variable in the population with an almost linear association with CVD. This is seen even in glucose concentrations below that used to diagnose diabetes. DECODE, an epidemiologic study in Europe, looked at over 25,000 subjects and demonstrated that mortality was increased not just in patients with diabetes but also in those with impaired glucose tolerance (IGT). The study also demonstrated that IGT carries a greater risk than impaired fasting glucose ((IFG), a finding of practical importance as glucose tolerance testing is often not carried out in patients at possible risk [11]. Norhammer et al. demonstrated that in patients with established CAD, IGT is common and may be missed [12]. This has led to recommendations for more widespread use of GTTs. In the AusDiab study, there is a graded increase in both all-cause and cardiovascular mortality from normal glucose tolerance to known diabetes [13]. Therefore, patients at risk for dysglycemia should be screened early and have risk factor management early, and those with CVD should be screened for dysglycemia.

Similarly, the EPIC-Norfolk study demonstrated that HbA1c in the normal range is also associated with increased CVD and mortality [14]. The relationship of CVD with HbA1c needs to be studied further given the importance of protein glycation in the pathogenesis of complications. In recent months, the use of HbA1c as an initial test for diagnosis of diabetes has been accepted by the American Diabetes Association (ADA).

Treatment of hyperglycemia in patients with prediabetes may have an impact on the risk for CVD. In the STOP-NIDDM study [15], patients with prediabetes were treated with acarbose. At the end of 3 years, patients treated with acarbose had a lower risk of developing diabetes and having a CV event.

In patients with known diabetes, treatment of hyperglycemia reduces the risk of CVD. Early prospective studies such as DCCT and UKPDS [16, 17] showed improvement in microvascular complications in patients with type 1 and type 2 diabetes respectively. When these patients were followed, a decrease in macrovascular complications was also demonstrated [18, 19]. The EDIC trial [18], describes long-term follow-up of the patients in the DCCT trial. In EDIC, lower HgBA1c while the patients were actively enrolled in the DCCT trial appeared to correlate with improved cardiovascular outcomes. It is important to recognize that the DCCT and UKPDS trials enrolled relatively young patients with a short duration of DM. In addition, after the original DCCT and UKPDS trials were terminated, the patients no longer maintained their randomization. Despite this, there appeared to be an improvement in CVD outcomes in intensively treated patients during long-term follow-up. In three recent large studies (ACCORD, ADVANCE, and VADT) where the patients studied were older than those in UKPDS and had DM for a longer duration, tight blood sugar control did not improve CV outcomes in the short term. Those with long-standing DM may have already developed atherosclerosis and management of non-glycemic factors takes on more importance.

The evidence supports the notion that elevated blood sugars do increase risk for CVD and control of hyperglycemia does improve that risk. The control of other risk factors also appears to be important, especially in those with long-standing type 2 diabetes.

What are other risk factors for cardiovascular disease? How should they be managed?

Before the development of type 2 diabetes, patients at risk often have evidence of insulin resistance. These patients may be obese with normal glucose levels and hyperinsulinemia or they may have IGT/IFG. In addition, other metabolic derangements may be present. These metabolic alternations may help with early identification of these patients. In the San Antonio Heart study [2], over 600 Mexican American patients who were hyperinsulinemic were followed for 8 years. Patients that developed diabetes over that period had higher triglycerides, lower HDL, higher systolic pressures, and higher fasting glucose and insulin levels. The investigators concluded that these patients were developing CVD even before they developed overt DM.

Treating multiple risk factors has resulted in improved risk for CVD. In the STENO-2 study [20], multifactorial intervention such as modifying lifestyle, reducing total cholesterol (LDL 126 mg/dl vs. 83 mg/dl), lowering blood pressure (systolic blood pressure 146 vs. 131 mmHg), and improving glycemic control (HbA1c 9.0% vs. 7.9%) was studied in patients with type 2 diabetes. At the end of that time, intensive treatment of risk factors resulted in reduction in the primary composite end point (nonfatal MI, cardiovascular death, revascularization, nonfatal stroke and amputation). The hazard ratio for the intensively treated group was 0.47 ($p = 0.01$)

How do we "risk stratify" patients?

The metabolic syndrome (MS) represents an attempt to capture patients who may have an increased risk for diabetes and cardiovascular disease. Patients with MS may have more than one risk factor that is known to be atherogenic. As the number of risk factors accumulate, the risk of CVD increases. There are multiple difficulties with the use of MS as a risk stratification tool. First, there are multiple definitions of the syndrome. Second, we do not know if the presence of some of the factors results in greater risk than others. The definitions give all risk factors equal weight.

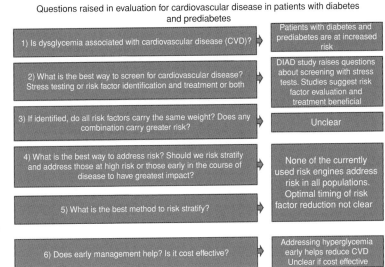

Questions raised in evaluation for cardiovascular disease in patients with diabetes and prediabetes

1) Is dysglycemia associated with cardiovascular disease (CVD)?	Patients with diabetes and prediabetes are at increased risk
2) What is the best way to screen for cardiovascular disease? Stress testing or risk factor identification and treatment or both	DIAD study raises questions about screening with stress tests. Studies suggest risk factor evaluation and treatment beneficial
3) If identified, do all risk factors carry the same weight? Does any combination carry greater risk?	Unclear
4) What is the best way to address risk? Should we risk stratify and address those at high risk or those early in the course of disease to have greatest impact?	None of the currently used risk engines address risk in all populations. Optimal timing of risk factor reduction not clear
5) What is the best method to risk stratify?	
6) Does early management help? Is it cost effective?	Addressing hyperglycemia early helps reduce CVD Unclear if cost effective

FIG 4.2 Clinical questions related to the screening for cardiovascular disease in patients with prediabetes and diabetes.

Third, the syndrome is present if three of five risk factors are present. There is no graded estimate of risk based on the number of risk factors present. Finally, the definitions do not include well-established risk factors for CVD such as LDL cholesterol.

Risk calculators have also been used to stratify patients with CVD risk factors. An early calculator was developed from the Framingham data [21]. It is easy to use and widely distributed. Since the number of diabetics in the Framingham study was small, the risk calculation for diabetics may not reflect true risk in these patients. A risk engine was developed from the UKPDS data [22]. It may be helpful for assessing risk in younger patients with a short duration of DM. Its accuracy in those with patients with type 1 DM or those with type 2 diabetes for a longer duration is not clear. All patients with diabetes do not have the same risk for CVD. The early risk engines have been modeled on data that are not inclusive of the range of patients with diabetes that we see in our practice.

A new model called ARCHIMEDES may address the limitations of the earlier risk engines [23]. It is described by the authors as a mathematical model written at a "deep level of biological, clinical and administrative detail." It attempts to account for a variety of interacting variables that can together affect a patient's risk for disease. Using data from multiple studies, it assesses risk on a continuum as opposed to discrete states. For our current purpose, it would take into account the type of diabetes, duration, presence, or absence of risk factors but also what we know about vascular biology in the presence of these risks. It also has the capacity to include clinical features such as adherence to medical regimens, etc. It has been validated against clinical trials and has a remarkable degree of concordance of its prediction to the outcomes from the trials.

As with a number of issues related to screening for CVD in prediabetes and diabetes, there is ongoing evaluation of risk stratification (see Figure 4.2).

Traditional risk factors

Several risk factors have been associated with CVD. The INTERHEART study evaluated a number of these risks and tried to assess the contribution of these risk factors to the presence of CVD [24]. It was a multicountry case control study. Over 15,000 patients who had acute myocardial infarction and closely matched controls were studied. Nine commonly recognized risk factors (smoking, abnormal lipids (apolipoprotein B1/apolipoprotein A1 ratio), HTN (self-reported), diabetes, abdominal obesity, psychosocial factors) were evaluated. The apolipoprotein B1/apolipoprotein A1 ratio was used since apolipoproteins can be checked in non-fasting blood samples unlike low-density lipoprotein levels that would require fasting samples. The authors of the INTERHEART study also cite a paper that shows that this ratio was able to predict CVD events. The percent attributable risk (PAR) for each risk factor was calculated. In other words, these risks accounted for 90% of the risk for CVD. The vast majority of risk is accounted for by what have come to be termed "traditional risk factors."

Nontraditional risk factors

Although the majority of CVD appears to be explained by traditional risk factors, there is residual risk that may be due to the presence of other factors. These have been termed "nontraditional" risk factors. These may be useful in determining risk in patients who by history would be at high risk for CVD but have normal values for the traditional risk factors. As our understanding of the mechanisms of CVD in diabetes has improved, the role of inflammation in the development of both DM and CVD has been recognized. In addition, abnormal fibrinolysis, endothelial function, alteration in adipokine release, and vascular wall abnormalities may all play a role in vascular dysfunction in patients with diabetes [25]. As these mechanisms are investigated, novel risk factors have been identified. A number of interventions we institute for traditional risk factors such as statins and ACE-I appear to improve these nontraditional risk factors.

Although promising, the nontraditional factors are not ready for routine use in all patients. There are multiple reasons for this, such as lack of standardized commercially available tests, lack of data on CVD event reduction following risk improvement, and so on. Of all the novel risks, hsCRP and coronary calcium scores may be the only ones that are currently clinically applicable.

Highly sensitive C-reactive protein (hsCRP)

As a marker of inflammation, hsCRP has been shown in large prospective epidemiologic studies to be associated with an increased incidence of vascular disease and increased mortality. This association was seen in those with and without a known history of CVD and independent of other traditional risk factors. The utility of hsCRP may be in patients at intermediate risk for CVD who have LDL levels at goal. In the Air Force/Texas Coronary Atherosclerosis Prevention Study [26], 6605 patients with dyslipidemia were treated with lovastatin. Patients who had low-density lipoprotein (LDL) levels above median (159 mg/dl) benefitted from the statin. In addition, those with LDL levels below the median but hsCRP levels above median (1.62 mg/L) also benefitted. In contrast, those with hsCRP and LDL levels below the median did not appear to benefit from the use of the statin. The recent JUPITER trial [27], conducted in 26 countries, evaluated >17,000 healthy individuals with no prior history of CVD, who had an LDL <130 mg/dl and hsCRP >2 mg/L. They were treated with Rosuvastatin 20 mg a day and followed for occurrence of the combined primary end point of myocardial infarction, stroke, arterial revascularization, hospitalization for unstable angina, or death from CVD. The trial was stopped after a median follow up of 1.9 years. The main composite end point was reduced by 44% in the treated group compared to placebo. Interestingly, patients traditionally considered low risk (non smokers, absence of metabolic syndrome, Framingham Risk Score of 10% or less) benefitted from Rosuvastatin treatment.

The JUPITER trial demonstrates that in patients considered low risk by measurement of traditional risk factors but have evidence of low-grade inflammation, significant improvement in CVD risk can be achieved by treating with a statin.

Coronary Artery Calcium Scoring (CAC)

Another novel risk factor receiving greater attention has been the Coronary Artery Calcium Scoring (CAC). Coronary calcium is a measure of atherosclerotic plaque development. The 2007 guidelines by the American Heart Association and other groups suggested that the utility of CAC may be greatest in those with intermediate 10-year risk for CVD [28]. Calcium scores are higher in patients with diabetes than in normoglycemic patients with other CVD risk factors. In correlation with clinical findings, CAC scores in symptomatic patients with diabetes appear to match scores in patients who do not have diabetes but do have a history of CAD. Raggi et al. have reported on >10,000 asymptomatic patients of whom about 900 had DM [29]. These patients had screening for CAD by CT ordered by the primary care physicians. They were followed for an average of 5 years. The all-cause mortality increased as calcium score increased, and for any given score, mortality was higher among patients with diabetes. Of particular interest was the finding that the absence of coronary calcium was predictive of low short-term risk of death (1% in 5 years) in those with or without a history of DM. The CAC may be used clinically to predict both a positive and negative risk for a CV event.

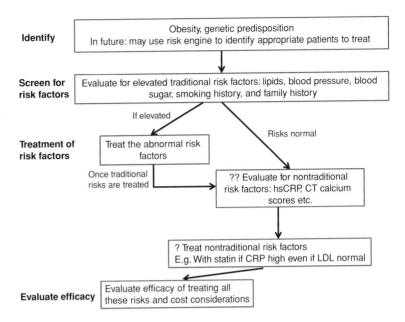

FIG 4.3 Approach to patient who may be at increased risk for cardiovascular disease.

Although intriguing, prospectively conducted long-term studies will have to be conducted before management of patients with diabetes can be altered based on CAC scores.

Summary

Patients with diabetes are at increased risk for cardiovascular disease. Screening with cardiac imaging in asymptomatic individuals may not be as efficacious as "screening" for and treating risk factors. Data regarding evaluation and management of "traditional risk factors" are available for patients with a known history of diabetes but less well established in those with prediabetes. For those with diabetes, screening for and treating traditional risk factors appears to improve outcomes. In patients with diabetes who have normal traditional risk factors, consideration can be given to evaluating and treating nontraditional risk factors such as hsCRP, although long-term outcomes are not available (see Figure 4.3).

A number of unanswered questions remain, including optimal risk stratification of patients. Although we do know that patients with prediabetes have increased risk of CVD, it is not known if early management of risk factors to goals suggested for diabetes will improve outcomes. It is also not clear if all patients with prediabetes should have nontra-

ditional risk factors checked, although the JUPITER trial seems to suggest that even "healthy" patients with evidence of low-grade inflammation may benefit from treatment. There is not enough data to make specific recommendations at this time.

References

1. Buse JB, Ginsberg HN, Bakris GL, et al. Primary prevention of cardiovascular diseases in people with diabetes mellitus:a scientific statement from the American Heart Association and the American Diabetes Association. *Diabetes Care.* 1: 162–172, 2007.
2. Haffner SM, Stern MP, Hazuda HP, Mitchell BD, Patterson JK. Cardiovascular risk factors in confirmed prediabetic individuals. Does the clock for coronary heart disease start ticking before onset of clinical diabetes? *JAMA.* **263**(21): 2893–2898, 1990.
3. Haffner SM, Lehto S, Ronnemaa T, Pvorala K, Laasko M. Mortality from coronary heart disease in subjects with type 2 diabetes mellitus and in nondiabetic subjects with and without prior myocardial infarction. *N Engl J Med.* **339**(4): 229–234, 1998.
4. ADA. American Diabetes Association: Consensus development conference on the diagnosis of coronary heart disease in people with diabetes:10–11 February 1998, Miami, Florida.. *Diabetes Care.* 21:1551–1559, 1998.

5. Sigan RJ, Kenny GP, Wasserman DH, Castaneda-Sceppa C. Physical activity/exercise and type 2 diabetes. *Diabetes Care.* 27(10):2518–2539, 2004.

6. Bax JJ, Young LH, Frye RL, Bonow RO, Steinberg HO, Barrett EJ. Screening for coronary artery disease in patients with diabetes. *Diabetes Care.* 30(10):2729–2736, 2007.

7. Wackers FJ, et al. Detection of silent myocardial ischemia in asymptomatic diabetic subjects. The DIAD study. *Diabetes Care.* 27(8):1954–1961, 2004.

8. Wackers FJ, Chyun DA, Young LH, et al. Resolution of asymptomatic myocardial ischemia in patients with type 2 diabetes in the Detection of Ischemia in Asymptomatic Diabetics (DIAD) study. *Diabetes Care.* 30(11):2892–2898, 2007.

9. Young LH, Wackers FJ, Chyun DA, et al. Cardiac outcomes after screening for asymptomatic coronary artery disease in patients with type 2 diabetes: the DIAD study: a randomized controlled trial. *JAMA.* 301(15):1547–1555. 2009.

10. Boden WE, O'Rourke RA, Teo KK, et al. Optimal medical therapy with or without PCI for stable coronary disease. *N Engl J Med.* 356(15):1503–1516, 2007.

11. The Decode Study Group. Is the current definition for diabetes relevant to mortality risk from all causes and cardiovascular and noncardiovascular disease. *Diabetes Care.* 26(3):688–696, 2003.

12. Norhammer A, Tenerz A, Nilsson G, et al. Glucose metabolism in patients with acute myocardial infarction and no previous diagnosis of diabetes mellitus: a prospective study. *Lancet.* 359(9324):2140–2144, 2002.

13. Barr EL, Zimmet PZ, Welborn TA, et al. Risk of cardiovascular and all-cause mortality in individuals with diabetes mellitus, impaired glucose tolerance, and impaired glucose tolerance. The Australian Diabetes, Obesity, and Lifestyle (AusDiab). *Circulation.* 116:151–157, 2007.

14. Khaw KT, Wareham N, Luben R, et al. Glycated haemoglobin, diabetes, and mortality in men in Norfolk cohort of European Prospective Investigation of Cancer and Nutrition (EPIC-Norfolk). *BMJ.* 322(7277):15–18, 2001.

15. Chiasson JL, Josse RG, Gomis R, et al. Acarbose treatment and the risk of cardiovascular disease and hypertension in patients with impaired glucose tolerance. The STOP-NIDDM trial. *JAMA.* 290(4):486–494, 2003.

16. The Diabetes Control and Complications Trial Research Group. The effect of intensive treatment of diabetes on the development and progression of long-term complications in insulin-dependent diabetes mellitus. *N Engl J Med.* 329(14):977–986, 1993.

17. UK Prospective Diabetes Study (UKPDS) Group. Intensive blood sugar control with sulphonylureas or insulin compared with conventional treatment and risk of complications in Patients with type 2 Diabetes (UKPDS 33). *Lancet.* 352:837–853, 1998.

18. The Diabetes Control and Complications Trial/Epidemiology of Diabetes Interventions and Complications (DCCT/EDIC) Study Research Group. Intensive diabetes treatment and cardiovascular disease in patients with type 1 diabetes. *N Engl J Med.* 353(25):2643–2653, 2005.

19. Holman RR, Paul SK, Bethel AM, et al. 10-year follow-up of intensive glucose control in type 2 diabetes. *N Engl J Med.* 359(15):1577–1589, 2008.

20. Gaede P, Vedel P, Larsen N, et al. Multifactorial intervention and cardiovascular disease in patients with type 2 diabetes. *N Engl J Med.* 348(5):383–393, 2003.

21. Stevens RJ, Kothari V, Adler AI, Stratton IM, Holman RR. The UKPDS risk engine: a model for the risk of coronary heart disease in type II diabetes (UKPDS 56). *Clin Sci.* 101:671–679, 2001.

22. Wilson PW, D'Agostino RB, Levy D, et al. Prediction of coronary heart disease using risk factor categories. *Circulation.* 97:1837–1847, 1998.

23. Eddy DM, Schlessinger L. Validation of the archimedes diabetes model. *Diabetes Care.* 26(11):3102–3110, 2003.

24. Yusuf S, Hawken S, Ounpuu S, et al. Effect of potentially modifiable risk factors associated with myocardial infarction in 52 countries (the interheart study): case-control study. *Lancet.* 364(9438):937–952, 2004.

25. Fonseca V, Desouza C, Asnani S, Jialal I. Nontraditional risk factors for cardiovascular disease in diabetes. *Endocr Rev.* 25(1):153–175, 2004.

26. Ridker PM, Rifai N, Clearfield M, et al. Measurement of C-reactive protein for the targeting of statin therapy in the primary prevention of acute coronary events. *N Engl J Med.* 344(26):1959–1965, 2001.

27. Ridker PM, Danielson E, Fonseca FA, et al. Rosuvastatin for vascular prevention in men and women with elevated C-reactive protein. *N Engl J Med.* 359(21):2195–2207, 2008.

28. Greenland P, et al. ACCF/AHA 2007 clinical expert consensus document on coronary artery calcium scoring by computed tomography in global cardiovascular risk assessment and in the evaluation of patients with chest pain. *JACC.* 49(3):378–402, 2007.

29. Raggi P, Shaw LJ, Berman DS, Callister TQ. Prognostic value of coronary artery calcium screening in subjects with and without diabetes. *JACC.* 43(9):1663–1669, 2004.

PART II
Initial Evaluation and Management of Diabetes

5 · What is the role of self-monitoring in diabetes? Is there a role for postprandial glucose monitoring? How does continuous glucose monitoring integrate into clinical practice?

Rami Almokayyad[1] and Robert Cuddihy[2]

[1] Endocrine Fellow, Division of Endocrinology, Department of Medicine, University of Minnesota Medical School, University of Minnesota, Minneapolis, MN, USA

[2] Medical Director, International Diabetes Center, World Health Organization Collaborating Center for Diabetes Education, Translation and Computer Technology, Minneapolis, MN, USA

LEARNING POINTS

- There is general consensus that the use of SMBG in most individuals with T1DM or those with T2DM treated with insulin is of benefit.

- The benefit of SMBG in individuals with T2DM, not on insulin therapy, remains inconclusive and controversial.

- The role of postprandial glucose monitoring has previously been firmly established in gestational diabetes but remains controversial in T1DM or T2DM.

- Continuous Glucose Monitoring (CGM) devices have documented benefit in adults with T1DM on an insulin pump therapy who use the data it provides to modify their therapy.

- There is a clear need for well-controlled clinical trials to assess the value of SMBG in T2DM for those on other than insulin therapy.

- The lack of a simple universal output of SMBG and CGM data are an impediment to their appropriate uptake and use in primary care.

Self-monitoring of blood glucose

Self-monitoring of blood glucose (SMBG) can be considered one of the bigger advances in diabetes management after the discovery of insulin and oral agents.

Bedside measurement of plasma glucose was introduced in the mid-1920s as a necessity, after the discovery and use of the first insulin. At that time, the only modality to monitor diabetes control was qualitative urine glucose measurements, which only gave patients an estimate of their levels over the proceeding 1–2 days, revealing hyperglycemia only when serum glucose had exceeded the renal threshold (~200 mg/dl) resulting in glycosuria. The procedure of measuring glucose would typically take 20 minutes, as described by Maclean in his book *Modern Methods in the Diagnosis and Treatment of Glycosuria and Diabetes*, published in 1924 [1]. The use of this method was limited to use by the clinician.

By the early 1940s, semiquantitative urine glucose measurement kits became commercially available for home use, and they became the major modality for glucose self-monitoring at home.

In the mid-1960s, reagent strips were introduced as a semiquantitative method of measuring capillary whole blood glucose; a drop of blood was added to these reagents that utilized a glucose oxidase reaction to effect a colorimetric change. The resultant color from the reaction could then be compared with a standard chart and this would give a rough estimate of the blood glucose level. These strips were initially limited to office and hospital use, with limited patient access for home use.

Clinical Dilemmas in Diabetes, First Edition. Edited by Adrian Vella and Robert A. Rizza
© 2011 Blackwell Publishing Ltd. Published 2011 by Blackwell Publishing Ltd.

By the late 1960s reflectance meters were introduced that utilized the same type of reagent strips where a light source was reflected on the strip (instead of reading them manually) enabling the reflected light to be read by a photoelectric cell, which in turn gave a readout of the estimated glucose (using a swinging needle at that time). In the late 1970s meters were developed for patient use.

With advances in technology, electrochemical meters were introduced, and as the technology evolved, improvements were made to reduce the size of these meters, reduce their reaction and reading times, simplify blood sampling techniques, and to reduce the discomfort associated with blood sampling [2]. Today, glucose meters have a central role in diabetes management, with nearly 70% of all patients with diabetes performing some SMBG [3].

Long-term follow-up of participants in the Diabetes Complication and Control Trial (DCCT) as part of the Epidemiology of Diabetes Interventions and Complications (EDIC) in type 1 diabetes mellitus (T1DM), and the 10-year follow-up of the United Kingdom Prospective Diabetes Study (UKPDS) in type 2 diabetes mellitus (T2DM) provide clear evidence that the early and intensive control of hyperglycemia reduces the long-term risks of microvascular and macrovascular complications in diabetes. The effect of good glycemic control seems to persist for years, to some extent independently of subsequent glycemic control. This phenomenon is referred to as "metabolic memory" or "the legacy effect" [4–6]. However, tight glycemic control does come at a cost, which is a threefold increased risk of severe hypoglycemia seen in the DCCT trial (T1DM), as well as the Action to Control Cardiovascular Risks in Diabetes (ACCORD) trial in T2DM [7, 8]. ACCORD also suggested an increased mortality risk with assignment to a strategy aiming to achieve near normoglycemia. However, somewhat surprisingly, this risk was inversely proportional to the rate of fall in HbA1c, being lowest in those individuals who rapidly corrected their HbA1c and highest in those who lowered their HbA1c slowly, or not at all, and the highest mortality in both the standard and intensive glycemic control arms of ACCORD occurred in those patients with higher HbA1c [publically presented ACCORD data with REF coming out in Diabetes Care online within 1 week—Matt Riddle, doi: 10.2337/dc09-1278, *Diabetes Care*, May 2010, vol. 33, no. 5, 983–990]. The available evidence would suggest that in most patients with diabetes one should maintain "tight" glycemic control as early in the course of the disease as possible and to continue to maintain this level of control as tightly as possible

[9], generally targeting an A1c level < 7.0% by ADA guidelines (or < 6.5% by IDF or AACE guidelines), if this can be accomplished safely without exposing the patient to undue risk of severe hypoglycemia.

SMBG therefore can play a pivotal role, when used properly, as an adjunctive tool to enhance patient self-management of their diabetes. SMBG provides day-to-day data on glycemic control; it provides an immediate feedback about the effect of nutrition, physical activity, and medications on blood glucose. It allows prompt determination of hypoglycemia or hyperglycemia that not only can improve patient safety, but also can motivate individuals to make appropriate changes in diet, exercise, and medications.

By shaping meal and activity patterns and providing feedback on medication dosing or titration while simultaneously providing useful information on the potential occurrence or risks of hypoglycemia, the information gleaned from SMBG monitoring can help optimize the delicate balance between the benefits and risks of tight glycemic control.

In this section, we will discuss the utility of SMBG in diabetes management, and we will discuss the evidence behind its use in different patient groups.

SMGB in type 1 DM and insulin-requiring T2DM patients

The use of SMBG in patients with type 1 diabetes and in those with type 2 diabetes treated with intensive insulin therapies or multiple daily insulin injections (MDI) appears logical for several reasons, is supported by clinical trial data, and thus is not controversial.

First, SMGB will provide day-to-day information that can help adjust insulin dose to optimize the overall glycemic control. Patients on bolus ("prandial or meal-related") insulin use the premeal SMBG data to adjust the dose of their prandial insulin, correcting it for the amount of carbohydrate consumed, as well for any variance of the premeal glucose above or below the desired target range (so-called corrective dose insulin). While various insulin adjustment methods may differ in their specific titration schemes, they all utilize premeal SMBG values as an actionable item aiding in appropriately adjusting the insulin dosing before a meal so as to achieve tighter glycemic control.

One of the earliest studies that demonstrated the effectiveness of SMBG in improving glycemic control was conducted in 1982 [10]. This concept was emphasized in the Diabetes Complication and Control Trial, in which intensive insulin therapy has shown to improve glycemic control and reduce microvascular complications, and this was achieved by intensifying insulin regimens utilizing SMBG [7].

Also, SMBG is an important safety tool in insulin treated patients to detect hypoglycemia, especially in patients with hypoglycemia unawareness.

The recommendation from the DCCT was to perform SMBG at least four times per day; however, observational studies have shown that most patients with type 1 diabetes on intensive (physiological) insulin regimen fall short of these recommendations [11].

SMBG in non-insulin-requiring T2DM

Although SMBG is now widely accepted as a part of the management of patients with non-insulin-treated type 2 diabetes, its efficacy and rationale is more controversial. Most of the existing data for the efficacy of SMBG in these subjects come from cross-sectional and retrospective studies, which slightly favored more frequent SMBG [12–14].

Many randomized clinical trials (RCTs) have been carried out in small groups of patients. Participants were not recruited from representative populations in the community and the strategies for use of the results from SMBG were not clearly defined. The relative benefit in terms of HbA1c reduction typically was modest, even in those randomized clinical trials which did show benefit, in the range from a one-quarter to two-thirds of 1%, and most meta-analysis of various combinations of these RCTs favor SMBG. Epidemiologic studies utilizing large patient databases have generally noted improved glycemic control in individuals with diabetes who monitor more often, but such studies can only implicate an association between more frequent SMBG and improved glycemic control, but not a causal relationship. Selection biases and other confounding variables may also affect these results [15]. Other cross-sectional studies, such as the Fremantle Diabetes Study, do not show benefit in terms of glycemic control with SMBG [16].

The Cochrane Collaborative best-evidence-based review of SMBG use in patients with T2DM on non-insulin therapies also appears to favor SMBG but noted that more evidence is needed [17].

Recently, Farmer and colleagues conducted a randomized controlled trial (Diabetes Glycaemic Education and Monitoring [DiGEM] study) that aimed to test whether SMBG, used with or without instruction in incorporating findings into self-care, can improve glycemic control in non-insulin-treated diabetes patients compared with standardized usual care [18]. A total of 453 patients were individually randomized to one of three groups: (1) standardized usual care with 3-monthly HbA1c (control); (2) blood glucose self-testing with patient training focused on clinician interpretation of results in addition to usual care (less intensive self-monitoring); or (3) SMBG with additional training of patients in interpretation and application of the results to enhance motivation and maintain adherence to a healthy lifestyle (more intensive self-monitoring).

There was no evidence of glycemic benefit between the three groups at the end of 12 months (no difference in the primary outcome; Hemoglobin A1C). In addition, there was no evidence of a significantly different impact of self-monitoring on glycemic control when comparing subgroups of patients defined by duration of diabetes, therapy, and diabetes-related complications. Patients who were in the more intensive SMBG arm detected more hypoglycemia. The economic analysis suggested that SMBG resulted in extra health care costs and was unlikely to be cost-effective if used routinely. There was an initial negative impact associated with more frequent use of SMBG on the quality of life [19].

The potential clinical ramifications from this study have been huge and called into question the utility, cost-effectiveness, and effect on quality of life of SMBG individuals with T2DM who are not on insulin therapy. In an era of tightening financial resources, an epidemic of T2DM, and attempts to curb health care expenditures in general, this and subsequent reports from the DiGEM study had lead to a wide reappraisal of benefits or SMBG in individuals who are not yet treated with insulin. Reappraisal of the need to cover SMBG testing supplies for individuals with T2DM not treated with insulin by payers and national groups such as the National Health Service in the U.K. and the Centers for Medicare and Medicaid Services (CMS) in the United States have reportedly taken place. Thus, a careful look at some of the potential concerns or criticism of the DiGEM study is warranted.

This study enrolled individuals with relatively recent onset of diabetes (median duration of 3 years) treated with diet or oral agents with reasonably good glycemic control (mean HbA1c of 7.5%), and specifically selected individuals who were either not monitoring SMBG at all or monitoring no more than a single one-time SMBG per week. Thus, the study may have inadvertently selected a biased population less geared toward, or less compliant with, SMBG monitoring and with potentially less to gain from improvements in glucose control. Of concern is the case that it was in the intensive SMBG cohort that more individuals quit SMBG monitoring than the less intensive cohort. Also, for those who were to utilize the SMBG data to modify their lifestyle or medication, a delineation of a specified action plan in response to the SMBG data is lacking and not delineated. While there was a minimal decline in HbA1c by 0.17 % in this group, it was not statistically significant. Of potential concern was the issue that the reduction in HbA1c in this study was far less than those reported from the majority of other RCT evaluating the effect of SMBG.

Criticisms aside, this study was a careful attempt to get at the issue of the value of SMBG in terms of improvements in glycemic control in such a population of individuals and at least raises the stakes for proponents of SMBG to prove its worth in non-insulin-treated populations. Several groups have formed to attempt to outline the necessary components of a large scale RCT to better evaluate the role and utility of SMBG in T2DM [15, 20].

From a philosophical standpoint it is of vital importance to understand the use of SMBG as a useful diagnostic tool to enhance patient self-management of diabetes rather than as a direct therapeutic intervention targeting glucose levels. As such, there are multiple aspects of the use of SMBG that must be in place for the data it generates to be accurate, beneficial to glycemic control and, most importantly, used by the patient. Important potential barriers to appropriate SMBG include proper technique, correct coding of glucose meters to match the testing strips, correct setting of the time and date of the meter to aid in SMBG review of downloaded meter data and, most importantly, appropriate patient education and understanding of the timing of SMBG and the use of the data derived from it to modify the patient's self-management. The data can then become an actionable item leading to modification in therapy (whether leading to changes in diet or activity through behavioral change, or adjustment in medication). Ideally, to maximize the impact of SMBG, the patients themselves should be educated on how to appropriately use SMBG. Such a tool could be used at various time points to optimize management throughout the day, uncovering needed behavioral modifications in diet and activity, providing feedback for potential problematic periods of marked hyperglycemia or hypoglycemia, and providing the patient an early detection of worsening overall glycemic control due either to situational factors such as intercurrent illness or steroid usage, or the progressive nature of T2DM itself. Such information would indicate the need to titrate therapy to reestablish target levels of glycemic control in a timely manner.

There is a great need for specific algorithms instructing patients what do in terms of altering their management or therapy in response to their SMBG data. Some early preliminary data suggest that patient-driven algorithms based on SMBG can be more effective in helping them reach target than management that relies on the patient's health care provider or clinician to review the data and recommend changes in therapy. For example, in the commonly seen patient with good control of AM fasting blood glucose (BG), but HbA1c's above target, it is likely that BG values are higher at other time points throughout the day.

Bergenstal et al showed that utilizing an algorithm for titrating premeal insulin solely based on preprandial SMBG values, rather than utilizing strict carbohydrate counting with matching insulin to carbohydrate dosing, was equally effective in controlling glycemic levels in insulin-treated individuals with T2DM [21].

The technical aspects of glucose meters that serve as barriers are the easiest to correct and, in fact, meters that do not require coding of the meter to match the testing strips are beginning to enter the market. Time and date stamping of SMBG values will become automated. Meal markers are available on some units to aid in interpreting fasting or premeal glucose patterns from postprandial patterns. Many meters can inform the patient if the blood sample is inadequate for an accurate test result.

The lack of patient education and training in diabetes self-management, including proper use of SMBG, remains a significant barrier that requires more effort to correct. In clinical practice, one frequently encounters patients treated with lifestyle modification and Metformin monotherapy who have been instructed to perform SMBG and dutifully obtain one fasting blood glucose value each morning. No alternative testing schema is offered if the AM fasting glucoses are within goal but the HbA1c remains above goal. Clearly, rather than obtain seven "normal fasting readings" per week the utility of SMBG would be markedly enhanced if such patients were educated to use these same seven weekly readings in a more dispersed fashion, sampling once daily, but at alternating times each day. Perhaps obtaining AM fasting blood glucose on Monday, 2-hour postprandial BG after breakfast on Tuesday, prelunch BG on Wednesday, 2-hour post-lunch BG on Thursday, predinner BG on Friday, post-dinner BG on Saturday, and bedtime BG on Sunday would provide a wealth of actionable information? For instance a significant postprandial rise in BG following a specific meal could signal the patient to make modifications in the timing or quantity of carbohydrate consumed during the day or to add more physical activity prior to this meal. If unable to correct this issue with dietary or activity changes, such findings could lead the patient to engage their physician to consider the addition of another pharmacologic agent targeting postprandial BGs. The individual could "learn" from the response of SMBG just how various meals and meal composition affect their BGs and what the affect of various activities are on their BGs, acting as a useful tool and reinforcement for beneficial behavioral modification. If the postprandial BG rise was more pronounced following one specific meal, then the pattern of SMBG monitoring might temporarily change while the individual "works on that particular problem area," perhaps using many of their weekly SMBG determinations before and after that particular meal to assess the result of various attempted interventions, returning to a widespread surveillance pattern of SMBG once the "problem is solved" or corrected. This surveillance SMBG would then inform the individual if and where the next issue in fine-tuning glycemic control should occur.

If individuals are on agents that can cause hypoglycemia, such as a sulfonylurea (SU), then surveillance SMBG can indicate if there is a problematic period of increased risk of hypoglycemia during the day, such as the late afternoon or predinner period or overnight, which should ideally lead to corrective intervention to reduce this risk.

Utilizing SMBG for continuous surveillance and quality improvement of their diabetes self-management can help counteract the clinical inertia currently seen in our health systems, which are not properly designed to manage non-acute chronic diseases such as diabetes. Brown et al [22] have demonstrated how this inertia can result in patients' encountering 8–10 years of exposure to significant chronic hyperglycemia, with the increased risk for complications that this entails while their medical regimen is very slowly progressed through the different available therapies. Patients should be empowered to contact their health care provider as soon as they encounter problematic hyperglycemia that has not responded to their attempts at correction, as medication may need to be advanced. Rather than await their next regularly scheduled 3- to 6-month appointment before advancement in therapy is undertaken, the therapies could be quickly optimized until the glycemic goals or treatment targets are achieved.

Another barrier to the optimal use of patient derived SMBG data in diabetes management occurs in physician offices. In today's environment where health care providers have less and less time in which to see their patients, they are often forced to complete the entire visit in 15 to 20 minutes. In such a scenario, the use of the glucose logbook to look for patterns from which to make therapeutic recommendations is problematic. It is difficult to expect busy providers to visually scan often messy, hand-scribbled columns of individual glucose values and try and make some sense of any emerging pattern after flipping through several pages in a standard glucose logbook (Figure 5.1). The ability to download glucose meter data and present verified aggregate glucose data in an organized fashion, with basic statistical summaries, is certainly an improvement. However, the multitude of differing proprietary software programs needed to download the data from each company's meter and the slightly different presentation format of each of these software programs severely inhibit the broad generalizability of this important tool and thus limits its uptake in offices, especially in primary care settings. As opposed to another diagnostic tool, the electrocardiogram (ECG), which has the same standardized universal output, no such common format and universal output exists for SMBG data. Thus, while the standard 12-lead ECG tracing enjoys widespread use in clinical practice, SMBG use remains most widely relegated to the use of a handwritten glucose logbook. This is a major gap in our ability to teach glycemic pattern recognition to our patients and fellow clinicians, severely impeding the great potential of SMBG to help shape therapeutic interventions and improve overall levels of control. The representation of all SMBG data expressed as a single day over 24 hours was an attempt to have some more common output from the multitude of meters, many of which do allow data to also be expressed in this form (Figure 5.2). Unfortunately, the widespread use of such a modal day output never became commonplace, especially in primary care practice where they may be most useful.

The many barriers to the proper use of SMBG and the controversy still remaining around the utility of SMBG in patients with T2DM who are not on insulin have given rise to an interesting question. Given that many available therapies including dietary and activity modification, or pharmacologic agents such as metformin, dipeptidyl peptidase-IV (DDP-4) inhibitors, glucagon-like peptide -1 (GLP-1) receptor agonists, and thiazolidinediones (TZDs) all can improve overall glycemic control and do not result in increased risks for hypoglycemia, could many patients use these therapies singly or in combination without the need for any SMBG?

These patients could be followed by period HbA1c measurement to be sure that they are achieving their overall

Date	Night BG	BREAKFAST			LUNCH			DINNER			BEDTIME		Notes/Ketones	SMBG values tranlated in mmol/L
		BG (mg/dL)	Med	BG	BG	Med	BG	BG (mg/dL)	Med	BG	BG (mg/dL)	Med		
2/24	179							199			272			9.9-11.0-15.1
2/25	198							177			189		Shopping	11.0-9.8-10.5
2/26	165							188			182			9.2-10.4-10.1
2/27	195							209			248			10.8-11.6-13.8
2/28	187							225						10.4-12.5
3/1	153							167			288		20 min walk	8.5-9.3-16.0
3/2	182							159			219			10.1-8.9-12.1
3/3	197							155			203			10.9-8.6-11.3
3/4	189							182			199		20 min walk	10.5-10.1-11.1
3/5	210							153			262		20 min walk	11.7-8.5-14.6
3/6	173													9.6
3/7														

FIG 5.1 Typical patient glucose logbook with self-reported data.

glycemic targets. The cost savings based on forgoing the need for expensive glucose testing strips one or many times daily, as well as the ease of daily self-management of their diabetes and potential perceived improvement in quality of life, might justify such an approach?

Thus, there remains an urgent and ongoing need for properly designed, well-controlled RCTs to evaluate just what is the benefit of SMBG in those individuals with T2DM treated with non-insulin therapies. This population, given their greater numbers, likely makes up the lion's share of the SMBG market and thus this question has enormously important ramifications for general public health care policy in dealing with the growing diabetes epidemic.

Postprandial SMBG

The role of postprandial SMBG is firmly established in women with gestational diabetes mellitus (GDM).

Adjusting insulin therapy in mothers with GDM, based on postprandial BG, resulted in improved HbA1c, lower birth weights (i.e., less macrosomia), less neonatal hypoglycemia and less need for a cesarean section at delivery [23].

Meal-based SMBG is a valuable tool for improving outcomes in pregnancy complicated by diabetes and has been shown to improve fetal perinatal outcomes [24]. This is more evident in insulin-treated patients, and less clear with diet-controlled patients [25], although such monitoring may be useful in providing feedback for behavioral modification and surveillance as to the adequacy of glucose control and the need to intensify therapies if not within target. Also, it encourages patients to actively participate in their own care.

The role of postprandial SMBG in T1DM and especially in T2DM is controversial. The landmark trials, such as the DCCT-EDIC and UKPDS and its 10-year follow-up trials clearly showed that improving overall glycemic control, thus reducing chronic exposure to hyperglycemia as measured by the HbA1c, reduced the risks of microvascular and macrovascular complications [4–7]. Thus, the current recommendations by the ADA to target an HbA1c of <7% in most individuals with diabetes [26]. These trials did not typically require postprandial SMBG, nor compare the effects of targeting fasting and

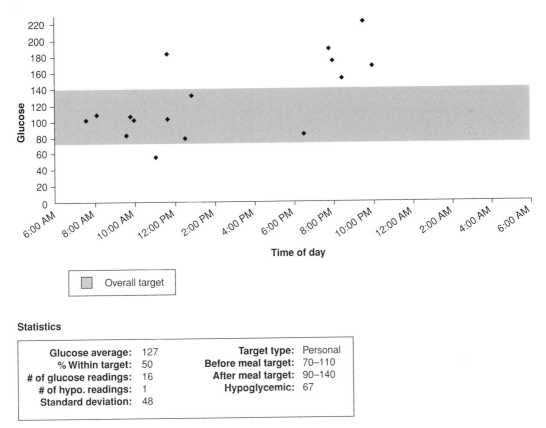

Statistics

Glucose average:	127	Target type:	Personal	
% Within target:	50	Before meal target:	70–110	
# of glucose readings:	16	After meal target:	90–140	
# of hypo. readings:	1	Hypoglycemic:	67	
Standard deviation:	48			

FIG 5.2 Modal Day presentation of downloaded meter with SMBG data.

premeal SMBG versus postprandial SMBG in reducing complications.

In T1DM it is not uncommon for individuals to monitor postprandial SMBG regularly to assess the adequacy of control exerted by their premeal short- or rapid-acting insulin on an MDI program or their bolus, if they are on insulin-pump continuous subcutaneous insulin infusion (CSII) therapy. Monitoring postprandial SMBG provides these individuals with feedback both on insulin dosage and self-management behavior such as carbohydrate counting and their insulin to carbohydrate ratio. Nonetheless, it remains a common clinical practice for many individuals with either T1DM or T2DM to use their next or following premeal SMBG, rather than a 2 hour PPG, to gauge the efficacy of their previous premeal insulin dose or other therapy directed toward glycemic control. This assumes that if the next premeal SMBG is within target, then the postprandial glucose values were likely "acceptable." While this method does provide a crude, indirect estimate of glycemic control

over this period, it cannot guarantee glucose excursions, or overall glycemic exposure, are well controlled. Thus, while this method is less labor intensive and may be an appropriate compromise in terms of "quality of life" for the individual, more intensive SMBG monitoring, including PPG, should be considered if HbA1c is not within the desired target range.

In T2DM the role of postprandial SMBG is even less clear. T2DM usually has a more indolent onset, slowly progressing through phases of glucose intolerance to frank diabetes, and is closely associated with the metabolic syndrome and the increased cardiovascular risk that this entails. There have been several studies, such as the *DECODE*, and others, that have found correlations with elevated postprandial glucoses and cardiovascular disease risk extending from impaired glucose tolerance right down into the normal range for glucose, and in fact indicate greater association with risks of cardiovascular disease for elevations in postprandial glucose (PPG) than fasting plasma glucose (FPG) [27, 28].

Again, most of the trials correlated improvement in chronic glucose exposure as measured by HbA1c with decreased risk of long-term complications. Some studies suggest a closer correlation of postprandial or post-challenge glucose with HbA1c and mortality than fasting glucose [29], but this remains controversial and is not seen in yet other studies. Therapies that specifically target PPG such as Acarbose have been shown to reduce CV disease and all-cause mortality in the Stop-NIDDM trial [30, 31]. Studies by Ceriello, and others, have provided indirect evidence that glycemic variability or excursions (typically most marked in the immediate postprandial period) directly contribute to diabetic complications through oxidative stress, and the generation of free radical formation, activation of the polyol pathways, and generation of PKC β and advanced glycosylation end products (AGES) [32, 33]. The role PPG plays in the development of long-term diabetic complications remains very controversial. One often-referenced paper, used to support this evidence that PPG plays a role in complications in T1DM, noted that in the DCCT trial those individuals in the intensive glycemic treatment arm suffered from less diabetes-related complications than did their counterparts in the standard arm, even when matched for HbA1c, which is actually incorrect [34]. This was actually a hypothesized extrapolation or modeling of the data and not directly representative of the clinical data itself [35]. While the controversy continues to rage, some groups like the International Diabetes Federation (IDF) have published guidelines for the control of PPG [36].

Given the relative lack of strong RCT data comparing the benefits of postprandial SMBG versus fasting and immediate premeal SMBG measurement, why might postprandial SMBG measurement be of importance in individuals with T2DM who are not treated with insulin? It may be necessary to target PPG to get more of these individuals to their glycemic goal. Monnier et al have shown in a population of individuals with T2DM not treated with insulin that the contribution of PPG to overall glycemic exposure rises progressively the closer one approaches a target HbA1c < 7% [37]. At HbA1c < 7.6% the contribution of PPG to overall glycemic exposure totals approximately 70%. This, in turn, may help to explain why in several RCTs that targeted interventions aimed at achieving an AM fasting blood sugar within a specific goal range (typically less than 100 mg/dL), many individuals who have achieved this target still have HbA1c that remains above 7%. With nearly 40% of the U.S. population not in target in terms of HbA1c, more focus on PPG through proper postprandial SMBG monitoring and patient education on what action to take if they are not in target may be necessary! As noted, the IDF has published a guideline of the targeting of postprandial SMBG [36], and the ADA and AACE guidelines give recommended postprandial target glucose levels.

A reasonable approach may be to recommend targeted PPG or intensification of SMBG in individuals who are either not within their goal range for HbA1c on their stabilized maintenance diabetes regimen, or in newly treated patients with initially high HbA1c's, as their HbA1c's are lowered by initial therapies and are approaching 7%. The key is to use SMBG when it serves a discreet purpose either as an actionable item to potentially modify therapy or in surveillance to ensure adequate glycemic control is being maintained.

Continuous glucose monitoring systems

The relatively recent advent of commercially available subcutaneous continuous glucose monitoring (CGM) systems that continuously measure interstitial fluid glucose has added to the armamentarium of tools potentially useful for the self-management of diabetes. Devices from three manufactures are currently available and licensed as an adjunctive tool for diabetes management, most commonly in T1DM for persons on MDI or CSII insulin regimens. The FDA has mandated that these devices not be used for directly calculating an insulin dose based on the most current CGM reading, as their accuracy in comparison to those from approved glucose meters measuring capillary venous whole blood has not been firmly established. Rather, the data generated from CGM can be useful in guiding necessary SMBG testing by delineating the real-time trending in sequential glucose values, either indicating worsening hyperglycemia that may result in the need to confirm with SMBG and potentially take an added supplemental dose of insulin; or in indicating rapid glucose lowering that may result in eventual hypoglycemia, warranting treatment. These systems also make available alarms that can call one's attention to developing hyperglycemia or hypoglycemia prompting corrective action.

Most studies of CGM to date have utilized this tool in patients with T1DM on MDI or CSII insulin therapies, taking advantage of the real-time glucose trending data to fine-tune insulin therapy. Just as with SMBG, CGM is but a tool to help guide one's diabetes self-management, and not an antihyperglycemic intervention in and of itself. The effects of CGM on HbA1c have been relatively mild but real. The recent JDRF CGM study [38] showed that the use of CGM in patients with T1DM on CSII did improve HbA1c in adult patients (over 25 years of age), but not in children and teenagers who had much higher rates of non-adherence with proper CGM use (i.e., wearing a sensor) or using the provided data for decision making.

The Star 1 trial [39] did not demonstrate dramatic HbA1c lowering in individuals with T1DM using CSII who used CGM. It did suggest that in those who used the CGM, the increased usage was associated with an increased probability of HbA1c lowering. Many other moderate-sized trials (*n* of 100–200) assessing CGM use have come to similar conclusions, i.e., increased use of the CGM devices and the data they provide are associated with higher probability of HbA1c lowering.

The soon-to-be completed Star 3 trial is intended to demonstrate that CGM use with CSII is superior to MDI therapy in patients with T1DM.

Like almost any intervention, there has been a "downside" occasionally noted in some individuals with T1DM who use a CGM. In some individuals there is a tendency to "overbolus" in response to continuing high readings viewed on the device. This occurs when individuals feel compelled to frequently re-bolus with a short- or rapid-acting insulin when high glucose readings are viewed on the CGM device, most of which provide a new reading every 1–5 minutes. This impatience, upon frequently viewing high glucose following an intervention that has not yet had adequate time to work, can lead to "insulin stacking." This phenomenon occurs where the effect of the most recent insulin dose is in addition to ("on top of") the ongoing insulin effect from the residual insulin on board from the previous injection, resulting in hypoglycemia. Proper education and training of individuals as well as careful patient selection is required in choosing individuals who will benefit from CGM.

Another effect that has been seen is "sensor burnout," where it becomes difficult to maintain the ongoing effort required to respond to the wealth of data provided by a device in "real time," which may or may not require an action on the individual's part. In some studies utilizing CGM the HbA1c can be seen to improve over the first 3–9 months only to regress toward the mean after more prolonged follow-up because the information is no longer being used with the same intensity.

Currently, there is much research attempting to eventually link the continuous data derived from a CGM device to an insulin pump. Such a system might to able to respond to the continuous data communicated to the pump by the CGM device and respond with automated changes in the insulin infusion. Such a "closed loop" device has been the holy grail of diabetes therapies, short of an actual cure for the disease.

The potential future growth of CGM may well depend largely on its intermittent use for collection and summary of large quantities of glucose data for "glycemic pattern recognition" in individuals with T2DM (or T1DM). The use of periodic CGM in this way would function as a "diagnostic biopsy" providing much more detailed and potentially more useful information than an HbA1c. This glycemic pattern data would aid in targeting appropriate therapeutic changes as well as delineating the optimal and appropriate timing of SMBG once the short period of CGM monitoring is concluded.

However, just as with SMBG, similar barriers are arising with CGM, as each company promotes its own proprietary software for data downloading. With no standardized universal output and at least three competing and differing software outputs, the widespread adoption of CGM tools in T2DM, especially in primary care, will face similar barriers as the proper use of SMBG. Its use will inevitably be retarded by the increased effort, logistical issues, and more complicated training and education the widespread use of such varying outputs in the CGM will require of busy physician practices. These issues are made even more complex by the sheer amount of data generated by CGM devices (up to 15K glucose values over a 2-week period) making even organizing the data as modal day challenging to make clinically relevant sense of (Figure 5.3).

Future applications of CGM may make graphical organization of this immense amount of data more feasible to be used in the busy office setting, perhaps allowing for quick pattern recognition of summarized glycemic data, rather than a laborious and time-consuming review of each glucose data point. Mazze et al, at the International Diabetes Center in Minneapolis, have developed a universal output from the three currently available commercial CGM devices that has the added advantage of summarizing and smoothing the immense amount of data from such devices in both a quantitative statistical manner as well as in an intuitive graphic display (Figure 5.4). The ambulatory glucose profile (AGP) readily aids in rapid assessment and pattern

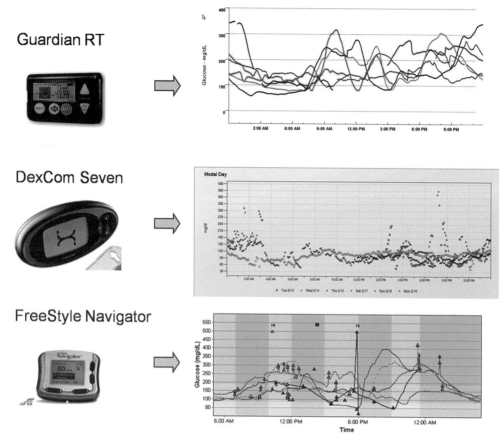

FIG 5.3 Varying outputs from commercially available CGM devices.

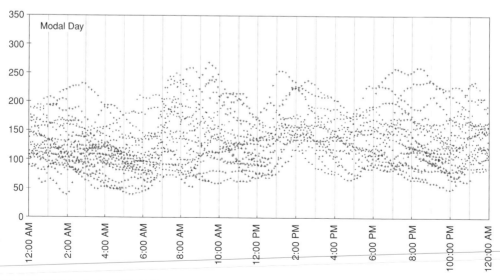

FIG 5.4 CGM device output as a Modal Day.

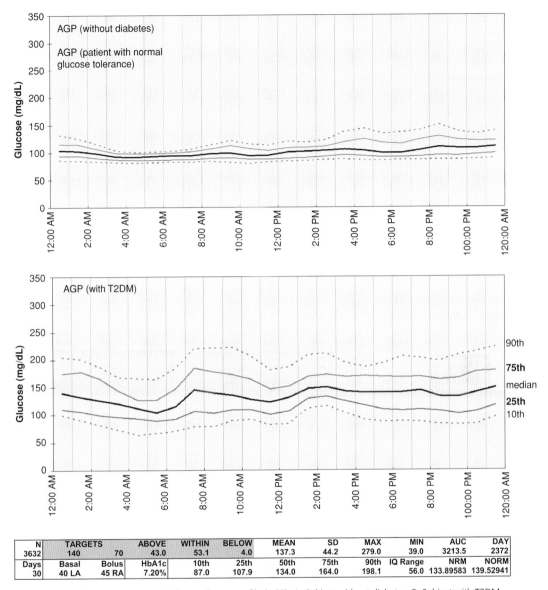

FIG 5.5 Universal CGM output as ambulatory glucose profile (AGP). A. Subject without diabetes. B. Subject with T2DM

N	TARGETS		ABOVE	WITHIN	BELOW	MEAN	SD	MAX	MIN	AUC	DAY
3632	140	70	43.0	53.1	4.0	137.3	44.2	279.0	39.0	3213.5	2372
Days	Basal	Bolus	HbA1c	10th	25th	50th	75th	90th	IQ Range	NRM	NORM
30	40 LA	45 RA	7.20%	87.0	107.9	134.0	164.0	198.1	56.0	133.89583	139.52941

recognition of the individual patient's stable daily glycemic pattern (Figure 5.5). Much like the standardized tracings of an EGC, the universal graphic output of an AGP may aid in its utility as a tool for the time-pressed primary care physician who is attempting to complete an office visit, an assessment of multiple medical issues, and devise a therapeutic plan for their patients with diabetes within the context of a 15 to 20 minute office visit. In such a scenario the office or

practice would own and reuse the CGM device after proper cleaning and disinfection of the device between patient uses. The patient or his or her payer would only pay for a single sensor (about $55) and perhaps an interpretation fee (much like an ECG). Thus, if use of this data to generate an AGP allowed the treating physician to rapidly and more accurately assess the patient's current glycemic control pattern, select an appropriate therapy, and guide the timing and intensity of targeted SMBG in follow-up, it would appear to be time saving. Combine this with the potential ability for this method to allow more rapid and targeted titration of interventions or medication until therapeutic glycemic targets are reached, and this future approach may be relatively cost effective.

It is important to keep in mind that both SMBG and CGM are but tools to aid in diabetes self-management and to provide actionable data for patients and their caregivers. They are not a therapeutic intervention expected to improve overall glycemic control in and of themselves. To optimize the benefits of SMBG or CGM, it must be used with appropriate understanding of how the information gleaned from these tools is to be used to monitor, and if need be alter, one's current therapies. These tools need to be viewed in the larger context of the patient's knowledge, abilities, financial resources, and desire to utilize these tools appropriately. Current data, especially on the use of SMBG in patients with T2DM not utilizing insulin therapy remains fraught with controversy. Opinions are driven by contradictory conclusions from multiple small, sometimes poorly designed clinical trials, as well as various meta-analysis. There remains a real need for well-controlled, thoughtfully designed randomized clinically controlled trials to help answer these questions. Groups are now attempting to define those important characteristics to be included in such trials [15, 20].

References

1. MacLean H. *Modern Methods in the Diagnosis and Treatment of Glycosuria and Diabetes.* Constable, London, 1924.
2. Dufaitre-Patouraux L, Vague P, Lassmann-Vague V. History, accuracy and precision of SMBG devices. *Diabetes Metab.* **29**(2 Pt 2):S7–14, 2003.
3. Centers for Disease Control and Prevention. MMWR self-monitoring of blood glucose among adults with diabetes — United States, 1997—2006. *Morb Mortal Wkly Rep.* **56**(43):1133–1137, 2007.
4. The Diabetes Control and Complications Trial/ Epidemiology of Diabetes Interventions and Complications (DCCT/EDIC) Study Research Group. Intensive diabetes treatment and cardiovascular disease in patients with type 1 diabetes. *N Engl J Med.* **353**:2643–2653, 2005.
5. The Diabetes Control and Complications Trial/ Epidemiology of Diabetes Interventions and Complications Research Group. Sustained effect of intensive treatment of type 1 diabetes mellitus on development

and progression of diabetic nephropathy. *JAMA.* **290**: 2159–2167, 2003.
6. Holman RR, Paul SK, Bethel MA, et al. 10-year follow-up of intensive glucose control in type 2 diabetes. *N Engl J Med.* **359**:1577–1589, 2008.
7. The Diabetes Control and Complications Trial Research Group. The effect of intensive treatment of diabetes on the development and progression of long-term complications in insulin-dependent diabetes mellitus. *N Engl J Med.* **329**:977–986, 1993.
8. The Action to Control Cardiovascular Risk in Diabetes Study Group. Effects of intensive glucose lowering in type 2 diabetes. *N Engl J Med.* **358**:2545–2559, 2008.
9. Del Prato S, LaSalle J, Matthaei S, Bailey CJ, on behalf of the Global Partnership for Effective Diabetes Management. Tailoring treatment to the individual in type 2 diabetes practical guidance from the Global Partnership for Effective Diabetes Management. *Int J Clin Pract.* **64**:295–304, 2010.
10. Schiffrin A, Belmonte M. Multiple daily self-glucose monitoring: its essential role in long-term glucose control in insulin-dependent diabetic patients treated with pump and multiple subcutaneous injections. *Diabetes Care.* **5**:479–484, 1982.
11. Hansen MV, Pedersen-Bjergaard U, Heller SR, et al. Frequency and motives of blood glucose self-monitoring in type 1 diabetes. *Diabetes Res Clin Pract.* **85**(2):183–188. Epub 2009 Jun 3, 2009.
12. Evans JM, Newton RW, Ruta DA, et al. Frequency of blood glucose monitoring in relation to glycaemic control: observational study with diabetes database. *BMJ.* **319**(7202):83–86, 1999.
13. Davidson PC, Bode BW, Steed RD, Hebblewhite HR. A cause-and-effect-based mathematical curvilinear model that predicts the effects of self-monitoring of blood glucose frequency on hemoglobin A1c and is suitable for statistical correlations. *J Diabetes Sci Technol.* **1**(6):850–856, 2007.
14. Murata GH, Shah JH, Hoffman RM, et al. Intensified blood glucose monitoring improves glycemic control in stable, insulin-treated veterans with type 2 diabetes: the Diabetes Outcomes in Veterans Study (DOVES). *Diabetes Care.* **26**(6):1759–1763, 2003.
15. Klonoff DC, Bergenstal R, Blonde R, et al. Consensus report of the coalition for clinical research – self-monitoring of blood glucose. *J Diabetes Sci Technol.* **2**(6):1030–1053, 2008.
16. Davis WA, Bruce DG, Davis TME. Does self-monitor of blood glucose improve outcome in type 2 diabetes? The Fremantle Study. *Diabetologia.* **50**:510–515, 2007.
17. Welschen LMC, Bloemendal E, Nijpels G, et al. Self-monitoring of blood glucose in patients with type 2 diabetes mellitus who are not using insulin. *Cochrane*

Database Syst Rev. 2005, Issue 2. Art. No.: CD005060. DOI: 10.1002/14651858.CD005060.pub2.

18. Farmer A, Wade A, Goyder E, et al. Impact of self monitoring of blood glucose in the management of patients with non-insulin treated diabetes: open parallel group randomized trial. *BMJ.* **335**(7611):132, 2007.

19. Farmer A, Wade A, French DP, et al. Blood glucose self-monitoring in type 2 diabetes: a randomised controlled trial *Health Technol Assess.* **13**(15), 2009.

20. Hirsch IB, Bode BW, Childs BP, et al. Self-Monitoring of Blood Glucose (SMBG) in insulin- and non-insulin-using adults with diabetes: consensus recommendations for improving SMBG accuracy, utilization, and research. *Diabetes Technol Ther.* **10**(6):419–439, 2008.

21. Bergenstal R, Johnson M, Powers M, et al. Adjust to target in type 2 diabetes. *Diabetes Care.* **31**(7):1305–1310, 2008.

22. Brown LB, Nichols GA, Perry A. The burden of treatment failure in type 2 diabetes. *Diabetes Care.* **27**:1535–1540, 2004.

23. DeVeciana M, Major C, Morgan M, et al. Postprandial versus preprandial blood glucose monitoring in women with gestational diabetes mellitus requiring insulin therapy. *N Engl J Med.* **333**(19):1237–1241, 1995.

24. Wecher DJ, Kaufmann RC, Amankwah KS, et al. Prevention of neonatal macrosomia in gestational diabetes by the use of intensive dietary therapy and home glucose monitoring. *Am J Perinatol.* **8**:131–134, 1991.

25. Homko CJ, Sivan E, Reece EA. The impact of self-monitoring of blood glucose on self-efficacy and pregnancy outcomes in women with diet-controlled gestational diabetes. *Diabetes Educ.* **28**(3):435–443, 2002.

26. 2010 ADA Clinical Practice Recommendations.

27. The DECODE Study Group. Glucose tolerance and mortality: comparison of WHO and American Diabetes Association diagnostic criteria. The DECODE study group. European Diabetes Epidemiology Group. Diabetes Epidemiology: Collaborative analysis of Diagnostic criteria in Europe. *Lancet.* **354**:617–621, 1999.

28. Ohkubo Y, Kishikawa H, Araki E, et al. Intensive insulin therapy prevents the progression of diabetic microvascular complications in Japanese patients with non-insulin-dependent diabetes mellitus: a randomized prospective 6-year study. *Diabetes Res Clin Pract.* **28**:103–117, 1995.

29. Avignon A, Radauceanu A, Monnier L. Nonfasting plasma glucose is a better marker of diabetic control than fasting plasma glucose in type 2 diabetes. *Diabetes Care.* **20**: 1822–1826, 1997.

30. Chiasson JL, Josse RG, Gomis R, et al. Acarbose treatment and the risk of cardiovascular disease and hypertension in patients with impaired glucose tolerance: the STOP-NIDDM trial. *JAMA.* **290**:486–494, 2003.

31. Hanefeld M, Cagatay M, Petrowitsch T, et al. Acarbose reduces the risk for myocardial infarction in type 2 diabetic patients: meta-analysis of seven long-term studies. *Eur Heart J.* **25**(1):10–16, 2004.

32. Ceriello A, Ihnat M, Thorpe J. Clinical review 2: The "metabolic memory": is more than just tight glucose control necessary to prevent diabetic complications? *Journal Of Clinical Endocrinology And Metabolism [serial on the Internet].* **94**(2):410–415, 2009, [cited February 1, 2010]. Available from: MEDLINE with Full Text.

33. Brownlee M, Hirsch I. Glycemic variability: a hemoglobin A1c-independent risk factor for diabetic complications. *JAMA [serial on the Internet].* **295**(14):1707–1708, 2006, [cited February 1, 2010]. Available from: MEDLINE with Full Text.

34. DCCT Study Group. The relationship of glycemic exposure (HbA1c) to the risk of development and progression of retinopathy in the diabetes control and complications trial. *Diabetes.* **44**:968–983, 1995.

35. Lachin JM, Genuth S, Nathan DM, Zinman B, Rutledge BN and for the DCCT/EDIC Research Group. Effect of glycemic exposure on the risk of microvascular complications in the diabetes control and complications trial—Revisited. *Diabetes.* **57**:995–1001, 2008.

36. *Guideline for Management of Postmeal Glucose.* International Diabetes Federation, www.idf.org, 2007.

37. Monnier L, Lapinski H, Colette C. Contributions of fasting and postprandial plasma glucose increments to the overall diurnal hyperglycemia of type 2 diabetic patients: variations with increasing levels of HbA1c. *Diabetes Care.* **26**:881–885, 2003.

38. Juvenile Diabetes Research Foundation Continuous Glucose Monitoring Study Group. Continuous glucose monitoring and intensive treatment of type 1 diabetes. *N Engl J Med.* **359**:1464–1476, 2008. DOI: 10.1056/NEJMoa0805017.

39. Hirsch IB, Abelseth J, Bode BW, et al. Sensor-augmented insulin pump therapy: results of the first randomized treat-to-target study. *Diabetes Technol Ther.* **10**:377–383, 2008.

6 The optimal diet for diabetes is?

Maria L. Collazo-Clavell

Associate Professor of Medicine, Division of Endocrinology, Diabetes, Metabolism & Nutrition, Mayo Clinic, Rochester, MN, USA

LEARNING POINTS

- The goals of medical nutrition therapy (MNT) are to achieve metabolic goals, treat or prevent diabetes related complications, minimize other health risks, respect personal and cultural preferences.

- For the individual with a normal BMI (18.5–24.9 kg/m^2) and stable weight, no discrete daily calorie amount need be advised. For the individual who is overweight (BMI 25–29.9 kg/m^2) or obese (BMI > 30 kg/m^2), weight loss is advised with a calorie restricted diet.

- Carbohydrate intake in patients with diabetes should adhere to the following guidelines: the total amount of carbohydrate in meals or snacks has a greater impact on glycemia than source or type of carbohydrates; carbohydrate intake should be from whole grains, fruits, vegetables and low-fat dairy products; sucrose and sucrose-containing foods need to be limited to <10% of total calories; there is no long-term benefit on weight management by following a low-carbohydrate diet (<35% of total calories).

- Protein intake should represent ≤ 20% of total calories. Protein restriction (0.8–1.0 g/kg or 16% of total calories) may be associated with protection of renal function in people with type 1 or 2 diabetes and microalbuminuria and people with type 1 diabetes and macroalbuminuria.

- Fat intake should focus on healthy fats, monounsaturated (MUFAs) and polyunsaturated fats (PUFAs) with avoidance of trans-fatty acids, restriction of saturated fats to 10% of total calories and restriction of dietary cholesterol intake to 300 mg/day.

- Weight management should focus on lifestyle changes with calorie restriction through healthy eating habits and regular physical activity. The initial goal should be a weight loss of 5–10% of initial body weight. Many patients would benefit by participating in a comprehensive structured lifestyle program promoting behavioral change.

Medical nutrition therapy (MNT) remains a cornerstone in the management of the patient with diabetes mellitus. Unfortunately, many patients seek sources of nutritional information that have little scientific merit while evidence-based nutritional recommendations are ignored or deemed too difficult to implement. Our responsibility as medical practitioners is to remain knowledgeable as to the proven dietary principles that protect the health of our patients with diabetes while being supportive as these changes are being implemented.

So what is the optimal diet for the patient with diabetes? In principle, MNT should protect the health of our patients by helping them achieve desired metabolic goals, treat or prevent diabetes-related complications, minimize other health risks while respecting personal and cultural preferences [1].

Goals of MNT:

- *Achieve metabolic goals*
- *Treat or prevent diabetes-related complications*
- *Minimize other health risks*
- *Respect personal and cultural preferences*

Clinical Dilemmas in Diabetes, First Edition. Edited by Adrian Vella and Robert A. Rizza
© 2011 Blackwell Publishing Ltd. Published 2011 by Blackwell Publishing Ltd.

TABLE 6.1 Classification of overweight and obesity by Body Mass Index (BMI kg/m^2)

Normal	18.5–24.9
Overweight	25–29.9
Obesity	
Class I	30–34.9
Class II	35–39.9
Class III	>40

Starting with the basics: Calories

Calorie recommendations will vary depending on the goals of energy balance: weight maintenance, weight loss, or weight gain. Weight maintenance would be recommended for individuals that are at a healthy weight range according to Body Mass Index (BMI) criteria (Table 6.1). Weight loss is desired for those who meet criteria for overweight and obesity in order to minimize the impact of obesity on insulin resistance and lower the risk for other weight-related medical complications [2].

Accurate methods for measuring total caloric energy requirements are expensive and not easily incorporated into clinical practice. These include indirect calorimetry to mea-sure basal metabolic rate, whole-room calorimetry or dou-bly labeled water to measure total energy expenditure and heart rate or activity monitors to measure physical activity [3]. Instead, daily calorie recommendations are often gen-eralized according to sex, age, and weight. Estimated caloric needs can also be determined by utilizing various formulas, one of the most common being the Harris Benedict equa-tion (HBE) (Table 6.2). This formula determines resting energy expenditure (REE): the number of calories required to maintain current weight at rest. In controlled trials, the HBE has been found to be accurate in determining REE amongst groups, although there may be inaccuracies when estimating individual REE. An activity factor is added to account for calories spent in activities of daily living and exercise. This activity factor is generally in the order of 30–50% of REE. This activity factor can be an additional source for inaccuracy, since patients may often overestimate their activity level. However, caloric estimates based on the HBE equation are well accepted [2–4].

For the individual with a normal BMI (Table 6.1), and whose weight is stable, specific calorie amounts need not be recommended. However, for the individual who is overweight or obese, the recommendation is weight loss through calorie restriction [2, 5]. A calorie restriction from

TABLE 6.2 Dietary recommendations for the patient with diabetes mellitus

Calorie recommendations using Harris Benedict equation (HBE)	
	HBE + (30–50% activity factor) = kcal/day
Men	HBE = 66 + 13.8(weight in kg) + 5.0 (height in cm) – 6.8 (age in years)
Women	HBE = 655 + 9.5(weight in kg) + 1.9 (height in cm) – 4.7(age in years)
Overweight/obesity	
	HBE (1.3) – (250–500 kcal) = kcal/day
Carbohydrate intake	45–55% of total calories
Protein intake	20% of total calories
Fat intake	25–35% of total calories
Saturated fat	<10% of total calories
Cholesterol	<300 mg/day
Trans fatty acids	0 mg/day
PUFAs	<10% of total calories
MUFAs	
Micronutrients	
Sodium	<2,400 mg/d
Calcium	1000–1500 mg/d
Sodium	<2400 mg/day
Folic acid	
Reproductive age women	400 mcg/day
Alcohol	
Men	2 alcohol-containing beverages/day
Women	1 alcohol-containing beverage/day

HBE(1.3) of 250–500 kcal can be advised depending on patient preference and motivation. Although greater calorie restriction will be associated with greater initial weight loss, the patient faces the risk of lower long-term adherence with the greater calorie restriction [1, 2].

- *For the individual with a normal BMI (18.5–24.9 kg/m²) and stable weight, no discrete daily calorie amount need be advised.*
- *For the individual who is overweight (BMI 25–29.9 kg/m²) or obese (BMI > 30 kg/m²), weight loss is advised with a calorie-restricted diet*
  Daily caloric intake = HBE(1.3) – (250–500 kcal)

Breaking down calories: Macronutrients

Carbohydrates

Carbohydrates are the foundation of most diets. This is particularly true for patients with diabetes. Food carbohydrates can be categorized as sugars, starch, and fiber. Controversies continue regarding the amount of carbohydrates that are optimal for the patient with diabetes. The most recent recommendations by the American Diabetes Association (ADA) do not provide specific percentages of total calories to be ingested as carbohydrates. Several factors can impact our recommendations for carbohydrate intake to our patient with diabetes (e.g., the type of insulin regime, activity levels in athletes). However, there are many misconceptions regarding carbohydrate intake that should be addressed. The medical literature supports the following recommendations for carbohydrate intake:

- *Total amount of carbohydrate in meals or snacks has a greater impact on glycemia than source or type of carbohydrate [1, 2, 6, 7].*
- *Optimal health benefits are observed when carbohydrate intake is from whole grains, fruits, vegetables, and low-fat dairy products [1, 2, 6, 7].*
- *Sucrose and sucrose containing foods do not need to be restricted in people with diabetes nor do they affect glycemia differently than an isocaloric amount of starch. They need to be incorporated as part of the overall meal plan but limited to <10% of total calories [1, 2, 6, 7].*
- *For weight management, calories and not nutrient composition is the most important factor for success. There is no long-term benefit on weight management by following a low-carbohydrate diet (<35% of total calories) [8, 9].*

TABLE 6.3 General recommendations for food intake in patients with diabetes

Foods to be encouraged
MUFAs (replacing saturated fats)
  Olive oil and canola oil
    Used in spreads, food preparation, and cooking
PUFAs
  Limit to 10% of total calories
  Oily fish meal 1–2/week
    Salmon, herring, halibut, trout, and tuna
  Corn, sunflower, and soybean oils
    Used in spreads, food preparation, and cooking
High-fiber foods
  Fruits, vegetables, legumes, and whole grains

Foods to be discouraged
Trans-fatty acids
  Hydrogenated vegetable oils
  Pies, pastries, biscuits, and cakes
Saturated fats and cholesterol
  Animal-based products
    Butter, mayonnaise, regular fat milk, and lard

Generally, in people with diabetes carbohydrates represent 45–55% of total calories recommended. This flexibility can accommodate personal and cultural preferences [1–3].

Fiber

High intake of fiber-containing foods is preferred in patients with diabetes. High fiber diets have been shown to confer benefits on glycemic control, hyperinsulinemia, and lipids in patients with both type 1 and type 2 diabetes. However, a specific daily amount is not included in the recent recommendations by the ADA [1, 7].

Intake of high-fiber foods are associated with metabolic health benefits, however, no specific daily amount is recommended.

Protein

Recommendations for protein intake in patients with diabetes are generally based on expert consensus. Some studies suggest a higher protein requirement in patients with both type 1 and type 2 diabetes as a result of increased protein turnover. However, this higher protein requirement is easily met by the average protein intake currently reported by most adults of 20% of total calories ingested. Lower protein intakes of less than 20% of total calories have not been associated with additional health benefits, particularly for the prevalence of nephropathy in patients with diabetes mellitus. The impact of higher protein intake, greater than 20% of total calories, on the prevalence of nephropathy have not been studied but is generally not recommended. Patients with type 1 or type 2 diabetes and microalbuminuria may benefit from protein restriction (0.8–1.0 g/kg or 16% of total calories). This degree of protein restriction has been shown to improve glomerular filtration rates and reduce albuminuria. Protein restriction has also been shown to reduce the decline in glomerular filtration rates in people with overt nephropathy and type 1 diabetes [1, 2].

- *Protein intake should represent ≤ 20% of total calories* [1, 2, 6, 7].
- *Protein restriction (0.8–1.0 g/kg or 16% of total calories) may be associated with protection of renal function in people with type 1 or 2 diabetes and microalbuminuria* [1, 2, 6, 7].
- *Protein restriction (0.8 g/kg) can protect renal function in people with type 1 diabetes and macroalbuminuria* [1, 2, 6, 7].

Fats

The strongest consensus regarding intake of dietary fat for patients with diabetes is no different than that for the general population and includes:

- *Avoidance of trans-fatty acids*
- *Restriction of saturated fats to 10% of total calories*
- *Restriction of dietary cholesterol intake to 300 mg/day*

These recommendations are supported by a large body of evidence supporting the effect of saturated fat/trans-fatty acid intake on LDL cholesterol and risk for cardiovascular events [1, 2, 6, 7].

There is controversy regarding the amount of daily calories to be consumed as fat. In the past, the recommendation was to restrict the intake of dietary fat to less than 30% of total calories. However, this recommendation has been challenged by evidence supporting the potential benefits of monounsaturated (MUFAs), polyunsaturated fatty acids (PUFAs: Omega-3 and Omega-6) on lipid profiles and cardiovascular events. Replacing saturated fats by monounsaturated or polyunsaturated fats instead of carbohydrates is associated with favorable lipid profiles with higher levels of HDL cholesterol and lower serum triglycerides. Omega-3 fatty acids mainly found in oily fish and fish oils may offer additional cardiovascular benefits. Cardioprotective effects

have been reported with dietary consumption of 1–2 servings of fish high in Omega-3 fatty acids per week. A 38% decrease in coronary artery disease (CAD) mortality has been reported with weekly intakes of fish high in Omega-3 fatty acids (Table 6.2) more than five times per week [10–12].

Therefore, if adhering to the recommended daily intake of saturated fat and cholesterol, a higher intake of "healthier" fat may not be associated with additional health risk and need not be as strictly restricted as previously recommended. Intake of dietary fat of up to 35% of total calories is acceptable [6]. Polyunsaturated fat intake should be limited to 10% of total calories. Higher intakes may be associated with lowering of the cardioprotective effects of HDL cholesterol [1, 6, 7]. The only caution to be acknowledged is the caloric density associated with dietary fat, even "healthier fats," in the patient who is trying to manage their weight. Restriction of dietary fat is an effective way of limiting caloric intake and should be a strong determinant in the recommendations provided to a patient with diabetes who is trying to manage their weight [1].

- *There is lack of consensus regarding the intake of calories as fat; it is generally recommended that it be limited to <35% of total calories.*
- *The intake of MUFAs and PUFAs over saturated fats has been shown to provide cardiovascular health benefits.*
- *Intake of PUFAs should be limited to <10% of total calories.*

Micronutrients

A well-balanced diet should provide daily requirements for most micronutrients [1, 7]. The medical literature does not support a clear benefit to multivitamin and mineral supplementation in the general population or in patients with diabetes mellitus [1]. However, special consideration should be given to the following circumstances:

Folic acid supplementation in pregnant women has been shown to lower the risk for neural tube defects. The current recommendation for folic acid intake is 400 mcg/day for all women capable of becoming pregnant [1]. This is the amount present in multivitamin preparations.

Calcium requirements are frequently not met by most individual's eating habits. This requirement would be fulfilled by daily intakes of 3–4 servings of a dairy product. As a result, most individuals would benefit from additional calcium supplementation. Daily intakes of calcium of 1000–1500 mg are recommended [1].

Sodium restriction has been shown to lower blood pressure in individuals with and without established hypertension. Current recommendations are to limit sodium intake to <2400 mg/day [1].

A daily multivitamin and mineral preparation can be recommended to those individuals following restrictive diets either in their efforts at weight management or special dietary preferences [1].

Specific micronutrient recommendations:

Folic acid (women in reproductive years)	*400 mcg/day*
Calcium	*1000–1500/day*
Sodium	*<2400 mg/day*

Alcohol

Recommendations for alcohol intake in people with diabetes are the same as in the general population. For men, the recommendation is two alcohol-containing beverages per day and for women one alcohol-containing beverage per day. Abstinence is advised for individuals with medical conditions adversely affected by alcohol intake such as severe hypertriglyceridemia. The cardiovascular benefits attributed to alcohol intake are not restricted to specific alcoholic beverage [1, 2, 6, 7].

Recommended alcohol intake

For men	*2 alcohol-containing beverages/day*
For women	*1 alcohol-containing beverage/day*

Sweeteners

Common sweeteners are sucrose, fructose, and sugar alcohols. Several studies have confirmed that sucrose consumption does not lead to a greater rise in postprandial blood glucose when compared to an isocaloric amount of another carbohydrate. Hence, they need not be restricted but should be incorporated as part of the carbohydrate intake in a meal plan. Since there are no nutritive benefits to sucrose intake, it should be limited to 10% of total calories [1, 2].

Compared to sucrose, fructose is associated with a lower postprandial glucose rise. Despite this benefit, a large intake of fructose can lead to weight gain and unfavorable lipid profiles with elevated fasting triglycerides and LDL cholesterol. There is no proven benefit to the use of fructose over

sucrose as a sweetener. However, the intake of naturally occurring fructose such as fruits need not be restricted [1, 2, 6].

Sugar alcohols such as sorbitol and xylitol are associated with lower postprandial glucose rise and lower calorie content compared to sucrose. However, large amounts of sugar alcohols, 30–49 g, can be associated with osmotic diarrhea. There have been no proven advantages to the use of sugar alcohols as a sweetener [1, 2, 6].

Nonnutritive sweeteners can provide benefits for individuals trying to follow a calorie-restricted diet. Despite safety concerns, several studies have not confirmed any health risk associated to their use [1, 2, 6, 7].

- *Sucrose intake need not be restricted but limited to 10% of total calories.*
- *There are no proven benefits to the use of fructose or sugar alcohols over sucrose as sweeteners.*
- *Nonnutritive sweeteners can be used safely and be helpful for individuals trying to follow a calorie restricted diet.*

Hypoglycemia

Hypoglycemia is a common complication in the management of the patient with diabetes. Treatment involves the intake of glucose or carbohydrate-containing food. The severity of hypoglycemia will dictate the amount of glucose or carbohydrate to be ingested to resolve the hypoglycemia. Intakes of 10–20 g of carbohydrate can raise blood glucose levels by 40–60 mg/dl in 30–45 minutes [1, 6].

In the treatment of hypoglycemia, intakes of 10–20 g of carbohydrate can raise blood glucose levels by 40–60 mg/dl in 30–45 minutes.

Special considerations

Pregnancy

Prepregnancy nutrition counseling should focus on individual meal planning to meet metabolic goals by the time of conception. During pregnancy, modification of nutritional therapy is necessary to continue to achieve metabolic goals but also allow for appropriate weight gain and meet additional nutritional requirements. Increased caloric requirements are noted during the second and third trimester. This is only in the order of an additional 300 kcal/day. Recommended protein intake is 0.75 g/kg per day plus an additional 10 g/day. Folic acid supplementation (400 mcg/day) is recommended to lower the risk for neural tube defects [1].

During pregnancy, modification to nutritional therapy includes:

Additional 300 kcal/day during the second and third trimester
Protein intake of 0.75 g/kg plus 10 g
Folate supplementation of 400 mcg/day

Children and adolescents

Nutrient requirements for children and adolescents with both type 1 and type 2 diabetes are the same as nondiabetic children of the same age. A healthy lifestyle with regular physical activity should be emphasized in both. Determining energy (caloric) requirements need to take into consideration a child's usual intake as well as daily activity routine. In children with type 1 diabetes, meal planning needs to account for insulin regime being used and is best accomplished with the guidance of a registered dietitian. Intensive insulin regimes can allow flexibility for children and adolescents with diabetes allowing for variability in mealtimes and schedules. In children with type 2 diabetes, avoidance of excessive weight gain is desirable by promoting healthy eating and regular physical activity [1].

• *Nutrient requirements are not different for children with type 1 and type 2 diabetes compared to similar age children and adolescents.*
• *In children and adolescents with type 1 diabetes, meal planning must take into consideration insulin regime.*
• *In children with type 2 diabetes, weight maintenance should be encouraged by promoting a healthy lifestyle.*

Weight management

Weight management with either avoidance of weight gain or weight loss is often a recommendation for people with diabetes and BMI values above 25 kg/m^2 [1, 2]. This can be particularly challenging for the patient with diabetes, since glucose-lowering therapy, most notable insulin, is often associated with weight gain [5]. For the patient with type 2 diabetes, this is an important consideration for the treating physician as they choose a medication. Another fact to remember is that the process of pursuing weight loss, improvement of eating habits, and regular physical activity,

is associated with many health benefits, despite only achieving weight maintenance [13]. Hence, the focus should be on lifestyle changes.

An initial weight loss goal is a weight loss of 5–10 % of initial body weight [1, 5, 6, 13]. This degree of weight loss has been shown to provide many health benefits with improvement in metabolic parameters [13, 14]. Although initially this degree of weight loss can be easily achieved, it is often difficult to maintain [13]. Patients pursuing weight management would benefit from ongoing support promoting lifestyle changes. Structured lifestyle programs often include frequent visits with a dietitian for MNT, physical activity recommendations, and educational sessions promoting behavioral change toward a healthier lifestyle [1, 6, 14]. Additional interventions, such as pharmacotherapy or surgery for weight loss, should be considered in the patient meeting accepted criteria [1, 5].

There has been controversy regarding dietary recommendations to prescribe for weight loss. At present, the main recommendation is to focus on modest calorie restriction (250–500 kcal/day) from usual caloric intake [1, 2]. Activity recommendations include 30 minutes of an aerobic activity most days of the week [13]. Achieving this activity recommendation will often involve helping the patient identify obstacles in order to overcome them.

• *Weight management should focus on lifestyle changes with calorie restriction through healthy eating habits and regular physical activity.*
• *Initial goal should be a weight loss of 5–10% of initial body weight.*
• *Many patients would benefit by participating in a comprehensive structured lifestyle program promoting behavioral change.*

Implementation

Putting dietary recommendations into practice is challenging for most patients with diabetes mellitus. Despite the existence of these recommendations for years, patients with diabetes have not made progress at improving their eating habits. In fact, for those age groups in which the prevalence of diabetes is high (45–65 years) higher calorie consumption mainly in the form of carbohydrates has been reported [15].

The physician plays a central role in the care of the patient with diabetes. It is imperative that he/she be well informed regarding general principles of the nutritional guidelines recommended. They should continually encourage changes in eating habits that have been proven to provide health benefits. The physician should be able to dispel common myths regarding the eating habits for patients with diabetes. For the patient taking insulin, especially the patient on an intensive insulin program, the physician must recognize how nutritional recommendations will influence insulin dosing. As a result, a more detailed nutritional assessment is often required [1, 7]. This can be provided through an individual MNT session with a registered dietitian or with the dietitian being a member of a DSMT program [16].

An MNT visit can help individualize dietary recommendations. Areas for potential change in current eating habits can be identified and changes toward recommended guidelines be encouraged while respecting the patient's cultural/dietary preferences [1, 16]. Other resources to promote dietary change can be discussed such as learning to read food labels, use of recipe books, and access to online nutritional information for frequently visited food establishments to aid our patients make better choices. A nutritional assessment can also explore the best method for dietary instruction. Patients may be interested in learning more about carbohydrate counting or glycemic index.

Carbohydrate counting

Carbohydrate counting is a meal planning method focusing on the amount of carbohydrate present in foods consumed. Although the popularity of carbohydrate counting has increased over the past decade, this concept is not new. There are references to carbohydrate counting dating back to the 1920s and it was one of four meal planning techniques used during the Diabetes Control and Complications Trial. Some consider carbohydrate counting a simpler method of meal planning, since it focuses on one macronutrient. Patients with all types of diabetes may benefit from using carbohydrate counting in their meal planning but should be selected after a nutritional assessment is completed [17, 18].

Carbohydrate counting has two main assumptions: carbohydrate is the main macronutrient affecting postprandial glucose rise and carbohydrates are quickly converted to glucose after a meal. Three levels of carbohydrate counting instruction have been proposed. The concept of carbohy-

drate counting is introduced in Level 1. Patients learn about the carbohydrate content of foods and may start counting grams of carbohydrates. They learn about the impact of carbohydrate intake on their postprandial glucose levels. They are encouraged to practice consistency in the amount of carbohydrate consumed in meals and snacks in order to achieve metabolic goals. Hence, keeping a diet record becomes an important tool in the learning process. The amount of carbohydrate recommended to a patient for meals and snacks is ultimately determined by metabolic goals and patient preferences [17].

Level 2 focuses on pattern management. As a result of continued record keeping, individuals can learn to recognize how their blood glucose is affected by food, medications, and physical activity. This can guide additional modification to meal planning, activity levels, and medication to achieve metabolic goals [17].

Level 3 is generally for patients on intensive insulin therapy via multiple daily injections or insulin infusion via an insulin pump. At this level, patients start to use insulin to carbohydrate ratios to match the amount of rapid-acting insulin required before a meal to control postprandial glucose rise. In order to succeed patients need to feel confident in their estimation of carbohydrate amount in foods consumed. An example for insulin/carbohydrate ratio is 1 unit of rapid-acting insulin per 15 g of carbohydrate. Patients would benefit from continued visits to a registered dietitian, as they learn how to estimate the carbohydrate content of foods, practice portion control, and recognize the need to change carbohydrate to insulin ratio to better control postprandial glucose levels [17].

It is important to remember that although protein and fats are not incorporated in this meal planning technique, they are important macronutrients with nutritional and caloric value. Learning appropriate portion control of these macronutrients can help avoid weight gain that can occur when the amount of calories as fat consumed is disregarded.

- *Carbohydrate counting*
- *Carbohydrates are the main macronutrient affecting postprandial glucose rise*
- *Carbohydrates are quickly converted to glucose after a meal*
  Level 1: Introduction of basic concepts
  Level 2: Pattern recognition
  Level 3: Use of insulin to carbohydrate ratios for premeal insulin dose

Glycemic index

Some patients with diabetes may be interested in the glycemic index (GI) for their meal planning. The GI quantifies the postprandial glycemic response of a food compared to the glycemic response of a standard food, 50 g of glucose, or a white bread challenge. Low GI foods cause a lower postprandial glucose response compared to a high GI food. Many factors affect the GI value of a food. For example, the type of sugar and/or starch in the food, food processing, cooking, and other meal components will affect the GI of a food. Fiber, fat, and protein content tend to be associated with lower GI indexes. At present, there is not enough evidence to support the use of GI principles in the meal planning for all patients with diabetes. Most studies available are short in duration limiting conclusions regarding long-term benefits [1, 2, 17, 18]. However, the interested patient should be referred to a registered dietitian for further education.

Summary

Medical nutrition therapy remains the foundation in the management of the patient with diabetes mellitus. Despite the overwhelming availability of nutritional recommendations, it is important that we adhere to the basic nutritional principles that have been shown to benefit our patients. Implementation of these principles is often challenging and we should support our patients in their efforts utilizing resources available.

References

1. American Diabetes Association. Nutrition principles and recommendations in diabetes. *Diabetes Care.* **27**(Suppl 1): S36–S46, 2004.
2. Ha TKK, Lean MEJ. Technical review: recommendations for the nutritional management of patients with diabetes mellitus. *Eur J Clin Nutr.* **52**:467–481, 1998.
3. Lin PH, Proschan MA, Bray GA, et al. Estimation of energy requirements in a controlled feeding trial. *Am J Clin Nutr.* **77**:639–645, 2003.
4. Kien CL, Ugrasbul F. Prediction of daily energy expenditure during a feeding trial using measurements of energy expenditure, fat free mass, or Harris Benedict equations. *Am J Clin Nutr.* **80**:876–880, 2004.
5. Albu J, Rhaja-Khan N. The management of the obese diabetic patient. *Prim Care Clin Off Pract.* **30**:465–491, 2003.
6. Vaughn L. Dietary guidelines for the management of diabetes. *Nurs Stand.* **19**(44):56–64.
7. Choudhary P. Review of dietary recommendations for diabetes mellitus. *Diabetes Res Clin Pract.* **65**(Suppl 1):S9–S15, 2004.
8. McAuley KA, Hopkins CM, Smith KJ, et al. Comparison of high-fat and high-protein diets with a high-carbohydrate diet in insulin – resistant women. *Diabetologia.* **48**:8–16, 2005.
9. Mann J, McAuley K. Carbohydrates: is the advise to eat less justified for diabetes and cardiovascular health? *Curr Opin Lipidol.* **18**(1):9–12, 2007.
10. Mozaffarian D, Katan MB, Ascherio A, Stampfer MJ, Willett WC. Trans fatty acids and cardiovascular disease. *N Engl J Med.* **354**: 1601, 2006.
11. Mata P, et al. Effects of long-term monounsaturated vs. polyunsaturated- enriched diets on lipoproteins in healthy men and women. *Am J Clin Nutr.* **55**:846, 1992.
12. Jacobson TA. Beyond lipids: the role of Omega-3 fatty acids from fish oil in the prevention of coronary heart disease. *Curr Atheroscler Rep.* **9**:145–153, 2007.
13. Tuomilehto J, Lindstrom J, Eriksson JG, et al. Prevention of type 2 diabetes mellitus by changes in lifestyle among subjects with impaired glucose tolerance. *N Engl J Med.* **344**: 1343–1350, 2001.
14. Franz MJ, Warshaw H, Daly AE, et al. Evolution of diabetes medical nutrition therapy. *Postgrad Med J.* **79**:30–35, 2003.
15. Oza-Frank R, Cheng YJN, Venkat KM, Gregg EW. Trends in nutrient intake among adults with diabetes in the United States: 1988–2004. *J Am Diet Assoc.* **109**(7):1173–1178, 2009.
16. Daly A, Michael P, Johnson EQ, et al. Diabetes white paper: defining the delivery of nutrition services in medicare medical nutrition therapy vs. medicare diabetes self-management training programs. *J Am Diet Assoc.* **109**:528–539, 2009.
17. Gillespie SJ, Kulkarni KD, Daly AE. Using carbohydrate counting in diabetes clinical practice. *J Am Diet Assoc.* **98**(8): 897–905, 1998.
18. Kelley DE. Sugars and starch in the nutritional management of diabetes mellitus. *Am J Clin Nutr.* **78**(Suppl):858S–64S, 2003.

7 How to determine when to pursue lifestyle change alone versus pharmacotherapy at diagnosis?

Galina Smushkin[1] and F. John Service[2]

[1] Fellow, Mayo Clinic, Division of Endocrinology, Rochester, MN, USA
[2] Professor of Medicine, Mayo Clinic College of Medicine, Rochester, MN, USA

LEARNING POINTS

- Current guidelines list both lifestyle intervention and metformin as core initial therapies, but warn that the high rate of weight gain after an initial successful moderate weight loss, limits the role of lifestyle modifications in controlling glycemia long term.

- Pharmacotherapy at diagnosis should be considered when there is a concurrent use of medications known to induce hyperglycemia, such as glucocorticoids, atypical antipsychotics, or immunosuppressants related to organ transplantation.

- Early pharmacotherapy should be initiated if a patient has symptoms such as weight loss, polyuria and polydipsia, evidence of microvascular complications at diagnosis, or severe concomitant hypertriglyceridemia.

- Benefits of intentional weight loss, caloric restriction, and exercise training in type 2 diabetes have been established in a number of trials.

- A large-scale Look AHEAD trial currently in progress is designed to examine the effect of lifestyle interventions similar to the Diabetes Prevention Program (DPP) on cardiovascular outcomes in people with type 2 diabetes.

- Lifestyle modification can be recommended as monotherapy with greater confidence if there is access to a multidisciplinary program either in one's own practice, by way of an enrollment in a trial or through the community-based initiatives.

In a world idealized by evidence-based-medicine aficionados, selection of therapy appropriate for each and every medical contingency would be prescriptive and not subject to debate: a specific treatment matched to a unique clinical profile would have been identified from previously conducted clinical trials. In actuality such a medical utopia will never be realized for the management of diabetes because no series of studies could possibly encompass the wide range of patient demographics and the permutations and combinations of the multiple medications available for the management of diabetes. In many respects, the choice implied in the title is misleading, since an accommodation in lifestyle, even if it is the minimal effort entailed in taking a tablet once a day, is an accompaniment of the presence of diabetes. The thrust of this debate is the determination that lifestyle change alone in lieu of concomitant medication may be sufficient to control diabetes.

Whereas the diagnostic criteria for diabetes appear to undergo convulsive disruption about every 20 years or so, the clinical management of diabetes seems to undergo frequent changes in recommendations. In contrast to the situation with type 1 diabetes where the selection of therapy is not controversial but its implementation is difficult, the reverse is true for type 2 diabetes, where the taking of the medication is easy but the selection from the various drugs available is complex.

In patients with type 2 diabetes, intensive lifestyle modification is a valuable adjunct to pharmacotherapy and in some patients may eliminate the need for pharmacotherapy entirely. Current guidelines from the ADA and the EASD list both lifestyle intervention and metformin as well-validated core initial therapies, but warn that the high rate of weight gain after an initial successful moderate weight loss, limits the role of lifestyle modifications in controlling glycemia long term [1]. Metformin on the other hand is an agent that

Clinical Dilemmas in Diabetes, First Edition. Edited by Adrian Vella and Robert A. Rizza
© 2011 Blackwell Publishing Ltd. Published 2011 by Blackwell Publishing Ltd.

has withstood the test of time, demonstrating efficacy and relative safety. It improves fasting glycemia by decreasing hepatic glucose production and thereby improves HbA1c by 1.0–2.0% on average. Even greater glycemic improvement may be observed in a patient who has been treatment-naïve. The appeal of metformin is that these results may be achieved without weight gain or hypoglycemia, as long as it is not used in patients with significant renal, hepatic or gastrointestinal dysfunction, or decompensated heart failure. Such a favorable benefit–risk profile certainly justifies the recommendation to use metformin as a first-line agent, but does its initiation right at the diagnosis of type 2 diabetes detract the focus from weight loss efforts? At the time of diagnosis, how does a clinician select patients for whom it is appropriate to postpone pharmacotherapy in favor of lifestyle changes? In some clinical situations, the choice of initial management is obvious, whereas others present the health care provider with substantial dilemmas. This chapter addresses a number of such scenarios.

Pharmacotherapy should be considered when there is significant blood glucose elevation from concurrent use of medications known to induce hyperglycemia, such as glucocorticoids, atypical antipsychotics, or immunosuppressants related to organ transplantation. The odds ratio for developing diabetes on glucocorticoid therapy ranges 1.3–2.3 [2–4] and is dose dependent. The hyperglycemia is more severe in the postprandial period and is related to the reduction in insulin sensitivity [5]. To what extent dietary changes and increased physical activity can attenuate these adverse glycemic effects of glucocorticoids has not been systematically studied. In general, the underlying medical conditions for which steroids are prescribed present significant barriers to increasing physical activity and the appetite-stimulating effects of steroids make dietary management challenging. For this reason, early initiation of pharmacotherapy is appropriate, particularly if the duration of steroid use is anticipated to be prolonged or high doses are used. Many of the currently available oral therapies for type 2 diabetes have been suggested for the treatment of steroid-induced hyperglycemia. However, there are scant published data on the efficacy of oral agents in this setting, and the concomitant medical conditions in patients requiring glucocorticoid therapy, such as renal or liver dysfunction, represent a contraindication to the use of agents such as metformin or sulfonylureas. In general, insulin is a safe and effective treatment for steroid-induced diabetes. In particular, NPH insulin can be used successfully as a once-daily injection, since it has an action profile that parallels the time course of prednisone effects on glucose, peaking at 4–6 hours and lasting approximately 12 hours.

There has been debate whether the higher prevalence of diabetes in persons affected by schizophrenia reflects an increased risk from this disease per se, the associated lifestyle and family history, or the adverse metabolic effects of the antipsychotic medications. Prospective randomized clinical trials are few [6, 7], but data from pharmacoepidemiologic studies suggest that there is an increased risk of diabetes with olanzapine and clozapine compared to typical antipsychotics or other atypical agents such as aripiprazole or risperidone [8]. Weight gain related to the use of these agents likely accounts for the majority of cases of new-onset diabetes occurring during treatment. However, there may be a substantial proportion of patients in whom rapid, dramatic development of hyperglycemia occurs independent of adiposity, likely reflecting direct impairment of the β-cell function by the antipsychotic drug. It has been proposed that this effect may be mediated by antagonistic actions on the M2 muscarinic receptors in the pancreas [9]. Given these forces at work, early institution of pharmacotherapy should be considered in a patient newly diagnosed with diabetes who is also taking atypical antipsychotics. Communication with the patient's treating psychiatrist is also appropriate, as consideration should be given to switching to a different antipsychotic agent. In terms of the choice of initial glucose-lowering therapy for a patient with psychiatric comorbidities, evidence is limited. A recent systematic review of eight randomized double-blind, placebo-controlled trials concluded that metformin will attenuate weight gain in adults and adolescents without diabetes, treated with atypical antipsychotics [10]. Intuitively, one would expect a lower incidence of diabetes to result, but the trials were too short in duration to confirm this. The severity of presentation of newly-diagnosed diabetes in a setting of antipsychotic drug use should direct the choice of initial pharmacotherapy used. Thus, if there is evidence of extreme hyperglycemia and hyperosmolar state, initiation of insulin therapy is imperative.

The incidence of new-onset diabetes after solid organ transplantation is increasing and is linked most closely to immunosuppressive therapy with corticosteroids, calcineurin inhibitors, and sirolimus [11]. Weight gain is a common predisposing factor, but there is evidence of direct β-cell toxicity from calcineurin inhibitors. Animal studies as well as in vitro studies of human pancreatic islets have demonstrated decreased beta-cell volume, insulin content, and insulin release with cyclosporin treatment [12, 13]. Tacrolimus and sirolimus may be even more diabetogenic than cyclosporin, with some studies showing 70% higher incidence of diabetes in the two years after a kidney transplant, compared to non-tacrolimus-based immunosuppression [14]. For these reasons, post-transplant status requiring immunosuppressive therapy should lower the physician's threshold for initiation of pharmacotherapy at the time of diagnosis of diabetes. No single choice of therapy has been proven to be more effective in this clinical scenario, so the traditional approach of using oral agents as first line is generally used. Depending on the transplanted organ and its function, there may be specific contraindications to the use of certain oral agents, and thus treatment may require even a greater degree of individualization than in a person with diabetes but without a history of organ transplantation.

The degree of glucotoxicity and the extent of β-cell decompensation at the time of diagnosis should be factored into the decision of whether immediate pharmacologic intervention is needed. Glucotoxicity refers to the concept that continuous elevation of glucose exerts damaging effects on the β-cell, further impairing its ability to produce and secrete insulin. There is in vitro evidence from cultured β-cell lines and pancreatic islets that, under the conditions of persistent hyperglycemia, there is a decrease in insulin mRNA, insulin content, and release. Mechanisms are likely multiple and have not been completely elucidated [15]. It has been proposed that excess glucose is shunted into pathways producing reactive oxygen species, which subsequently decrease the activity of insulin gene promoter leading to a decreased expression of the insulin gene. In vitro data from cultured islets and in vivo measurements of oxidative stress markers in subjects with diabetes support this notion, but to date the effectiveness of potent antioxidants in improving β-cell function in people with diabetes has not been conclusively demonstrated. In vitro experiments suggest that the phenomenon of glucotoxicity is at least in part reversible, but reversibility is time dependent. Prolonged exposure to hyperglycemia triggers the expression of proapoptotic genes and if apoptosis ensues, β-cell mass may be lost irreversibly. For this reason, the higher the degree of glucotoxicity deemed to be present, the more pressing is the need to reverse hyperglycemia and the stronger the argument in favor of pharmacotherapy. Unfortunately, besides the measurement of plasma glucose, there are no other easily quantifiable markers of glucotoxicity.

For a given serum glucose level, there is likely a significant interindividual variability in the degree of impairment at the level of the β-cell. Nevertheless, extremes of glucotoxicity are reasonably easily recognized by the presence of symptoms and measurable, profound metabolic disturbances.

Symptoms such as polyuria, polydipsia, and weight loss at the time of diagnosis should prompt initiation of pharmacotherapy. Polyuria develops once the reabsorptive capacity of the kidney is overwhelmed at plasma glucose levels exceeding 180 mg/dl. The osmotic diuretic effect of urinary glucose contributes to dehydration, which further exacerbates hyperglycemia. Since calories are lost in the urine, weight loss ensues. Engaging in an intense exercise program under these conditions can worsen rather than improve hyperglycemia and increase the likelihood of ketosis, even in type 2 diabetes. Pharmacotherapy along with rehydration interrupts the hyperglycemia-generating forces and establishes conditions where lifestyle modification can be safely implemented.

Pharmacotherapy is mandatory when diabetes is diagnosed with ketoacidosis or hyperosmolar hyperglycemic state requiring management with insulin, initially administered intravenously via a drip and subsequently subcutaneously as multiple daily injections. Similarly, severe hypertriglyceridemia (triglycerides greater than 1000 mg/dl) at the time of the diagnosis of diabetes warrants immediate initiation of pharmacotherapy, which is usually insulin. As the glucotoxicity subsides following the treatment of the acute abnormalities, some patients with type 2 diabetes may transition to oral diabetic medications and if aggressive lifestyle modification is undertaken and maintained, there is evidence that a fraction of patients may be tapered off pharmacotherapy entirely. In a study from China, more than 300 patients newly diagnosed with type 2 diabetes were treated with aggressive insulin or oral drug therapy attaining euglycemia within 2 weeks of diagnosis and maintaining therapy for 2 weeks before discontinuation of all pharmacotherapy and initiation of aggressive lifestyle changes [16]. On a one-year follow-up 40–50% of the patients initially treated with insulin were maintaining adequate glycemic control with lifestyle interventions alone. Of note, patients in this study had significant hyperglycemia at the time of diagnosis with fasting glucose level 200 mg/dl and HgbA1C 9–10%, implying a significant degree of glucotoxicity.

The presence of microvascular complications at the time of diagnosis constitutes another situation where pharmacotherapy is favored. In the UKPDS cohort of patients with type 2 diabetes, 37% had retinopathy and 7% had nephropathy in the form of microalbuminuria or proteinuria at the time of the initial diagnosis [17, 18]. The robust reductions in the rates of progression of these complications seen with intensive management of glycemia support management with pharmacotherapy from the time of diagnosis to ensure a significant glycemic improvement. There has been no randomized clinical trial comparing the effects of intensive lifestyle modification alone versus pharmacotherapy on the progression of preexisting microvascular complications in people newly diagnosed with diabetes. It is reasonable to assume that if optimal glycemic control is achieved by diet and exercise alone, a similar reduction in the progression of microvascular complications should be expected as with pharmacotherapy initiated at diagnosis. Given the heterogeneity of results that patients achieve with lifestyle modification, clinicians may prefer the greater predictability of glycemic impact associated with pharmacotherapy in the initial management of such patients.

What about patients who are relatively asymptomatic, are diagnosed with type 2 diabetes on routine fasting glucose screening and have no evidence of microvascular disease at the time of diagnosis? Clinicians often utilize HgbA1C to guide management decisions, opting to start pharmacotherapy if the baseline value is greater than an arbitrarily selected value such as 7%. However, is this approach too cynical, based on an assumption that patients who arrived at this juncture after decades of physical inactivity, unhealthy food choices, and progressive weight gain are destined to fail at lifestyle modification? This view is not unfounded: research suggests that overweight patients with diabetes are less successful at weight loss maintenance than people without diabetes [19], and a meta-analysis of 22 studies of weight loss interventions in patients with type 2 diabetes over 5 years showed minimal improvements in weight [20]. Nevertheless, in the modern model of patient–physician relationship that is based on joint decision making, it is the physician's obligation to present the patient with specific information about the efficacy of lifestyle modifications and the intensity and the consistency of interventions needed to achieve favorable results. Simultaneously with giving information, a physician should elicit information about the patient's preparedness to embrace lifestyle changes and anticipate possible barriers. In the subsequent pages, we will address these aspects with the goal of enabling a clinician to counsel a newly diagnosed patient comprehensively about lifestyle modification.

The efficacy of lifestyle modification in primary prevention of type 2 diabetes was reported by the Diabetes Prevention Program (DPP), where the incidence of diabetes was reduced by 58% in the lifestyle intervention group compared to placebo after 3 years [21]. Early evidence that aggressive lifestyle changes are effective in secondary prevention comes from a 6-year Swedish study that included 41 patients with early-stage type 2 diabetes [22], where a combination of dietary intervention and increased physical activity resulted in a 3.7% weight loss and a 52% remission rate. Other studies report more modest glycemic effects, but in general, changes in HgbA1C correspond to changes in weight [20]. Thus, interventions that produce a more marked weight loss (10–15%) by means of combining a very low calorie diet, physical activity, and behavior modification result in a more significant HgbA1C improvement (2–2.5%) [23]. Observational studies suggest that weight loss also translates into a meaningful decrease in mortality: a substantial 25% reduction in mortality associated with a mean intentional loss of 11% of body weight (24 lbs) was reported in a 12-year observational follow-up of overweight patients with type 2 diabetes [24].

There is evidence that significant caloric restriction leads to substantial improvement in plasma glucose levels even before weight loss ensues. Anderson et al. summarized glucose and weight response in nine studies of very low energy diets in 192 obese people with type 2 diabetes [25]. The glucose improvement was more rapid than weight loss, with the values improving by 50% within two weeks, whereas it took 6 weeks to achieve an approximate 10% weight loss.

Additional evidence of the favorable effects of caloric restriction on glucose metabolism comes from the bariatric intervention outcomes. Serum glucose and insulin levels have been reported to drop dramatically within 3 weeks of Roux-en-Y gastric bypass before significant weight loss had occurred [26]. In many cases, patients with type 2 diabetes who are on insulin therapy are able to discontinue insulin within several days of the procedure. Similar observations of a rapid resolution of type 2 diabetes have been made with vertical banded gastroplasty and laparoscopic adjustable gastric banding [27, 28]. These reports emphasize the important role that excess energy intake plays in the pathogenesis of hyperglycemia in people with type 2 diabetes. Multiple mechanisms have been proposed to explain the drastic improvement in the glucose profile, but there are few systematic studies. High ketogenicity of very low energy diets may stimulate insulin secretion, improve insulin resistance, and directly suppress hepatic gluconeogenesis [29]. In the setting of bariatric intervention, an interruption of the enteroinsular axis by way of alteration of incretin levels has been suggested as a possible mechanism, but confirmatory studies are largely lacking.

Glycemic improvement can also be seen with exercise training alone, even in the absence of a significant change in body mass. Molecular mechanisms leading to improved insulin sensitivity with exercise are numerous and are beyond the scope of this chapter. A meta-analysis of 14 clinical trials on the effects of exercise in people with type 2 diabetes demonstrated a statistically significant mean decrease in HgbA1C of 0.7%, despite unchanged mean weight [30]. However, the majority of these clinical trials were relatively short in duration and long-term trials are needed to demonstrate sustained effects of lifestyle modification on meaningful outcomes in type 2 diabetes, such as microvascular and macrovascular complications.

An association between cardiorespiratory fitness (CRF) and all-cause mortality has been clearly established in people with type 2 diabetes, independent of the BMI. Thus, Wei et al. found that in 1263 men with diabetes, low CRF and physical inactivity were independent predictors of all-cause mortality, with 2.1- and 1.7-fold increased risk respectively [31]. More recently, a similar association between CRF and all-cause mortality was reported in women with impaired fasting glucose and undiagnosed diabetes [32]. Likewise, the protective effect of cardiorespiratory fitness held true for subjects with BMI > 25. In men with type 2 diabetes, mortality from cardiovascular disease has also been shown to be associated with cardiorespiratory fitness. Church et al. demonstrated a hazard ratio of 1.2 for each incremental 1-MET difference in fitness in 2316 men with type 2 diabetes followed for a mean of 16 years [33]. Importantly, there was no increased CVD risk in the overweight and obese men once their level of fitness was taken into account. In all these studies, regular physical activity was a major determinant of the level of cardiorespiratory fitness. This evidence underscores the importance of promoting regular physical activity and optimal fitness in patients with type 2 diabetes, even if this does not lead to weight loss. The goal of avoiding low-fitness category may be more obtainable and therefore better embraced by individuals who have grown frustrated with prior failures of achieving sustainable weight loss.

A large-scale Look AHEAD (Action for HEAlth in Diabetes) trial was launched in 2001 and is designed to examine the effect of lifestyle interventions similar to DPP on cardio-vascular outcomes in people with type 2 diabetes [34]. The study cohort includes over 5000 obese patients with a mean HgbA1C of 7.3%, some of whom have already had a cardiovascular event. Several lifestyle goals are more rigorous in Look AHEAD than in DPP, targeting 10% weight loss, 1200–1500 kcal/day diet for initial weights <250 lbs and up to 1800 kcal/day for weights >250 lbs, 175 minutes of physical activity per week. The interventions are delivered in groups and individually by professional teams comprising of dietitians, psychologists, and exercise specialists. The interim analysis after 1 year shows a mean 8.6% weight loss and a mean 0.6% decline in HgA1C, as well as improvements in a number of CVD risk factors including blood pressure and lipid profile [35]. The projected duration of the Look AHEAD is 12 years.

Setting specific attainable goals improves adherence to a lifestyle modification program [36] and therefore it is imperative that the physician quantitates the intensity of the recommended lifestyle changes. Table 7.1 lists common recommendations [37]. The specifics of necessary dietary changes are addressed in a separate chapter.

Once weight loss has been achieved, intensification of physical activity may be needed to prevent weight regain. Data from the National Weight Control Registry suggest that people who are successful at long-term maintenance of weight loss expend approximately 2800 kcal/week (or 60 minutes of brisk walking per day) [38].

Poor long-term adherence to lifestyle modifications often deters physicians from recommending this as monotherapy. Multiple individual, social, and economic barriers can affect

TABLE 7.1 Commonly recommended lifestyle changes

Weight loss	• Total 5–10% in the first year
	• 0.5–1 kg/week
Diet	• Initial caloric restriction by 500–1000 kcal/day from baseline caloric intake
	• 1000–1200 kcal/day diet to ensure continued weight loss
Exercise	• At least 150 min/week of moderate intensity aerobic activity Or
	• 90-min/week of vigorous aerobic activity
	• To be distributed over at least 3 days per week
	• No more than 2 consecutive days without activity

patients' motivation and impair their efforts. It is conceivable that the multitude and the complexity of these factors is greater than the determinants of compliance with any pharmacotherapy. Interventions employing assessment of the patients' motivational stage and subsequent individualized counseling approach tailored to the stage of preparedness are generally effective at promoting behavior change [39]. Additionally, follow-up to provide reinforcement is important [40]. Such comprehensive approach may be beyond the scope of available time and even expertise level of a busy clinician. Therefore, lifestyle modification can be recommended with greater confidence if there is access to a multidisciplinary program either in one's own practice, by way of an enrollment in a trial or through the community-based initiatives.

References

1. American Diabetes Association (ADA). Introduction. *Diabetes Care.* **32**(Suppl 1):S1–S2, 2009.
2. Conn JW, Fajans SS. Influence of adrenal cortical steroids on carbohydrate metabolism in man. *Metabolism.* **5**(2): 114–127, 1956.
3. Gulliford MC, Charlton J, Latinovic R. Risk of diabetes associated with prescribed glucocorticoids in a large population. *Diabetes Care.* **29**(12):2728–2729, 2006.
4. Owen OE, Cahill GF, Jr. Metabolic effects of exogenous glucocorticoids in fasted man. *J Clin Invest.* **52**(10):2596–2605, 1973.
5. Rizza RA, Mandarino LJ, Gerich JE. Cortisol-induced insulin resistance in man: impaired suppression of glucose production and stimulation of glucose utilization due to a postreceptor detect of insulin action. *J Clin Endocrinol Metab.* **54**(1):131–138, 1982.
6. Newcomer JW, Haupt DW. The metabolic effects of antipsychotic medications. *Can J Psychiatry.* **51**(8):480–491, 2006.
7. Lieberman JA, Phillips M, Gu H, et al. Atypical and conventional antipsychotic drugs in treatment-naive first-episode schizophrenia: a 52-week randomized trial of clozapine vs chlorpromazine. *Neuropsychopharmacology.* **28**(5): 995–1003, 2003.
8. Scheen AJ, De Hert MA. Abnormal glucose metabolism in patients treated with antipsychotics. *Diabetes Metab.* **33**(3): 169–175, 2007.
9. Johnson DE, et al. Inhibitory effects of antipsychotics on carbachol-enhanced insulin secretion from perifused rat islets: role of muscarinic antagonism in antipsychotic-induced diabetes and hyperglycemia. *Diabetes.* **54**(5):1552–1558, 2005.
10. Miller LJ. Management of atypical antipsychotic drug-induced weight gain: focus on metformin. *Pharmacotherapy.* **29**(6):725–735, 2009.
11. Bodziak KA, Hricik DE. New-onset diabetes mellitus after solid organ transplantation. *Transpl Int.* **22**(5):519–530, 2009.
12. Yagisawa T, et al. Effects of cyclosporine on glucose metabolism in kidney transplant recipients and rats. *Transplant Proc.* **19**(1 Pt 2):1801–1803, 1987.
13. Nielsen JH, Mandrup-Poulsen T, Nerup J. Direct effects of cyclosporin A on human pancreatic beta-cells. *Diabetes.* **35**(9):1049–1052, 1986.
14. Kasiske BL, et al. Diabetes mellitus after kidney transplantation in the United States. *Am J Transplant.* **3**(2):178–185, 2003.
15. Poitout V, Robertson RP. Glucolipotoxicity: fuel excess and beta-cell dysfunction. *Endocr Rev.* **29**(3):351–366, 2008.
16. Weng J, et al. Effect of intensive insulin therapy on beta-cell function and glycaemic control in patients with newly diagnosed type 2 diabetes: a multicentre randomised parallel-group trial. *Lancet.* **371**(9626):1753–1760, 2008.
17. Kohner EM. Microvascular disease: what does the UKPDS tell us about diabetic retinopathy? *Diabet Med.* **25**(Suppl 2): 20–24, 2008.
18. Bilous R. Microvascular disease: what does the UKPDS tell us about diabetic nephropathy? *Diabet Med.* **25**(Suppl 2): 25–29, 2008.
19. Guare JC, Wing RR, Grant A. Comparison of obese NIDDM and nondiabetic women: short- and long-term weight loss. *Obes Res.* **3**(4):329–335, 1995.
20. Norris SL, et al. Long-term effectiveness of lifestyle and behavioral weight loss interventions in adults with type 2 diabetes: a meta-analysis. *Am J Med.* **117**(10):762–774, 2004.
21. Knowler WC, et al. Reduction in the incidence of type 2 diabetes with lifestyle intervention or metformin. *N Engl J Med.* **346**(6):393–403, 2002.
22. Eriksson KF, Lindgarde F. Prevention of type 2 (non-insulin-dependent) diabetes mellitus by diet and physical exercise. The 6-year Malmo feasibility study. *Diabetologia.* **34**(12): 891–898, 1991.
23. Wing RR, et al. Effects of a very-low-calorie diet on long-term glycemic control in obese type 2 diabetic subjects. *Arch Intern Med.* **151**(7):1334–1340, 1991.
24. Williamson DF, et al. Intentional weight loss and mortality among overweight individuals with diabetes. *Diabetes Care.* **23**(10):1499–1504, 2000.
25. Anderson JW, Kendall CW, Jenkins DJ. Importance of weight management in type 2 diabetes: review with meta-analysis of clinical studies. *J Am Coll Nutr.* **22**(5):331–339, 2003.

26. Rubino F, et al. The early effect of the Roux-en-Y gastric bypass on hormones involved in body weight regulation and glucose metabolism. *Ann Surg*. **240**(2):236–242, 2004.

27. Deitel M. The early effect of the bariatric operations on diabetes. *Obes Surg*. **12**(3):349, 2002.

28. Segato G, et al. Weight loss and changes in use of antidiabetic medication in obese type 2 diabetics after laparoscopic gastric banding. *Surg Obes Relat Dis*. **6**(2):132–137, 2009.

29. Baker S, Jerums G, Proietto J. Effects and clinical potential of very-low-calorie diets (VLCDs) in type 2 diabetes. *Diabetes Res Clin Pract*. **85**(3):235–242, 2009.

30. Boule NG, et al. Effects of exercise on glycemic control and body mass in type 2 diabetes mellitus: a meta-analysis of controlled clinical trials. *JAMA*. **286**(10):1218–1227, 2001.

31. Wei M, et al. Low cardiorespiratory fitness and physical inactivity as predictors of mortality in men with type 2 diabetes. *Ann Intern Med*. **132**(8):605–611, 2000.

32. Lyerly GW, et al. The association between cardiorespiratory fitness and risk of all-cause mortality among women with impaired fasting glucose or undiagnosed diabetes mellitus. *Mayo Clin Proc*. **84**(9):780–786, 2009.

33. Church TS, et al. Cardiorespiratory fitness and body mass index as predictors of cardiovascular disease mortality among men with diabetes. *Arch Intern Med*. **165**(18):2114–2120, 2005.

34. Ryan DH, et al. Look AHEAD (Action for Health in Diabetes): design and methods for a clinical trial of weight loss for the prevention of cardiovascular disease in type 2 diabetes. *Control Clin Trials*. **24**(5):610–628, 2003.

35. Pi-Sunyer X, et al. Reduction in weight and cardiovascular disease risk factors in individuals with type 2 diabetes: one-year results of the look AHEAD trial. *Diabetes Care*. **30**(6): 1374–1383, 2007.

36. Estabrooks PA, et al. The frequency and behavioral outcomes of goal choices in the self-management of diabetes. *Diabetes Educ*. **31**(3):391–400, 2005.

37. Sigal RJ, et al. Physical activity/exercise and type 2 diabetes: a consensus statement from the American Diabetes Association. *Diabetes Care*. **29**(6):1433–1438, 2006.

38. Hill JO. Understanding and addressing the epidemic of obesity: an energy balance perspective. *Endocr Rev*. **27**(7): 750–761, 2006.

39. Kirk AF, et al. Promoting and maintaining physical activity in people with type 2 diabetes. *Am J Prev Med*. **27**(4):289–296, 2004.

40. Loveman E, Frampton GK, Clegg AJ. The clinical effectiveness of diabetes education models for type 2 diabetes: a systematic review. *Health Technol Assess*. **12**(9):1–116, iii, 2008.

8   Insulin sensitizers versus secretagogues as first-line therapy for diabetes: Rationale for clinical choice

Robert J. Richards[1], L. Yvonne Melendez-Ramirez[2], and William T. Cefalu[3]

[1] Associate Professor of Medicine, Joint Program on Diabetes, Endocrinology and Metabolism, Pennington Biomedical Research Center & LSUHSC School of Medicine, New Orleans, LA and Baton Rouge, LA, USA

[2] Assistant Professor of Medicine, Joint Program on Diabetes, Endocrinology and Metabolism, Pennington Biomedical Research Center & LSUHSC School of Medicine, New Orleans, LA & Baton Rouge, LA, USA

[3] Douglas L. Manship, Sr. Professor of Diabetes, Chief, Joint Program on Diabetes, Endocrinology and Metabolism, Pennington Biomedical Research Center & LSUHSC School of Medicine, New Orleans, LA and Baton Rouge, LA, USA

LEARNING POINTS

- As a rule, the secretagogues and sensitizers can potentially lower A1c in the range of 1–2% depending on the baseline A1c.
- Metformin is mostly weight neutral while thiazolidinediones and insulin secretagogues often lead to weight gain.
- Metformin and thiazolidinediones are unlikely to cause hypoglycemia.
- Thiazolidinediones are linked to bone loss in women, but the link is not well defined and requires more studies.
- Concern over the safety of rosiglitazone lead to the FDA severely restricting its use.

Introduction

The progress made over the recent past in providing new information on the pathophysiology of type 2 diabetes has been nothing short of astounding. It is hard to appreciate that within recent memory, available choices for treatment included only insulin or sulfonylureas. Although the biguanides, i.e., metformin, had been studied and available in other parts of the world, it wasn't until the last decade of the twentieth century that these agents were available in the United States. However, within the last decade, new pharmacologic agents have become available that address specific pathophysiologic defects with novel mechanisms of action. As a result, clinicians now have a variety of agents from at least seven classes at their disposal to address the pathophysiologic defects that characterize type 2 diabetes, i.e., insulin secretory dysfunction, insulin resistance, and hepatic glucose overproduction. In addition, agents are being actively investigated that address other mechanisms to improve glycemia, i.e., SGLT2 inhibitors, glucose kinase activators, inflammatory agents, etc. However, the downside of having so many choices is having to decide which drug offers the most advantages to the patient while limiting the untoward side effects. The ultimate choice will depend on factors such as patient phenotype, underlying comorbidities, physician experience, and cost, among others. For the purpose of argument and for this chapter only, we will discuss only these two general options: secretagogues (sulfonylureas and meglitinides) and sensitizers (metformin and thiazolidinediones). Other drugs such as incretin therapies that may impact insulin secretion or sensitization are covered elsewhere.

There is an ongoing debate whether type 2 diabetes is primarily a disorder of skeletal muscle insulin resistance, insulin insufficiency, or both. This debate is beyond the scope of this review. However, it has been observed for many years that the liver is also a key player in the pathogenesis. Studies also reveal the importance of the gastrointestinal

Clinical Dilemmas in Diabetes, First Edition. Edited by Adrian Vella and Robert A. Rizza

© 2011 Blackwell Publishing Ltd. Published 2011 by Blackwell Publishing Ltd.

TABLE 8.1 Comparison of insulin sensitizers and secretagogues with respect to various end-points

Issue	Secretagogues		Sensitizers	
	Sulfonylureas	Meglitinides	Metformin	TZD
Glucose				
HbA1c (%)	↓1–2	↓1–1.5	↓1–2	↓0.5–1.4
Fasting glucose (mg/dl)	↓40–50	↓20–70	↓40–50	↓40–60
Postprandial glucose (mg/dl)	↓20–60	↓60–110	↓50–140	↓60–70
Lipids				
Total cholesterol	No effect	No effect	Small decrease	Small decrease[3]
LDL	No effect	No effect	Small decrease	Small decrease[3]
HDL	No effect	No effect	Little effect	Small increase[3]
Triglycerides	No effect	No effect	Small decrease	Small decrease[3]
Adverse events				
Risk of hypoglycemia	Significant	Less likely	Minimal	Minimal
Body weight	↑2–5 kg	↑1–4 kg	Overall neutral	↑2–4 kg
Risk of edema	Minimal	Minimal	Minimal	Increased risk
Bone disease	None reported	None reported	None reported	Yes
Cancer[1]	Increased risk	Unknown	Decreased risk	Increased risk
Cardiovascular disease	Little impact	Unknown	Likely protective	Being debated
Cost/efficacy ratio ($ Per unit drop in A1c)[2]	<5[4]	100–200	<5	100–250

[1] Risk is based on a relatively few number of papers reporting mostly observational data.
[2] Relative costs are derived from www.drugstore.com. These reported costs are estimates only.
[3] The currently available agents, rosiglitazone and pioglitazone, exhibit differing effects.
[4] Cost used to determine efficacy is based on glipizide and glyburide.

tract in the pathophysiology. Thus, it is clear that type 2 diabetes is multifactorial. For the purposes as described in this chapter, we will primarily focus on the defects of insulin secretion and insulin resistance in providing the rationale as to why a provider should use either class of drugs (secretagogues or sensitizers) as a first-line choice. Of course, the answer is never easy. Each of these classes has advantages and disadvantages. The clinician must balance a host of arguments when selecting a treatment plan. We will attempt to summarize some of the arguments as they pertain to these two classes of agents. This summary is organized by issue rather than agent. A further summarization is presented in Table 8.1.

Glucose control

There is no single, perfect indicator of treatment effectiveness, but the most accepted and well validated indicator is HbA1c. Almost by definition, all agents used to treat diabetes have efficacy based on how they lower this indicator—some do so more than others. At least since the mid-1990s, the mantra has been to strive for glucose

control that is as near to normal as possible, but given the recent cardiovascular trials (see below), less stringent control may be indicated in individuals who are prone to more hypoglycemia, have prior cardiovascular events, or have other significant comorbidities. Both the ACCORD [1] and ADVANCE [2] studies demonstrated risks involved with aggressive glucose control.

The HbA1c lowering for each particular agent is in large part dependent on the baseline value: the higher the initial HbA1c, the greater the reduction, regardless of the agent used [3]. Nevertheless, the expected decrease in HbA1c is usually reported to be in the approximate ranges of 1–2% for sulfonylureas, 1–1.5% for meglitinides (repaglinide about 0.5% greater than nateglinide) [4], 1–2% for metformin, and 0.5–1.4% for thiazolidinediones [5]. For perspective, the estimated drop in HbA1c is 1–2% if lifestyle changes are made and are successful [5].

Reductions in fasting glucose are also partially dependent upon baseline levels [3, 6]. Nevertheless, one may expect a reduction in fasting glucose levels of about 40–50 mg/dl with sulfonylureas [7]. Metformin exhibits similar results [6], though some studies demonstrate a greater improvement [8]. The reduction in fasting glucose is similar with the thiazolidinediones [9] and the meglitinides [10].

Glucose levels after meals or after oral glucose loading are not widely reported for some agents. Metformin decreases glucose concentrations after an oral glucose load by about 50–60 mg/dl [6], while self-reported postprandial glucose drops by about 140 mg/dl [8]. The thiazolidinediones reduce post-challenge glucose by about 60–70 mg/dl [11]. Sulfonylureas decrease postprandial glucose on the order of about 20 mg/dl [12] to 60 mg/dl [13]. The main focus of the meglitinides is on postprandial glucose. They reduce it by about 60–110 mg/dl, with repaglinide showing greater efficacy [10]. However, the effectiveness of secretagogues versus sensitizers on postprandial control may primarily be based on how well they lower the fasting levels. Essentially, by lowering fasting levels, the absolute postprandial value may be reduced, but the increment between fasting and postprandial peak may not be markedly altered. Newer agents in the incretin class appear to be more effective on postprandial control than traditional agents such as secretagogues or sensitizers [14].

Effect on body weight

Weight gain is virtually inevitable in the treatment of diabetes. An increase of 2–5 kg may be commonly observed with sulfonylureas [15, 16]. Similar weight gain was reported by the UKPDS investigators regarding 750 overweight subjects treated with sulfonylureas compared to lifestyle intervention [17]. The benefit of metformin is that it is mostly weight neutral but favors a mild weight loss [18]. Fortunately, even a small amount of weight loss can significantly improve cardiovascular risk [19]. A major disadvantage of thiazolidinediones and meglitinides is the weight gain [18].

Lipid effects

The insulin sensitizers are associated with beneficial changes to lipids of varying degrees. A systematic review of randomized, controlled trials involving a total of 3000 subjects reported that metformin was associated with small declines in total cholesterol (−10 mg/dl), LDL (−8.5 mg/dl), and triglycerides (−11.5 mg/dl) [20]. Most clinicians expect to see small beneficial changes in lipid profiles with metformin.

The two currently available thiazolidinediones appear to have different effects on lipid profiles. In a randomized, blinded, crossover, head-to-head trial of rosiglitazone and pioglitazone that did not utilize a placebo, the different effects on lipids [9] were suggested by the authors as likely being due to different PPAR activities. With rosiglitazone, the total cholesterol increased by 28 mg/dl, LDL increased by 21 mg/dl, HDL increased by 2.4 mg/dl, and triglycerides increased by 13 mg/dl. With pioglitazone, the total cholesterol increased by 9 mg/dl, LDL increased by 12 mg/dl, HDL increased by 5.2 mg/dl, and triglycerides decreased by 52 mg/dl. Taken together as a class, the thiazolidinediones raise HDL by a mean of 3–5 mg/dl but raise LDL by a mean of 10 mg/dl [18].

The sulfonylureas and meglitinides do not significantly affect lipids [16, 18, 21].

Risk of hypoglycemia

A major difference between the insulin sensitizers and secretagogues is the rate of hypoglycemia. Secretagogues are well known to put patients at risk for hypoglycemia. The sensitizers have much lower rates of symptomatic hypoglycemia. The risk of hypoglycemia when using sulfonylureas has been reported to be about 2–4% [16]. The meglitinides confer a similar risk of hypoglycemia [18], but are suggested to be less likely to cause nocturnal hypoglycemia, due in part to a very short half-life, short duration of action, and the usual practice of drug administration only at the time of eating.

Risk of bone disease

A recent concern with the thiazolidinediones is a potential increase in the risk of fractures, which has been suggested to be a class effect [22]. The ADOPT study of over 4300 subjects reported the fracture risk was significantly increased with rosiglitazone compared to metformin and glyburide. This increased risk occurred among women, but not men, in both the lower and upper limbs [23].

Risk of developing cancer

Though controversial, diabetes has been reported to be a risk factor for development of cancer and for death from cancer. Both type 1 diabetes and type 2 were reported to be associated with an increased cancer risk, although the types of cancers are different [24]. Several investigators have suggested that treatment modalities may influence cancer risk in patients with type 2 diabetes [24]. However, this issue if far from settled. Additional work is required before the putative role of treatment is clear. Recently, there were reports regarding insulin glargine and increased cancer risk [24], but further discussion is beyond the scope of this review. However, the oral drugs are also being studied for possible risks. A retrospective study suggested an increased risk of cancer with sulfonylureas but a protective effect with metformin [25]. Another report added more evidence in favor of metformin [26]. The reports so far on thiazolidinediones have been mixed. Little or no information regarding the meglitinides and cancer have yet been reported. Any linkage between glucose-lowering drugs and cancer is subject to many confounders and prospective trials involving all hypoglycemic agents are needed before firm conclusions can be made [27]. So at this time, the association of specific cancer risk and antidiabetic treatment suffers from a paucity of data.

Cardiovascular disease

Patients with diabetes have a high risk for cardiac events. They exhibit a risk similar to that seen in nondiabetic patients with a prior history of myocardial infarction [28]. Patients with diabetes need to be treated similar to patients without diabetes but with known coronary artery disease—a well appreciated high-risk population. This is reflected in the treatment guidelines provided by the American Diabetes Association (ADA) [29], American Association of Clinical Endocrinologists (AACE) [30], American Heart Association (AHA) [31] and National Cholesterol Education Program (NCEP) [32].

Sulfonylureas

The effect of antidiabetic agents on cardiovascular disease (CVD) has been an area of interest for many years beginning with the controversial University Group Diabetes Program (UGDP). The initial concern regarding a linkage between cardiovascular disease and insulin secretagogues has not always borne out. For example, a systematic review demonstrated little evidence for such a risk [18], but large retrospective studies recently suggested there may be a small increased risk associated with sulfonylureas when compared to metformin [33]. The duration of follow-up is important. It may take many years before the beneficial effect of improved glycemia on the risk of CVD is realized. In

the UKPDS, subjects were followed for 10 years post-study without intervening in treatment decisions [34]. Though UKPDS did not initially demonstrate a statistically significant reduction in myocardial infarctions [35], the 10-year post-study follow-up did show a reduction [34].

Meglitinides

No long-term studies have yet been published examining cardiovascular disease with either repaglinide or nateglinide. This lack of long-term cardiovascular data provides yet another area requiring additional clinical research.

Metformin

Metformin has been investigated in many clinical studies, sometimes with mixed results. In a subset of subjects, all overweight, the UKPDS demonstrated that intensive treatment with metformin reduced the risk of several end points when compared to conventional treatment, primarily diet only. They were myocardial infarction, all macrovascular disease, and death from cardiovascular disease [17]. However, the same improvement in risk was seen in overweight subjects assigned to intensive treatment with insulin or sulfonylureas; metformin did not offer an advantage. Other end points in the same study were different. Metformin did prove significantly better than sulfonylurea or insulin for all-cause mortality and the aggregate of any diabetes-related end point, micro- or macrovascular.

In a different subset of UKPDS, defined as subjects of any weight who failed sulfonylurea therapy, adding metformin had no benefit on any clinical end point. Quite the contrary, adding metformin to these subjects actually increased the risk of diabetes-related death and all-cause mortality [17]. The investigators speculated that the increased risk seen with the combination of metformin and sulfonylurea therapy may represent "extremes of the play of chance." When the investigators combined the two subsets, the increase in risk was negated.

The UKPDS investigators later published a 10-year follow-up of all subjects originally randomized to conventional therapy, intensive therapy with metformin (only overweight subjects were originally randomized into this group), and intensive therapy with sulfonylurea-insulin [34]. Initial intensive treatment with either sulfonylurea-insulin or metformin (overweight subjects only) reduced the risk of myocardial infarction, death from any cause, and several other end points, some of which were not significantly different during the intervention phase of UKPDS. Duration of follow-up is key.

Though metformin is relatively contraindicated in patients with heart failure, there is little worry that metformin will cause heart failure, and it carries only a minimal risk of edema [18].

Based on considerable clinical experience, metformin is widely used without any overt evidence of danger and continues to be recommended as first-line drug therapy.

Thiazolidinediones

As recent studies have suggested, heart failure is very much a concern with this class. The thiazolidinediones worsen existing heart failure and may induce heart failure in susceptible patients. The drug is not approved for use in patients with class 3 or 4 heart failure (NYHA). Many clinicians also avoid the drug in patients with class 2 heart failure. The risk of developing heart failure is 1–4% [18].

In a meta-analysis, treatment with rosiglitazone was associated with a significantly increased risk of myocardial infarction [36]. However, the ACCORD and BARI-2D studies did not show increased CV events or mortality with rosiglitazone treatment [1, 37]. In high-risk type 2 DM patients, the addition of pioglitazone reduced the composite of all-cause mortality, nonfatal MI, and stroke [38]. Thus, studies have supported and refuted findings about rosiglitazone, while similar studies involving pioglitazone showed no increased risk but perhaps a small benefit. These issues are outlined in a consensus statement jointly issued by the ADA and the European Association for the Study of Diabetes (EASD) [5]. They recommend "caution." The thiazolidinediones remain an important class, but clinicians must consider potential cardiovascular risk. More studies are needed. The RECORD study indicated no increase in overall cardiovascular risk with rosiglitazone compared to therapy with metformin and sulfonylureas, but the increase in heart failure was significantly higher [39]. However, in 2010 evidence against rosiglitazone accumulated, and the FDA severely restricted its use. This effectively removes it from consideration by clinicians.

Overall, the effect of antidiabetic agents on CVD disease has been a topic of great debate based on observations to date. As such, the Food and Drug Administration (FDA) has suggested specific guidelines for assessing cardiovascular risk for new drugs in development. Specifically, any new agent needs to demonstrate that it does not increase cardiovascular risk before it can be considered for approval.

Other risks and benefits

Beta-cell preservation

The UKPDS estimated that about 50% of beta-cell function is lost by the time diabetes is diagnosed [40]. ADOPT followed beta-cell function over a period of about five years while treated with glyburide, metformin, or rosiglitazone [23]. During the first six months of treatment, beta-cell function increased. This initial increase was much greater with glyburide than with metformin or rosiglitazone. After the initial 6 months, all groups lost beta-cell function, but the rate of loss was greatest for the secretagogue.

Durability

More effective beta-cell function may be reflected in durability of effect. UKPDS showed 9-year monotherapy failure rates [41], indicated by fasting glucose >140 mg/dl and HbA1c ≥7%, to be quite high for all the modalities; i.e., insulin, sulfonylureas, metformin, and diet alone. Clearly these studies were landmark trials in defining the progressive nature of the disease. The ADOPT study examined durability of glycemic control with glyburide, metformin, and rosiglitazone [23]. The investigators measured the cumulative monotherapy failure rate at five years, defined as fasting glucose >180 mg/dl, and found it to be lowest for rosiglitazone (15%), intermediate for metformin (21%), and highest for glyburide (34%). Durability appears to be an advantage of the thiazolidinediones as compared to the other agents. Unfortunately, although the thiazolidinediones appeared to offer some benefits, the progression of disease was not halted. Treatment durability is of great interest to clinicians. The durability of newer therapies, such as incretins, is being studied.

Some agent specific risks

Metformin is associated with an increased risk of lactic acidosis. Fortunately, this risk is minimal when used appropriately. Use of the drug is absolutely contraindicated in the presence of renal dysfunction, as defined as a serum creatinine equal to or greater than 1.5 mg/dl in men and 1.4 mg/dl in women. Administration of nephrotoxic contrast media may cause acute renal failure, and metformin must be held until renal function is shown not to be affected. Metformin also has relative contraindications. The patient should exhibit adequate renal function, hepatic function, and heart function. The thiazolidinediones and insulin secretagogues are not as sensitive to renal dysfunction as is metformin. However, sulfonylureas exhibit a protracted duration of action in patients with significant renal disease. This is not the case for the meglitinides. The package inserts for repaglinide (current as of December 2009, last updated June 2006) and nateglinide (current as of December 2009, last updated July 2008) indicate approval for use in patients with creatinine clearances as low as 20 mL/min and 15 mL/min, respectively.

The thiazolidinediones have been associated with edema, heart failure, and fractures as discussed above. The risk of edema is 2–20% [18]. This class carries a risk of hepatotoxicity, but the risk is minimized when proper liver function is verified. These drugs must be used cautiously if ALT is elevated, not initiated if ALT >2.5 times the upper limit of normal (ULN), and discontinued if ALT >3 times the ULN. The risk of drug-induced pancreatitis is exceedingly low when patients are closely monitored. The anemia seen with this class is only partially explained by dilution, but is usually minor when present.

Cost-effectiveness

Efficacy and cost-effectiveness are important considerations when selecting a treatment strategy. The sulfonylureas and metformin are generic and inexpensive. They provide excellent ratios of cost:efficacy. The estimated cost-effectiveness is less than $5/month per one percentage point drop in HbA1c. In contrast, the cost:efficacy ratios are very variable for the meglitinides and thiazolidinediones, mainly due to variations in cost. Assuming a monthly cost of $100–200 for meglitinides and $100–250 for thiazolidinediones, their respective cost:efficacy ratios at the time of this publication are very roughly $60–200/month and $60–500/month per percentage point drop in HbA1c. No medical decision should ever be based solely on cost, but unfortunately cost is often a consideration, given the economic burden that diabetes has placed on our population. Most providers observe that patients with few resources are much more likely to be compliant with the less costly treatment alternatives. However, the initial cost of a drug is only one consideration. The initial drug chosen may be more expensive but have significant benefits on metabolic factors, i.e., glycemia, weight, and lipids. This benefit may be such that complication rates and other medical expenses are reduced years after diagnosis. Important considerations other than cost need to be factored into the treatment decision. Data on long-term benefits are vitally needed.

Conclusions

Based on the above rationale, there are benefits in choosing a sensitizer over a secretagogue in most clinical situations. In the majority of cases, clinicians will choose metformin as the first drug for treatment of type 2 diabetes unless it is contraindicated. Consensus statements and algorithms recommend metformin as the initial drug of choice along with lifestyle intervention [42]. Metformin appears to be effective, generally well tolerated, and has a very low risk for lactic acidosis when used properly. Most algorithms become very nonspecific after metformin. Arguments can be made for all of the other drugs approved for treating type 2 diabetes. Sulfonylureas have been used extensively and are well established. Unfortunately, the weight gain and hypoglycemia remain a concern. Clinicians also have considerable experience with the thiazolidinediones. The advantages are better durability, beneficial effect on lipids, and good insulin sensitizing effect. The disadvantages are weight gain, increased risk for heart failure in susceptible populations, and other cardiac events. But all glucose-lowering drugs exhibit different clinical profiles and have roles in the current treatment of diabetes. The choice of treatment is ultimately a decision between the clinician and the patient. As outlined in this review, there are many reasons supporting metformin as the initial choice. For purposes of this chapter, we primarily focused on the advantages and disadvantages of sensitizers versus secretagogues as requested by the editor. After initiating metformin, the agent of choice for the next step may include secretagogues or the newer agents in the incretin class or the addition of insulin. These agents are covered in other chapters.

References

1. The Action to Control Cardiovascular Risk in Diabetes Study Group. Effects of intensive glucose lowering in type 2 diabetes. *N Engl J Med.* **358**(24):2545–2559, 2008.
2. The ADVANCE Collaborative Group. Intensive blood glucose control and vascular outcomes in patients with type 2 diabetes. *N Engl J Med.* **358**(24):2560–2572, 2008.
3. Bloomgarden ZT, Dodis R, Viscoli CM, Holmboe ES, Inzucchi SE. Lower baseline glycemia reduces apparent oral agent glucose-lowering efficacy. *Diabetes Care.* **29**(9):2137–2139, 2006.
4. Raskin P. Comparison of repaglinide and nateglinide in combination with metformin. *Diabetes Care.* **26**(12): 3362–3363, 2003.

5. Nathan DM, Buse JB, Davidson MB, et al. Management of hyperglycemia in type 2 diabetes: a consensus algorithm for the initiation and adjustment of therapy. *Diabetes Care.* **31**(1):173–175, 2008.

6. DeFronzo RA, Goodman AM, The Multicenter Metformin Study Group. Efficacy of metformin in patients with non-insulin-dependent diabetes mellitus. *N Engl J Med.* **333**(9):541–549, 1995.

7. Bloomgarden ZT. Approaches to treatment of type 2 diabetes. *Diabetes Care.* **31**(8):1697–1703, 2008.

8. Kooy A, de Jager J, Lehert P, et al. Long-term effects of metformin on metabolism and microvascular and macrovascular disease in patients with type 2 diabetes mellitus. *Arch Intern Med.* **169**(6):616–625, 2009.

9. Goldberg RB, Kendall DM, Deeg MA, et al. A comparison of lipid and glycemic effects of pioglitazone and rosiglitazone in patients with type 2 diabetes and dyslipidemia. *Diabetes Care.* **28**(7):1547–1554, 2005.

10. Rosenstock J, Hassman DR, Madder RD, et al. Repaglinide versus nateglinide monotherapy. *Diabetes Care.* **27**(6): 1265–1270, 2004.

11. Miyazaki Y, DeFronzo RA. Rosiglitazone and pioglitazone similarly improve insulin sensitivity and secretion, glucose tolerance and adipocytokines in type 2 diabetic patients. *Diabetes Obes Metab.* **10**(12):1204–1211, 2008.

12. Derosa G, D'Angelo A, Fogari E, et al. Nateglinide and glibenclamide metabolic effects in naïve type 2 diabetic patients treated with metformin. *J Clin Pharm Ther.* **34**(1):13–23, 2009.

13. Vakkilainen J, Mero N, Schweizer A, Foley JE, Taskinen M-R. Effects of nateglinide and glibenclamide on postprandial lipid and glucose metabolism in type 2 diabetes. *Diabetes Metab Res Rev.* **18**(6):484–490, 2002.

14. Cefalu WT, Richards RJ, Melendez-Ramirez LY. Redefining treatment success in type 2 diabetes mellitus: comprehensive targeting of core defects. *Cleve Clin J Med.* **76**(Suppl 5):S39–S47, 2009.

15. Inzucchi SE. Oral antihyperglycemic therapy for type 2 diabetes: scientific review. *JAMA.* **287**(3):360–372, 2002.

16. Mizuno CS, Chittiboyina AG, Kurtz TW, Pershadsingh HA, Avery MA. Type 2 diabetes and oral antihyperglycemic drugs. *Curr Med Chem.* **15**(1):61–74, 2008.

17. UK Prospective Diabetes Study (UKPDS) Group. Effect of intensive blood-glucose control with metformin on complications in overweight patients with type 2 diabetes (UKPDS 34). *Lancet.* **352**(9131):854–865, 1998.

18. Bolen S, Feldman L, Vassy J, et al. Systematic review: comparative effectiveness and safety of oral medications for type 2 diabetes mellitus. *Ann Intern Med.* **147**(6):386–399, 2007.

19. Hermansen K, Mortensen LS. Bodyweight changes associated with antihyperglycaemic agents in type 2 diabetes mellitus. *Drug Saf.* **30**(12):1127–1142, 2007.

20. Wulffelé MG, Kooy A, Zeeuw D, Stehouwer CDA, Gansevoort RT. The effect of metformin on blood pressure, plasma cholesterol and triglycerides in type 2 diabetes mellitus: a systematic review. *J Intern Med.* **256**(1):1–14, 2004.

21. Lund SS, Tarnow L, Frandsen M, et al. Impact of metformin versus the prandial insulin secretagogue, repaglinide, on fasting and postprandial glucose and lipid responses in non-obese patients with type 2 diabetes. *Eur J Endocrinol.* **158**(1):35–46, 2008.

22. Dormuth CR, Carney G, Carleton B, Bassett K, Wright JM. Thiazolidinediones and fractures in men and women. *Arch Intern Med.* **169**(15):1395–1402, 2009.

23. Kahn SE, Haffner SM, Heise MA, et al. Glycemic durability of rosiglitazone, metformin, or glyburide monotherapy. *N Engl J Med.* **355**(23):2427–2443, 2006.

24. Smith U, Gale EA. Does diabetes therapy influence the risk of cancer? *Diabetologia.* **52**(9):1699–1708, 2009.

25. Currie C, Poole C, Gale E. The influence of glucose-lowering therapies on cancer risk in type 2 diabetes. *Diabetologia.* **52**(9):1766–1777, 2009.

26. Landman GWD, Kleefstra N, van Hateren KJJ, Groenier KH, Gans ROB, Bilo HJG. Metformin associated with lower cancer mortality in type 2 diabetes. *Diabetes Care.* **33**(2):322–326, 2010.

27. Gerstein HC. Does insulin therapy promote, reduce, or have a neutral effect on cancers? *JAMA.* **303**(5):446–447, 2010.

28. Schramm TK, Gislason GH, Kober L, et al. Diabetes patients requiring glucose-lowering therapy and nondiabetics with a prior myocardial infarction carry the same cardiovascular risk: a population study of 3.3 million people. *Circulation.* **117**(15):1945–1954, 2008.

29. American Diabetes Association. Executive summary: standards of medical care in diabetes – 2009. *Diabetes Care.* **32**(Suppl 1):S6–S12, 2009.

30. Rodbard HW, Blonde L, Braithwaite SS, et al. American Association of Clinical Endocrinologists medical guidelines for clinical practice for the management of diabetes mellitus [published correction appears in Endocr Pract 2008;14:802-803]. *Endocr Pract.* **13**(Suppl 1):1–68, 2007.

31. Grundy SM, Howard B, Smith S, Jr., Eckel R, Redberg R, Bonow RO. Prevention Conference VI: Diabetes and Cardiovascular Disease: Executive Summary: Conference Proceeding for Healthcare Professionals From a Special Writing Group of the American Heart Association. *Circulation.* **105**(18):2231-2239, 2002.

32. Expert Panel on Detection Evaluation and Treatment of High Blood Cholesterol in Adults. Executive summary of

the third report of the National Cholesterol Education Program (NCEP) expert panel on detection, evaluation, and treatment of high blood cholesterol in adults (Adult Treatment Panel III). *JAMA.* **285**(19):2486–2497, 2001.

33. Tzoulaki I, Molokhia M, Curcin V, et al. Risk of cardiovascular disease and all cause mortality among patients with type 2 diabetes prescribed oral antidiabetes drugs: retrospective cohort study using UK general practice research database. *BMJ.* **339**:b4731, 2009.

34. Holman RR, Paul SK, Bethel MA, Matthews DR, Neil HAW. 10-year follow-up of intensive glucose control in type 2 diabetes. *N Engl J Med.* **359**(15):1577–1589, 2008.

35. UK Prospective Diabetes Study (UKPDS) Group. Intensive blood-glucose control with sulphonylureas or insulin compared with conventional treatment and risk of complications in patients with type 2 diabetes (UKPDS 33). *Lancet.* **352**(9131):837–853, 1998.

36. Nissen SE, Wolski K. Effect of rosiglitazone on the risk of myocardial infarction and death from cardiovascular causes. *N Engl J Med.* **356**(24):2457–2471, 2007.

37. The BARI 2D Study Group. A randomized trial of therapies for type 2 diabetes and coronary artery disease. *N Engl J Med.* **360**(24):2503–2515, 2009.

38. Dormandy JA, Charbonnel B, Eckland DJA, et al. Secondary prevention of macrovascular events in patients with type 2 diabetes in the PROactive Study (PROspective pioglitAzone Clinical Trial In macroVascular Events): a randomised controlled trial. *Lancet.* **366**(9493):1279–1289, 2005.

39. Home PD, Pocock SJ, Beck-Nielsen H, et al. Rosiglitazone evaluated for cardiovascular outcomes in oral agent combination therapy for type 2 diabetes (RECORD): a multicentre, randomised, open-label trial. *Lancet.* **373**(9681):2125–2135, 2009.

40. U.K. Prospective Diabetes Study Group. U.K. prospective diabetes study 16. Overview of 6 years' therapy of type II diabetes: a progressive disease. *Diabetes.* **44**(11):1249–1258, 1995.

41. Turner RC, Cull CA, Frighi V, Holman RR, for the UK Prospective Diabetes Study Group. Glycemic control with diet, sulfonylurea, metformin, or insulin in patients with type 2 diabetes mellitus: progressive requirement for multiple therapies (UKPDS 49). *JAMA.* **281**(21):2005–2012, 1999.

42. Rodbard HW, Jellinger PS, Davidson JA, et al. Statement by an American Association of Clinical Endocrinologists/American College of Endocrinology consensus panel on type 2 diabetes mellitus: an algorithm for glycemic control. *Endocr Pract.* **15**(6):540–557, 2009.

Are insulin sensitizers useful additions to insulin therapy?

John W. Richard III[1] and Philip Raskin[2]

[1] Endocrinology Fellow, Division of Endocrinology, Diabetes, Nutrition and Metabolism, University of Texas Southwestern Medical Center at Dallas, Dallas, TX, USA

[2] Professor of Medicine, Clifton and Betsy Robinson Chair in Biomedical Research, University of Texas Southwestern Medical Center at Dallas, Dallas, TX, USA

LEARNING POINTS

- Patients with type 2 diabetes often need higher doses of insulin because of obesity and decreased insulin sensitivity.

- Insulin sensitizing agents act as useful additions to insulin therapy to combat worsening insulin sensitivity.

- Metformin suppresses hepatic glucose production (gluconeogenesis) and increases peripheral tissue insulin sensitivity.

- Thiazolidinediones increase insulin-stimulated glucose uptake in peripheral tissues, hepatic insulin sensitivity, and insulin sensitivity in adipose tissue through suppression of fatty acid production.

- Insulin sensitizing agents have proven effectiveness at improving glucose control and lipid profiles, and reducing insulin dose requirements; however, these agents are not without side effects.

Insulin sensitizers

Insulin resistance is not a new phenomenon. In the 1930s British physician Harold Percival Himsworth coined the term "insulin insensitivity" to describe patients he observed with resistance to injectable insulin. Fifty years later, Dr. Gerald Reaven described metabolic syndrome X, a condition characterized by decreased insulin sensitivity, high insulin levels, high triglycerides, and low HDL cholesterol leading to type 2 diabetes and cardiovascular disease risk. Considering the role of insulin resistance in the development of these disease processes, insulin action at the target tissue level is an attractive therapeutic target in type 2 diabetes [1]. The biguanides (i.e., metformin) and the thiazolidinediones (TZDs) act directly to improve insulin sensitivity, and so are regarded as insulin sensitizing drugs.

Biguanides

In Europe, *Galega officinalis* (goat's rue or French lilac) was used for centuries to treat diabetes. This guanidine-rich substance later led to the development of several glucose-lowering guanidine derivatives in the 1920s. With the discovery of insulin these antidiabetic agents were forgotten until the 1950s when the biguanides: metformin, phenformin and buformin were reintroduced into diabetes treatment [1]. Phenformin was withdrawn in many countries and from the U.S. market in 1975 because of a high incidence of lactic acidosis. Buformin received only limited use in a few countries, making metformin the principal biguanide drug used in pharmacotherapy worldwide, especially with its improved safety profile and lower cost [1].

Mechanism of action

The mechanism of action of biguanides (i.e., metformin) is still not fully understood, but this agent is distinctly different from oral sulfonylureas. Biguanides do not stimulate pancreatic insulin secretion and only partial suppression of gluconeogenesis occurs in the liver, therefore, hypoglycemia with monotherapy is rare [2, 3]. Metformin has a variety of metabolic effects, some of which extend beyond glucose lowering (Table 9.1). At a cellular level, metformin improves insulin sensitivity through a mediated modification of post-receptor signaling in the insulin pathway. Recent data have suggested that a protein, adenosine $5'$-monophosphate protein kinase (AMPK), has been identified as a possible

Clinical Dilemmas in Diabetes, First Edition. Edited by Adrian Vella and Robert A. Rizza
© 2011 Blackwell Publishing Ltd. Published 2011 by Blackwell Publishing Ltd.

Case

A 52-year-old woman with obesity and a 9-year history of type 2 diabetes presents with complaints of fatigue and difficulty losing weight. She denies polyuria, polydipsia, polyphagia, blurred vision, or vaginal infections.

She states that she has gained an enormous amount of weight since being placed on insulin 6 years ago. Her weight has continued to increase over the past 5 years, and she is presently at the highest weight she has ever been. She states that every time she tries to cut down on her eating she has symptoms of shakiness, diaphoresis, and increased hunger. She does not follow any specific diet and has been so fearful of hypoglycemia that she often eats extra snacks.

Her health care practitioners have repeatedly advised weight loss and exercise to improve her health status. She complains that the pain in her knees and ankles makes it difficult to do any exercise.

Her blood glucose values on capillary blood glucose testing have been 170–200 mg/d1 before breakfast. Before supper and bedtime values range from 150 mg/dl to >300 mg/dl. Her current insulin regimen is 45 U of NPH plus 10 U of regular insulin before breakfast and 35 U of NPH plus 20 U of regular insulin before supper. This dose was recently increased after her HbA1c, was found to be 8.9% (goal <7.0 %).

Past medical history is remarkable for hypertension, hypertriglyceridemia, and arthritis. Current medications include only insulin, lisinopril (Prinivil), and hydrochlorthiazide (Dyazide) with triamterene.

On physical exam, her height is 5′ 1 $\frac{1}{2}$″ and her weight is 265 lb. Her blood pressure is 160/88 mmHg. The remainder of the physical exam is unremarkable.

On laboratory testing, chemistries, BUN, creatinine, and liver function tests are normal. Thyroid function tests and urine microalbumin are also normal.

After an explanation that the increasing insulin doses were contributing to her weight gain and that she would need to decrease her insulin dose along with her food intake to prevent hypoglycemia, the patient agreed to follow a restricted-calorie diet and to decrease her insulin to 30 U of NPH and 10 U of regular insulin twice daily. As she had no contraindications to metformin (Glucophage), she was also started on 500 mg orally and it was increased to twice daily after one week.

She returned to the clinic 3 months later, still on the same dose of insulin. She continued to complain of fear of hypoglycemia in the middle of the night and was overeating at night. Despite this she had lost 7 lb. Her blood glucose values were still elevated in a range of 120–275 mg/dl before meals.

She was reassured that further insulin reduction would prevent hypoglycemia. Her insulin dosage was decreased to 25 U of NPH and 5 U of regular insulin twice daily and metformin was increased to 500 mg three times daily. Two months later, she returned to the clinic with an average blood glucose level of 160 mg/dl. Her weight was now 246 lb, and her HbA1c was 7.5%. She was feeling much more energetic and was able to start a walking program.

Questions

1. Are insulin sensitizers useful additions to insulin therapy?

TABLE 9.1 Direct and indirect effects of metformin therapy

Decreases hyperglycemia
Improves diastolic function
Decreases total cholesterol levels
Decreases very low density lipoprotein cholesterol levels
Decreases low-density lipoprotein cholesterol levels
Increases high-density lipoprotein cholesterol levels
Decreases oxidative stress
Improves vascular relaxation
Decreases plasminogen activator inhibitor-1 levels
Increases tissue plasminogen activator activity
Decreases von Willebrand factor levels
Decreases platelet aggregation and adhesion

target of metformin [1]. The mainstay of action of metformin can be attributed to its hepatic effects. Hepatic sensitivity to insulin is increased by metformin, thereby reducing gluconeogenesis (Figure 9.1) as well as glycogenolysis, which contribute to the postprandial plasma glucose lowering effects. Skeletal muscle and adipocytes undergo upregulation of the insulin-sensitive GLUT-4 and GLUT-1 transporters to the cell membranes, thereby increasing glucose uptake [2]. Glucose metabolism in the splanchnic bed also increases through insulin-dependent mechanisms. Additional metabolic effects include the suppression of fatty acid oxidation (Figure 9.2) as well as a reduction in triglyceride levels in patients with hypertriglyceridemia

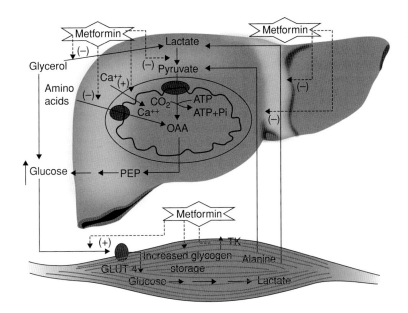

FIG 9.1 Mechanism of action of metformin on hepatic glucose production.

[1, 2]. Combined, the cellular effects of metformin counter insulin resistance and reduce the toxic metabolic effects of glucose toxicity and lipotoxicity in type 2 diabetes.

Pharmacokinetics

In normal subjects, studies demonstrate that metformin is excreted unchanged in the urine and does not undergo hepatic metabolism or biliary excretion. Because metformin is not metabolized, there is no interference with the metabolism of coadministered drugs. Renal clearance is approximately 3.5 times greater than creatinine clearance, which suggests that tubular secretion is the main route of metformin elimination. With an oral administration of metformin, patients with normal renal function have a plasma half-life of 2–5 hours, and almost 90% of an absorbed dose is eliminated within 12 hours [1].

Efficacy of combination therapy

Many people with type 2 diabetes are overweight and insulin resistant, making high doses of insulin often necessary to achieve adequate glucose control. However, insulin therapy is associated with weight gain, which could impede any progress in achieving glucose control that would normally be expected. In a double-blind, placebo-controlled study where patients were randomly assigned to receive placebo or metformin in combination with insulin for 24 weeks, the data showed that adding metformin to an intensified insulin regimen resulted in an 11% reduction in hemoglobin A1c compared to insulin therapy alone. The study also reported improved glucose control using 29% less insulin, and a less complicated insulin regimen with no increase in the occurrence of hypoglycemia or weight gain [4].

Further studies have verified these findings, like this randomized trial comparing insulin monotherapy to combined therapy with insulin and metformin, which showed clear benefit to using metformin with insulin compared to insulin alone. In this study, insulin as a monotherapy resulted in a reduction in HbA1c 8.7 ± 1.6 to 7.0 ± 1.0% with approximately 69% more insulin needed from baseline to achieve this effect. Patients in this arm of the study also required a more complicated insulin regimen in approximately 25% of the cases that became time consuming for both the patient and providers. These patients also gained 4.4 kg of weight. In the second arm of this study using insulin in combination with metformin resulted in a reduction in HbA1c of 8.8 ± 1.2 to 7.1± 1.0%, which was comparable to the monotherapy arm, however, these results were achieved without an increase in the total daily dose of insulin. In this arm, complexity of the insulin regimen was not affected, and there was virtually no weight gain or hypoglycemia reported. The only drawbacks were that two-thirds of patients

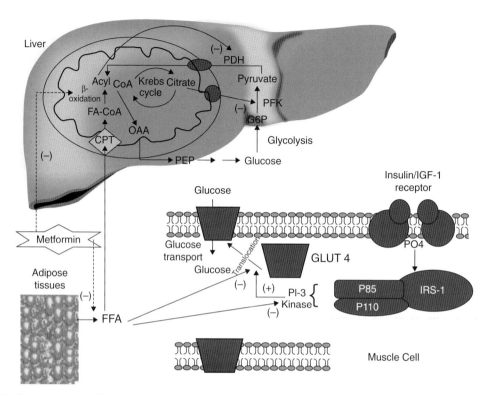

FIG 9.2 Metformin and fatty acids.

experienced gastrointestinal side effects, but they were mild and transient [5].

Because studies have shown that decreasing the required daily dose of exogenous insulin is associated with a decreased risk of cardiovascular disease, another placebo-controlled, randomized, double-blind trial was designed to look at effects on glucose control and insulin requirements when metformin was added in patients with type 2 diabetes intensively treated with insulin. After 16 weeks of combination therapy, the data showed that when metformin was compared with placebo use, there was a statistically significant improvement in glucose control shown by a hemoglobin A1c of 6.9 versus 7.6%. The data also showed that the use of metformin was associated with less weight gain (−1.6 kg compared with placebo) and with a small decrease in LDL cholesterol (− 0.19 mmol/l) [6].

Taken together, these data suggest that metformin can be an effective adjunct to insulin therapy. Studies have

shown that adding metformin to insulin therapy reduces hemoglobin A1c, total daily dose of insulin, and reduces or prevents the weight gain associated with intensive insulin treatment. However, metformin has gastrointestinal side effects that can hinder titration to its maximum effective dose, but these tend to be mild and transient.

Additional indications
Polycystic ovary syndrome. We now understand that the main feature of polycystic ovary syndrome (PCOS), as it relates to the use of insulin senitizers, is the decreased insulin sensitivity and compensatory hyperinsulinemia that is associated with the condition. Women suffering from PCOS have an increased risk of diabetes later in life, and an increased incidence of gestational diabetes if they conceive. The pathophysiology of the disorder is not fully understood, but the use of an insulin sensitizer appears to have a profound effect on many of the symptoms. In clinical studies,

women with PCOS being treated with insulin sensitizers like metformin saw a reduction in circulating insulin levels, a reduction in androgen levels, improvements in ovarian function, and improved lipid profiles and severity of hirsutism [7].

Contraindications

Metformin therapy is contraindicated in patients with liver failure, alcoholism, and active moderate to severe infection [1]; these conditions predispose to development of lactic acidosis, either by increased production or decreased metabolism of lactic acid [1]. Metformin is also contraindicated in people with kidney disorders (creatinine levels above 1.4 mg/dl in women and 1.5 mg/dl in men, depending on lean body mass [1], according to the package insert), and lung disease. Heart failure has long been considered a contraindication for metformin use, although a 2007 systematic review showed metformin to be the only antidiabetic drug *not* associated with harm in people with heart failure [8].

Current recommendations suggest that metformin should be temporarily discontinued before any radiographic study involving iodinated contrast, as contrast dye may temporarily impair kidney function, indirectly leading to lactic acidosis by causing retention of metformin in the body [9]. Once metformin is withheld, hydration should be maintained until preserved kidney function is documented at 24 and 48 hours after the intervention [1]. General anesthesia should be used cautiously to prevent hypotension, which leads to renal hypoperfusion and peripheral tissue hypoxia with subsequent lactate accumulation [1]. Metformin should also be used cautiously in the elderly, who's decreased lean body mass leads to reduced serum creatinine concentrations that often mask impaired glomerular filtration rates [1].

Adverse effects

Lactic acidosis. Lactic acidosis is a life-threatening complication of biguanide therapy that carries a mortality rate of 30–50% [1]. The estimated incidence of metformin-associated lactic acidosis is 0.03 cases per 1000 patient-years [1], which is 10 to 20 times lower than that seen with phenformin therapy [1], which was withdrawn because of an increased risk of lactic acidosis (up to 60 cases per million patient-years). Development of lactic acidosis is almost always related to coexistent hypoxic conditions that are probably responsible for the associated high mortality rate.

In one report, 91% of patients who developed lactic acidosis while being treated with metformin had a predisposing condition, such as congestive heart failure, renal insufficiency, chronic lung disease with hypoxia, or age older than 80 years [1]. Therefore, patients with impaired renal function or coexistent hypoxic conditions should not be given metformin. Excessive alcohol consumption may also potentiate the effect of metformin on lactate metabolism. A careful history of alcohol use is therefore important before starting metformin therapy [1].

Gastrointestinal. Side effects of metformin are mostly limited to digestive tract symptoms, such as diarrhea, flatulence, and abdominal discomfort [1, 10]. Approximately 5% of patients cannot tolerate treatment because of gastrointestinal side effects [1]. The mechanisms of these side effects remain unclear but probably are related to accumulation of high amounts of metformin in the intestinal tissue [2], with resultant elevation of local lactate production. These symptoms are dose dependent and can usually be avoided by slow titration and, in some cases, reduction of the dose [1]. Metformin therapy should be initiated with a single dose of medication (usually 500 mg) taken with the patient's largest meal to prevent gastrointestinal symptoms. These symptoms generally disappear within 2 weeks of treatment [11]. Medication doses should be increased in 500-mg increments given after meals every 1 to 2 weeks until a desirable blood glucose level or the maximal effective daily metformin dose of 2000 mg is reached [12].

Thiazolidinediones

The peroxisome-proliferator–activated receptors (PPARs) are a subfamily of super-receptors that regulate gene expression in response to ligand binding. [13] Three PPARs, identified as PPARα, PPARδ (also known as PPARβ), and PPARγ, have been discovered to date. PPARs regulate gene transcription by two mechanisms: transactivation, which is DNA-dependent and transrepression, which is DNA-independent and may explain the anti-inflammatory actions of PPARs [13].

PPARα is expressed mainly in the liver, heart, and muscle, as well as in the vascular wall [2]. Fibrates (i.e., fenofibrate) act as full or partial PPARα agonists. In general, the activation of PPARα enhances free fatty acid oxidation, controls how multiple genes regulate lipoprotein concentrations, and has anti-inflammatory effects (Table 9.2).

TABLE 9.2 Molecular targets of PPARγ and PPARα action

	Liver	Skeletal muscle	Adipose tissue	Vascular wall
PPARγ	• Decreased C-reactive protein	• Increased GLUT4 • Increased phosphatidyl 3-kinase • Decreased PDK-4	• Increased fatty acid transport protein-1 • Increased acyl–coenzyme A synthetase • Increased adiponectin • Increased LPL • Increased phosphatidyl 3-kinase • Increased GLUT4	• Decreased intercellular adhesion molecule-1 • Decreased vascular-cell adhesion molecule-1 • Decreased iNOS • Decreased interleukin-6
PPARα	• Decreased C-reactive protein • Decreased fibrinogen B			• Decreased vascular-cell adhesion molecule-1 • Decreased cyclooxygenase-2 • Decreased TNFα • Decreased interleukin-6 • Decreased tissue factor

Studies have shown that PPARα agonists can retard or even prevent atherosclerosis in both mice and humans [13].

PPARδ is expressed in several tissue types, with the most expression in the skin, brain, and adipose tissue. PPARγ is mainly found in adipose tissue but can also be found in pancreatic beta cells, vascular endothelium, and macrophages [13]. Its expression is low in tissues that express predominantly PPARα, such as the liver, the heart, and skeletal muscle. PPARγ was discovered as a target for thiazolidinediones only after testing many agents during multiple large clinical trials.

The first thiazolidinedione, troglitazone, was approved in 1997 for use in treating patients with type 2 diabetes in the United States. This glucose-lowering agent was subsequently withdrawn from the market, in March 2000, because of cases of hepatotoxicity. In 1999, two γ agonists, rosiglitazone and pioglitazone, were approved in the United States for use in treating hyperglycemia in type 2 diabetes. Currently, studies have linked rosiglitazone to increased risk of cardiovascular events, although this is certainly not clear cut [14].

Mechanism of action

The simulation of PPARγ is considered a major mechanism through which thiazolidinediones enhance insulin sensitiv-ity. As mentioned previously, PPARγ is mainly found in adipose tissue and less concentrated in skeletal muscle and liver. PPARγ is essential for normal adipocyte differentiation and proliferation as well as fatty acid uptake and storage [13]. Because PPARγ has such a profound effect on adipose tissue it has been postulated that thiazolidinediones achieve their insulin-sensitizing actions through direct means or indirectly, through altered adipokine release affecting insulin sensitivity beyond the adipose tissue itself. Basically, thiazolidinediones act directly by promoting fatty acid uptake and storage in adipose tissue (Figure 9.3). Through this process, there is an increase in adipose-tissue mass and other insulin-sensitive tissues, like skeletal muscle, the liver, and possibly pancreatic beta cells, are spared from the harmful effects of high concentrations of free fatty acids [13]. Therefore, thiazolidinediones keep fat in its proper place. Data from studies of PPARγ knockout mouse models supports the notion that thiazolidinediones act mainly on adipose tissue as long as normal amounts of adipose tissue exist [13].

Although thiazolidinediones keep fat in its proper place (in adipose tissue), there are still indirect processes that may be responsible for enhancing insulin sensitivity. Studies have shown that select thiazolidinediones (i.e., pioglitazone) regulate the expression of more than 100 genes

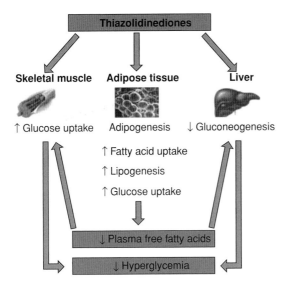

FIG 9.3 Effects of thiazolidinediones.

[8] and some of the established PPARγ target genes found in human adipose tissue are listed in Table 9.2. Several adipokines are regulated by PPARγ but we will focus mainly on adiponectin, an adiopocytokine produced exclusively by adipose tissue, because it has been shown to increase insulin sensitivity in rodents [13] Whether increases in adiponectin increases hepatic insulin sensitivity in humans is still not clear, only rodents have shown this effect of PPARγ on adiponectin levels.

Pharmacokinetics
The thiazolidinediones are absorbed completely and rapidly with peak concentrations achieved within 1–2 hours, but this may be slightly delayed when taken with food. Both rosiglitazone and pioglitazone are extensively metabolized by the liver. The metabolites of rosiglitazone are weakly active and are excreted mainly in the urine. Pioglitazone produces metabolites that are more active and are excreted mostly in the bile. Both thiazolidinediones are metabolized by the cytochrome P450 system and no clinically significant reduction in plasma concentrations of other drugs has been reported [15].

Efficacy of combination therapy
Studies have shown that thiazolidinediones used in combination with insulin therapy result in improved blood glucose control, reduced total daily insulin dose, and reduced

triglyceride levels. In a randomized, double-blind, placebo-controlled study of more than 300 insulin-treated type 2 diabetic patients, the addition of troglitazone at doses of 200mg and 600mg daily a reduction in HbA1c level of 0.8 and 1.4% resulted, while insulin dose was reduced by 11 and 29% respectively. On the other hand, subjects taking insulin and placebo experienced a decrease of 0.1% in HbAlc level and a 1% increase in insulin dose [16]. Subjects randomized to placebo therapy gained 1.5 kg, while those taking the study drug in 200mg and 600mg doses in combination with insulin gained 1.9 and 3.6 kg. Total cholesterol, LDL, and HDL cholesterol levels were found to be increased with troglitazone use at 600 mg/day. An open-label study showed that troglitazone had insulin-sparing effects that persisted up to 24 months [17]. In a randomized, double-blind, placebo-controlled study of more than 200 type 2 diabetic patients who were given troglitazone 400mg daily in combination with their baseline insulin dose, the results showed a significantly greater reduction in total daily dose of insulin and HbAlc level compared with those patients using insulin and placebo [18]. In this study, end points were defined as a 50% reduction in injected insulin or either a reduction in blood glucose by >15%, and only 7% of patients on insulin and placebo achieved these goals, while 22% of patients taking insulin and troglitazone 400 mg daily achieved these goals.

Studies using rosiglitazone or pioglitazone in combination with insulin therapy have yielded similar results. In a randomized control study of inadequately controlled insulin-treated type 2 diabetes patients, those receiving 26 weeks of treatment with rosiglitazone 4 and 8 mg experienced a reduction in HbAlc level of 0.6 and 1.2% respectively, as compared with virtually no change in the group taking insulin and placebo [19]. In this same study, insulin doses also decreased by 4.8 and 9.4% in the groups taking insulin plus study drug compared to a decrease of 0.6% in patients taking insulin and placebo. Total cholesterol, HDL, and LDL cholesterol levels were found to increase significantly on treatment with rosiglitazone. Unfortunately, significant weight gain occurred in the placebo, rosiglitazone 4mg, and rosiglitazone 8mg groups with corresponding values of 0.9 kg, 4.0 kg, and 5.3 kg. In a randomized, placebo-controlled study in patients receiving stable insulin therapy, when patients assigned to pioglitazone 15 or 30 mg daily in combination with their baseline doses of insulin for 16 weeks, HbAlc levels were reduced by 1.0 and 1.3% respectively, compared to a reduction of 0.3% in patients on insulin and placebo [13]. Those patients on insulin and pioglitazone gained 2.3 and 3.7 kg, compared with virtually no change in weight in those using insulin and placebo.

This data suggests that thiazolidinediones can be effective adjuncts to insulin therapy. However, with growing concerns about rosiglitazone and its association with increased myocardial infarction, CV-related deaths, and poor effect on lipid profile, pioglitazone appears to be the only remaining TZD to assist in achieving these desired effects of therapy [14]. A prospective, randomized trial of cardiovascular outcomes, called Prospective Pioglitazone Clinical Trial in Macrovascular Events (PROACTIVE) has looked at coronary and peripheral vascular events as a primary outcome and myocardial infarction, stroke, and death as secondary outcomes and the data support pioglitazone as having a favorable effect, especially on lipids, particularly triglycerides, more so than rosiglitazone [20]. In contrast to the previous study, the Rosiglitazone Evaluated for Cardiac Outcomes and Regulation of Glycemia in Diabetes (RECORD) trial, a long-term, multicenter, randomized, open-label study, found conflicting results when looking at cardiovascular outcomes in patients with type 2 diabetes treated with rosiglitazone plus metformin or sulfonylurea, as compared with the combination of metformin and sulfonylurea. The data showed that the rate of primary end points (hospitalization or death from cardiovascular causes) was low at 3.1% per year, while secondary end points like acute myocardial infarction, death from cardiovascular causes or any cause, or the composite of cardiovascular death, myocardial infarction, and stroke showed no statistically significant difference between the rosiglitazone group and the control group [21]. However, the fact remains that TZDs are still responsible for significant weight gain and increased peripheral edema.

Additional indications

Nonalcoholic fatty liver disease. Type 2 diabetes has a strong association with nonalcoholic fatty liver disease (NAFLD), which has a spectrum of liver damage that ranges from simple fatty liver (steatosis) to irreversible, advanced scarring of the liver (cirrhosis) [13]. There are an estimated 6.4 million adults in the United States diagnosed with NAFLD, which is the most common cause of elevated levels of liver enzymes [13]. Elevated levels of alanine amino-transferase (ALT) have been shown to predict type 2 diabetes independently of obesity [13]. Fatty liver disease is associated with decreased hepatic insulin sensitivity and correlates with

insulin requirements during insulin therapy in patients with type 2 diabetes [13].

Several recent studies have shown that thiazolidinediones actually reduce fat accumulation in the liver in patients with type 2 diabetes as well as in patients with lipodystrophy associated with the use of highly active antiretroviral therapy (HAART). Studies have also shown that liver enzymes actually decrease rather than increase during treatment with pioglitazone and rosiglitazone [13].

Polycystic ovary syndrome
The polycystic ovary syndrome is a disorder that affects approximately 4% of women of reproductive age [13]. Women with PCOS frequently develop insulin resistance and hence have an increased risk for type 2 diabetes [13]. Hyperinsulinemia, which accompanies insulin resistance, is thought to contribute to the hyperandrogenism that is seen in patients with PCOS [13]. Interventions with the role of reducing insulin levels, like weight loss and medications (i.e., metformin), can decrease hyperandrogenism and reduce insulin resistance [13]. A large-scale placebo-controlled trial of 410 women showed that the use of troglitazone showed significant improvements in ovulatory function, hirsutism, hyperandrogenism, and insulin resistance [13]. A more recent, small placebo-controlled study that randomized women to either rosiglitazone and placebo or to rosiglitazone and clomiphene has shown similar results. This study demonstrated that 56% of women previously resistant to clomiphene were able to ovulate [13]. Although metformin is considered safe for women who become pregnant, rosiglitazone and pioglitazone are classified as pregnancy category C, which indicates toxic effects in studies in animal models, but the results in human studies are inadequate. If these agents are used during pregnancy, then the potential benefit must justify the potential risk to the fetus. Polycystic ovary syndrome is currently not an approved indication for the use of TZDs.

Lipid lowering
Studies have shown that low-density lipoprotein (LDL) cholesterol levels have remained unchanged when monotherapy with pioglitazone or combination therapy with pioglitazone and sulfonylurea, metformin, or insulin has been used. However, some studies have shown increases in LDL cholesterol levels, between 8 to 16% higher with rosiglitazone use. Studies have also shown an approximate 10% increase in high-density lipoprotein (HDL)

cholesterol levels with the use of both drugs. The effects of TZDs on triglycerides have been more variable, with decreases in triglyceride levels having been observed more often with pioglitazone than with rosiglitazone [13]. In a direct comparison of rosiglitazone and pioglitazone, one study of 127 patients previously treated with troglitazone, supports the notion that both drugs have similar effects on glucose levels and body weight [13]. This same study supported the notion that pioglitazone is more effective than rosiglitazone at lowering LDL cholesterol and serum triglyceride levels. The difference in efficacy of these two drugs on lipids cannot be attributed to the effect they have on serum free fatty acid concentrations, which decreases by approximately 20 to 30% in both [13]. Pioglitazone appears to be a partial agonist of PPARα in vitro, and rosiglitazone appears to be a pure PPARγ agonist [13]. So far however, the data on mechanisms underlying the effects of the TZDs on lipids in humans is quite limited.

Lipodystrophies

The most common form of lipodystrophy is that associated with highly active antiretroviral therapy use in patients with human immunodeficiency virus (HIV) disease. After only 12 to 18 months of therapy with HAART, approximately half of patients develop a lipodystrophy-related symptom like facial lipoatrophy [13]. Facial lipoatrophy can be disfiguring and stigmatizing, especially since there is no pharmacologic therapy for this condition, which is usually accompanied by marked insulin resistance. Thiazolidinediones would seem to be a wonderful solution to insulin resistance and lipoatrophy caused by HAART because these drugs increase both insulin sensitivity and subcutaneous fat mass. Unfortunately, there has been only one placebo-controlled trial in which patients with HAART-associated lipodystrophy were treated with rosiglitazone 8 mg per day for six months, and there was no increase in adipose tissue or body weight, in contrast to studies in patients with type 2 diabetes [13].

Carotid intima-media thickness. Carotid IMT is a well-established surrogate marker for cardiovascular risk. A thickened carotid intima-media layer not only correlates with increased cardiovascular risk but also with the risk of future macrovascular events like myocardial infarction and stroke [22]. Several studies using multiple agents (i.e., ACE inhibitors, calcium channel blockers, β-blockers, and statins) have shown a reduction or even regression of carotid

IMT in patients without diabetes [22]. However, carotid IMT appears to be more significant in patients with type 2 diabetes reflecting a more dramatic cardiovascular risk in this patient population [22]. Limited data currently exists about the effect of intervention in type 2 diabetes on carotid IMT. However, a recent randomized control study of 192 patients showed that treatment with pioglitazone for 24 weeks led to a significant decrease in carotid IMT in patients with type 2 diabetes, and this was found to be independent of glucose control [22].

Contraindications

In patients with diabetes, hypertension and coronary artery disease occur frequently. These conditions are risk factors for the development of congestive heart failure (CHF) [23]. Diabetes can affect cardiac structure and systolic or diastolic function, independent of other established risk factors for CHF because of diabetic cardiomyopathy [23]. This phenomenon makes diabetes an independent risk factor for CHF, which was supported by an analysis of 9591 people with type 2 diabetes in the Kaiser Permanente Northwest Division that demonstrated that 11.8% of diabetic subjects had CHF at baseline, and an additional 7.7% developed CHF during a 30-month follow-up period [23]. This suggests that CHF may be present prior to physicians beginning therapy with TZDs or that this condition may develop during the course of treatment.

TZDs can still be used in patients with underlying asymptomatic heart disease, although its safety has not been fully established. The package inserts for both rosiglitazone and pioglitazone indicate that patients with more advanced heart disease (NYHA class III or IV) were excluded in premarketing clinical trials, and hence, these drugs are not recommended in such patients. Currently, there are no guidelines on the use of TZDs in patients with diabetes who have any degree of heart disease or for those already on a TZD who develop CHF. What makes this clinical dilemma more perplexing is the more common side effect of peripheral edema associated with TZDs, which makes the origin of the development of edema or weight gain more difficult to decipher.

Physicians should be cautious before prescribing TZDs to patients with diabetes who have been previously diagnosed with a condition that increases risk of bone fractures (i.e., osteoporosis, hyperparathyroidism, Paget's disease, etc.). Recent studies have shown a correlation between TZD use and an increased risk of bone fractures. In fact, according to data taken from the ADOPT study group and others, the relative risk of fractures with thiazolidinediones remained consistently elevated irrespective of age or menopausal status of women [24]. In addition, a recent meta-analysis showed that the long-term use of thiazolidinediones (rosiglitazone, pioglitazone or troglitazone) doubles the risk of fractures among women with type 2 diabetes, and the overall use of thiazolidinediones significantly increased the risk of fractures among patients with type 2 diabetes. Also identified in this meta-analysis was that thiazolidinedione use was also associated with significant changes in bone mineral density at the lumbar spine and the hip [24].

Adverse effects

A recent paper looked at multiple studies correlating weight gain and glycosylated hemoglobin with thiazolidinedione use and the paper showed that TZDs lead to an increase in body weight of 2 to 3 kg for every 1% decrease in glycosylated hemoglobin values. This increase in body weight was found to be the same irrespective of TZD use as a monotherapy or in combination with insulin or metformin in patients with type 2 diabetes. One of the mechanisms proposed to explain this phenomenon is that the increase in body weight is attributed to expansion of the subcutaneous fat depot, and in some patients to edema, whereas the mass of visceral fat remains unchanged or even decreases [13].

The use of TZDs is not only associated with weight gain, but some patients experience fluid retention and plasma volume expansion, which lead to the development of peripheral edema. The development of peripheral edema has been reported in 4 to 6% of patients undergoing treatment with TZDs as compared with 1 to 2% of those receiving placebo or other hypoglycemic therapies. Edema development appears to occur most when either of the TZDs is used in combination with insulin. Studies have shown that the use of rosiglitazone 4 or 8 mg per day in combination with insulin was associated with a 13.1% and 16.2% incidence of edema, respectively, compared with 4.7% in those taking insulin alone [19], and with pioglitazone used at 15 mg or 30 mg daily in combination with insulin resulted in a combined 15.3% incidence of edema, compared with 7.0% for insulin alone [23]. Edema appears to occur at a higher incidence when either of the TZDs is combined with insulin, as opposed to when TZDs are used in combination therapy with other oral hypoglycemic agents. This increase in body weight and edema has been associated with an increase in the incidence of congestive heart failure in patients treated with TZDs and insulin. As a result, the Food and Drug Administration added a warning in the drug packet information for those patients taking rosiglitazone and pioglitazone. The European Agency for the Evaluation of Medicinal Products actually considers insulin therapy a contraindication to the use of TZDs. According to the data this agency presents, the frequency of CHF was 2.5 times greater in combination therapy of insulin and thiazolidinediones than with insulin alone. However, the cause for this result remains unclear.

In a meta-analysis of 42 trials containing more than 27,000 patients, over 15,000 of them on treatment with rosiglitazone, the data showed an overall odds ratio of 1.43 for myocardial infarction (MI) and 1.64 for death from cardiovascular cause. From this meta-analysis, compared with placebo or with other hypoglycemic agents, treatment with rosiglitazone was associated with a significant increase in the risk of MI and with an increase in the risk of death from cardiovascular causes that was of borderline significance [14].

A recent study suggests an elevated risk of fracture associated with TZDs compared with other oral hypoglycemic agents. The risk of fracture with TZD use was present at multiple anatomic sites and these results were potentially clinically significant [25]. This suggests that caution should be taken when considering treatment of type 2 diabetic patients with TZDs who have an increased risk for fractures.

Discussion

So the question remains, "Are insulin sensitizers useful additions to insulin therapy?" Currently, the data suggest that metformin is a feasible option in all patients with type 2 diabetes and should be initiated at the onset of insulin therapy unless a specific contraindication to metformin use exists. The benefits of metformin therapy in these patients is an improvement in hemoglobin A1c, a reduction in total daily dose of insulin, and most importantly, a reduction in weight gain despite intensive insulin regimens [4–6]. The only potential disadvantage to metformin therapy is its side effect profile. This medication is contraindicated in patients with impaired renal function due to risk of lactic acidosis, but renal impairment can be a common condition in those with a prolonged diabetes course [1, 9]. The other disadvantage to metformin therapy relates to its gastrointestinal side effects which may impede titration to its maximal effective dose. However, these side effects are often mild and transient, and usually can be avoided by slow titration, and in some cases, reduction of the dose [1]. Therefore, metformin appears to be an appropriate choice when considering adding an inexpensive insulin sensitizer with few side effects to all patients with type 2 diabetes currently on insulin therapy or planning its initiation.

Similarly, studies have shown that thiazolidinediones used in combination with insulin therapy result in improved blood glucose control, reduced total daily insulin dose, and reduced triglyceride levels [16–19]. However, the side effects of these agents can prove to significantly reduce any benefit that may have been gained from their use. In studies, rosiglitazone has been associated with a significant increase in the risk of MI and with an increase in the risk of death from cardiovascular causes [14]. Rosiglitazone has also been found to significantly increase total cholesterol, HDL, and LDL cholesterol levels [13]. This data suggests that extreme caution should be used when treating patients with this medication, and likely even avoided. In addition, recent studies have suggested that TZDs have an elevated risk of bone fracture at multiple anatomic sites compared with other oral hypoglycemic agents [25]. Studies of pioglitazone have shown more favorable outcomes than rosiglitazone with less risk of myocardial infarction and other cardiovascular-related deaths, as well as a better lipid profile response, especially with triglycerides [14, 20]. However, a better track record still does not excuse the fact that each of these medications still causes significant weight gain and peripheral edema [13, 19]. With increased weight comes decreased insulin sensitivity, a hindrance to any benefit that this drug may afford the patient, and peripheral edema has its own disadvantages to maintaining medication compliance.

With dual therapy including insulin plus metformin or insulin plus thiazolidinediones, significant reductions have been shown in hemoglobin A1c, total daily dose of insulin, and weight gain. These results would suggest that triple therapy including insulin plus metformin and TZDs would produce an even more profound effect, and select studies have considered these combinations. For example, in this randomized study of 28 type 2 patients with diabetes using insulin monotherapy, 4 months of triple therapy was initiated by adding metformin to insulin, then troglitazone (TGZ) versus adding TGZ to insulin, then metformin. Researchers found that hemoglobin A1c decreased with dual therapy but improved more during triple therapy (insulin + metformin 7.0%, insulin + TGZ 6.2%; insulin + metformin, adding TGZ 6.1%, insulin + TGZ, adding metformin 5.8%). Total daily dose of insulin was significantly reduced in the insulin + TGZ group (–14.1 units), insulin + TGZ, adding metformin (–13.7 units), and the insulin + metformin, adding TGZ (–17.3 units), but not in the insulin + metformin group (–3.2 units). However, patients in the insulin + TGZ group experienced significant weight gain (4.4 kg), and those in the insulin + metformin, insulin + metformin, adding TGZ, and insulin + TGZ; adding metformin saw no weight gain. Thus, the order in which metformin and TZDs are added to the treatment regimen is important, especially as it relates to weight gain. Adding a TZD to a patient who is already on metformin seems to protect the patient from TZD-induced weight gain [26].

Ultimately, metformin is an excellent choice for all individuals with type 2 diabetes seeking to reach glucose and weight targets, and in fact, should always be used in combination with insulin unless there is some specific contraindication to its use. Thiazolidinediones, however, appear to be more problematic.

References

1. Krentz AJ, Bailey CJ. Oral antidiabetic agents current role in type 2 diabetes mellitus. *Drugs.* **65**, 2005.
2. Klip A, Leiter LA. Cellular mechanism of action of metformin. *Diabetes Care.* **13**(6):696–704, 1990.
3. Kirpichnikov D, McFarlane SI, Sowers JR. Metformin: an update. *Ann Intern Med.* **137**:25–33, 2002.
4. Aviles-Santa ML, Sinding J, Raskin P. Effects of metformin in patients with poorly controlled, insulin-treated type 2 diabetes mellitus. *Ann Intern Med.* 131:182–188, 1999.
5. Strowig SM, Aviles-Santa ML, Raskin P. Comparison of insulin monotherapy and combination therapy with insulin and metformin or insulin and troglitazone in type 2 diabetes. *Diabetes Care.* 25:1691–1698, 2002.
6. Strowig SM, Raskin P. Combination therapy using metformin or thiazolidinediones and insulin in the treatment of diabetes mellitus. *Diabetes Obes Metabol.* 7:633–641, 2005.
7. Muth S, Norman J, Sattar N, Fleming R. Women with polycystic ovary syndrome (PCOS) often undergo protracted treatment with metformin and are disinclined to stop: indications for a change in licensing arrangements? *Hum Reprod.* **19**:2718–2720, 2004.
8. Eurich DT, McAlister FA, Blackburn DF, et al. Benefits and harms of antidiabetic agents in patients with

diabetes and heart failure: systematic review. *BMJ.* **335**:497, 2007.

9. Weir J. Guidelines with regard to metformin-induced lactic acidosis and X-ray contrast medium agents. *R Coll Radiol.* **54**:29–33, 1999.

10. Garber AJ, Duncan TG, Goodman AM, Mills DJ, Rohlf JL. Efficacy of metformin in type II diabetes: results of a double-blind, placebo-controlled, dose response trial. *Am J Med.* 103:491–497, 1997.

11. Haupt E, Knick B, Koschinsky T, Liebermeister H, Schneider J, Hirche H. Oral antidiabetic combination therapy with sulphonylureas and metformin. *Diabetes Metab.* **17**:224–231, 1991.

12. DeFronzo RA, Goodman AM. Efficacy of metformin in patients with noninsulin-dependent diabetes mellitus. The Multicenter Metformin Study Group. *NEJM.* **333**:541–549, 1995.

13. Yki-Jarvinen H. Thiazolidinediones. *NEJM.* **351**:1106–1118, 2004.

14. Nissen SE, Nissen SE, Wolski K. Effect of rosiglitazone on the risk of myocardial infarction and death from cardiovascular causes. *NEJM.* **356**:2457–2471, 2007.

15. Baldwin SJ, Clarke SE, Chenery RJ. Characterisation of the cytochrome P450 enzymes involved in the in vitro metabolism of rosiglitazone. *Br J Clin Pharmacol.* **48**:424–432, 1999.

16. Schwartz S, Raskin P, Fonseca V, Graveline JF. Effect of troglitazone in insulin-treated patients with type II diabetes mellitus. *NEJM.* **338**:861–866, 1998.

17. Fonseca V, Foyt HL, Shen K, Whitcomb R. Long-term effects of troglitazone: open-label extension studies in type 2 diabetic patients. *Diabetes Care.* **23**:354–359, 2000.

18. Buse JB, Gumbiner B, Mathias NP, Nelson DM, Faja BW, Whitcomb RW. Troglitazone use in insulin-treated type 2 diabetic patients. The Troglitazone Insulin Study Group. *Diabetes Care.* **21**:1455–1461, 1998.

19. Raskin P, Rendell M, Riddle MC, Dole JF, Freed MI, Rosenstock J. A randomized trial of rosiglitazone therapy in patients with inadequately controlled insulin-treated type 2 diabetes. *Diabetes Care.* **24**:1226–1232, 2001.

20. Dormandy JA, Charbonnel B, Eckland DJ, et al. Secondary prevention of macrovascular events in patients with type 2 diabetes in the PROactive Study (PROspective pioglitAzone Clinical Trial In macroVascular Events): a randomized controlled trial. *Lancet.* **366**:1279–1289, 2005.

21. Home PD, Pocock SJ, Beck-Nielson H, et al. Rosiglitazone evaluated for cardiovascular outcomes – an interim analysis. *NEJM.* **357**:28–38, 2007.

22. Langenfeld MR, Forst T, Hohberg C, et al. Pioglitazone decreases carotid intima-media thickness independently of glycemic control in patients with type 2 diabetes mellitus: results from a controlled randomized study. *Circulation.* **111**:2525–2531, 2005.

23. Nesto RW, Bell D, Bonow RO, et al. Thiazolidinedione use, fluid retention, and congestive heart failure. *Diabetes Care.* **27**(1):256–263, 2004.

24. Loke YK, Singh S, Furberg CD. Long-term use of thiazolidinediones and fractures in type 2 diabetes: a meta-analysis. *CMAJ.* **180**:32–39, 2009.

25. Solomon DH, Cadarette SM, Choudhry NK, Canning C, Levin R, Sturmer T. A cohort study of thiazolidinediones and fractures in older adults with diabetes. *JCEM.* **94**:2792–2798, 2009.

26. Strowig SM, Aviles-Santa ML, Raskin P. Improved glycemic control without weight gain using triple therapy in type 2 diabetes. *Diabetes Care.* **27**:1577–1583, 2004.

Matheni Sathananthan[1] and Adrian Vella[2]

[1] Endocrinology Fellow, Division of Endocrinology, Diabetes, Nutrition and Metabolism, Mayo Clinic, Rochester, MN, USA

[2] Associate Professor of Medicine, Department of Endocrinology, Mayo Clinic, Rochester, MN, USA

LEARNING POINTS

- Glucagon-like peptide-1 (GLP-1) receptor agonists such as exenatide and liraglutide are powerful insulin secretagogues that also enhance satiety, delay gastric emptying, and produce some weight loss.

- Dipeptidyl peptidase-4 (DPP-4) inhibitors raise concentrations of endogenous GLP-1 but do not affect gastrointestinal function. They are less powerful insulin secretagogues than GLP-1 receptor agonists.

- Few studies have examined the use of incretin-based therapy in combination with insulin.

- A challenge to future clinical use of these combinations is the identification of patients who will benefit from these secretagogues, despite requiring insulin therapy.

Diabetes is a complex metabolic disorder characterized by chronic hyperglycemia arising because of a relative or absolute deficiency of insulin. Established type 2 diabetes is characterized by defective and delayed insulin secretion as well as abnormal postprandial suppression of glucagon. These two defects contribute to the defective suppression of endogenous glucose production after meal ingestion, leading to postprandial hyperglycemia. Additional contributors to postprandial hyperglycemia include an impaired ability of glucose and insulin to suppress endogenous glucose production and to stimulate glucose uptake.

The islets of people with long-standing type 2 diabetes have a characteristic appearance with prominent amyloid deposition and a decrease in functional β-cells [1]. These anatomical defects explain the decrease in insulin secretion, although defects in insulin secretion arise early in the pathogenesis of diabetes and likely precede any visible anatomic changes. Furthermore, common genetic variation that affects β-cell function and therefore insulin secretion in quantifiable ways increases the risk of progression from glucose intolerance to type 2 diabetes [2].

The defects in insulin action also arise early in the course of disease development and contribute to its pathogenesis [3]. Moreover, with progressive worsening of glucose tolerance, the impairment in insulin secretion worsens in concert with worsening defects in insulin action. Although a multitude of mechanisms have been invoked in the pathogenesis of impaired insulin action in prediabetes, a unifying mechanism remains elusive.

Lifestyle and dietary changes underpin the treatment of type 2 diabetes. Initiation of pharmacologic treatment is usually sequential; metformin is often first-line pharmacotherapy with a sulfonylurea added if glycemic goals are not achieved or maintained. The reasons for adopting such therapies include their relative safety, known efficacy and the fact that they are inexpensive. What has become less clear is what medications to use as third-line therapy when combination therapy with metformin and sulfonylureas is failing.

Thiazolidinediones, such as rosiglitazone and pioglitazone, are selective ligands of the peroxisome-proliferator-activated receptor gamma [4]. Thiazolidinediones improve insulin action in adipose tissue, skeletal muscle, and also the liver [5]. A major side effect of this class of drug is weight gain, due to fluid retention as well as increased adipose tissue mass [5]. In addition, thiazolidinediones are contraindicated in those with New York Heart

Association class III or IV heart failure. There has been considerable controversy regarding an increased risk of coronary events associated with rosiglitazone use—perhaps arising from its unfavorable effects on cholesterol concentrations. Moreover, there is an increased risk of fractures associated with thiazolidinedione use [6].

Incretin-based therapy is another potential adjunct to established therapies. Incretin hormones such as glucagon-like peptide-1 (GLP-1) and glucose-dependent insulinotropic polypeptide (GIP) are secreted by the enteroendocrine cells in response to meal ingestion and stimulate postprandial insulin secretion [7]. GLP-1 suppresses glucagon secretion and stimulates insulin secretion even after sulfonylureas are no longer effective [8]. Moreover, it decreases food intake and delays gastric emptying. However, it is rapidly inactivated in the circulation by an enzyme with wide distribution—dipeptidyl peptidase-4 (DPP-4)—so that its half-life is measured in minutes. Because of this, the hormone would need to be infused continuously for GLP-1 to be an effective therapy. Alternative approaches have focused on inhibition of DPP-4 to decrease clearance of endogenous GLP-1 or to develop GLP-1 receptor agonists that are resistant to degradation by DPP-4.

Exenatide was the first GLP-1 receptor agonist to be approved by the U.S. Food and Drug Administration (FDA) [9]. Exenatide is administered subcutaneously twice daily in doses of 5 or 10 µg [10]. Recently, Liraglutide, a once-daily GLP-1 receptor agonist has also been approved. There are several other GLP-1 receptor agonists currently under development including Albiglutide and Taspoglutide [10]. GLP-1 receptor agonists stimulate insulin secretion and inhibit glucagon secretion [11]. These actions are glucose-dependent, therefore minimizing the risk of hypoglycemia unless used in conjunction with a sulfonylurea [11]. Since their use is associated with a significant incidence of gastrointestinal side effects including nausea, many patients treated with these medications experience weight loss—at least in the short term [11].

In contrast, DPP-4 inhibitors, such as sitagliptin and saxagliptin, raise concentrations of endogenous GLP-1. Their effects on HbA1c lowering are less pronounced than that observed with GLP-1 receptor agonists. Moreover, their use does not cause weight loss. Whether this is due to the absence of gastrointestinal side effects or any discernible effect on gastric emptying and accommodation is unknown.

Another important adjunct to the treatment of patients who are failing first- and second-line therapy is insulin. Use of this intervention requires appropriate education and lifestyle intervention if hypoglycemia and/or weight gain are to be avoided. In such situations it is often used in conjunction with metformin. Usually, simple regimens of "basal" insulin are utilized first. However, there are certain circumstances where more elaborate "basal-bolus" regimens are utilized. These significantly increase the patient's participation in his or her care with more frequent monitoring, and daily adjustment/ supplementation. Utilizing insulin in combination with incretin-based therapy raises the possibility that simpler regimens can avoid meal-dosed insulin therapy and perhaps mitigate the weight gain associated with the initiation of insulin treatment.

A "basal" insulin regimen is often used in the treatment of people with type 2 diabetes. This often involves twice-daily injection of NPH insulin or the use of a single dose of long-acting insulin analogue. Insulin dosing is subsequently adjusted to ensure that appropriate control of fasting glucose concentrations is achieved. However, such regimens are limited by their ability to adequately control postprandial hyperglycemia and are unlikely to be effective in situations where dietary intake is unrestricted and / or β-cell function is severely impaired [12]. In patients failing metformin and sulfonylurea combination therapy, a GLP-1 receptor agonist appears to be an attractive alternative given the effects on postprandial glycemic control as well as weight. In a 26-week study where patients failing oral therapy were randomized to exenatide 10 µg twice daily or once-daily insulin glargine titrated to maintain fasting blood glucose levels less than 100, both therapies reduced HbA1c by 1.11%. Patients receiving exenatide experienced greater reduction in postprandial glucose excursions, and in weight, compared to the glargine-treated group who experienced a greater reduction in fasting glucose concentrations [12]. Nevertheless, there was a significant incidence of gastrointestinal side effects in the exenatide-treated group.

DPP-4 inhibitors exhibit synergistic actions with metformin and are effective in combination. They can reduce fasting and postprandial glucose concentrations with no significant increase in adverse effects (such as hypoglycemia). In a study of patients on metformin who were randomly assigned to receive sitagliptin 100 mg daily or placebo, results showed that sitagliptin treatment resulted in a reduction in hemoglobin A1c by 0.65% compared to placebo [13]. The utility of combination therapy with DPP-4 inhibitors and sulfonylureas is less clear with conflicting data as to the magnitude of HbA1c lowering when compared to the placebo arm. There is also uncertainty as to whether the combination is associated with increased risk of hypoglycemia and weight gain [14].

Although GLP-1 infusion has been shown to produce an insulin secretory response in patients who have experienced secondary failure of conventional oral therapy, it is possible that glycemic benefit observed in some patients arises more from the effects on gastric emptying and glucagon secretion than effects on insulin secretion. In these circumstances where β-cell function is significantly impaired, little additional benefit can be expected from therapy with a DPP-4 inhibitor since there is no significant effect on delaying gastric emptying or on weight. Although GLP-1 receptor agonists and DPP-4 inhibitors improve β-cell function, after cessation of treatments β-cell function returns to pretreatment levels [15].

Pramlintide is a synthetic analog of the peptide hormone amylin [16]. Amylin is co-secreted with insulin from pancreatic β-cells [17]. Type 2 diabetics have a relative deficiency in amylin while type I diabetics have essentially none [16]. Pramlintide is currently indicated as adjunctive therapy in the treatment of type 1 and type 2 diabetes [17]. It enhances satiety and reduces postprandial glucose fluctuations [17]. A study was done to assess the effect of mealtime pramlintide on weight control and long-term glycemic control in type 1 diabetics [18]. Patients were randomized to receive either placebo or pramlintide four times daily in addition to existing insulin regimens. Patients treated with pramlintide had a mean reduction in hemoglobin A1c of 0.67% compared to placebo (0.16% reduction) after 13 weeks of treatment. There was also a significant placebo-corrected treatment difference in hemoglobin A1c that was sustained through week 52 [18]. Both pramlintide and rapid-acting insulin analogs decrease postprandial hyperglycemia, but the side-effect profile is different for both [19]. Pramlintide may be associated with nausea and weight loss whereas rapid-acting insulin analogs have the added expense of risk of hypoglycemia and weight gain [19]. A 24-week open-label multicenter study was conducted in which patients were randomly assigned to either mealtime pramlintide or a titrated rapid-acting insulin analog, with basal insulin and prior oral antihyperglycemic medications [19]. The primary end point was the proportion of patients achieving a hemoglobin A1c of less than or equal to 7.0%

without weight gain or severe hypoglycemia [19]. This was achieved more in the pramlintide-treated group [19]. Neither group experienced severe hypoglycemia, which was defined as an event requiring administration of glucagon or IV glucose, or requiring the assistance of another person [19].

There are a limited number of studies evaluating combination therapy with insulin and GLP-1 receptor agonists. In one instance, the electronic medical records of three private practice endocrinologists who prescribed insulin and exenatide in patients with type 2 diabetes were reviewed [20]. Exenatide use resulted in a reduction of hemoglobin A1c despite a reduction or discontinuation of premeal insulin use [20]. However, in this study 36% of patients discontinued exenatide due to adverse side effects, namely gastrointestinal intolerance. In addition, 10% of patients experienced hypoglycemia [20]. A retrospective review of patients with diabetes mellitus type 2 treated in the outpatient setting revealed reductions in weight, hemoglobin A1c and prandial insulin requirements in patients who received exenatide in addition to insulin-based therapy [21]. In a retrospective analysis of obese type 2 diabetics treated with exenatide 5 mcg/day and insulin therapy, it was found that insulin requirements were decreased in those who were on split-mixed insulin as well as those on short-acting insulin [22]. The dosages of those on glargine or NPH insulin did not change significantly. Those treated with exenatide and insulin therapy experienced a reduction in hemoglobin A1c levels, triglycerides, and systolic blood pressure with the combination therapy [22].

Similarly, there are few studies assessing the use of DPP-4 inhibitors in combination with insulin therapy. A study in people with type 2 diabetes evaluating the efficacy of the addition of sitagliptin to insulin therapy alone, or in combination with metformin, showed a statistically significant reduction in hemoglobin A1c with the addition of sitagliptin to both treatment groups. However, there was an increased incidence of hypoglycemia in those treated with sitagliptin compared to placebo [23].

The treatment of diabetes is complex and with the availability of various treatment options, health care providers are faced with the difficult task of treating patients effectively, while minimizing side effects that could not only cause harm, but also prevent compliance with the therapy being prescribed. The place of incretin-based therapy in the conventional treatment algorithm is still the subject of considerable debate. Metformin is often considered to be first-line therapy for people with type 2 diabetes, however, DPP-4 inhibitors are often considered to be suitable adjuncts to metformin monotherapy. Their role in combination with a sulfonylurea is less certain.

On the other hand, GLP-1 receptor agonists are often considered as second or third-line agents, in part because parenteral administration is a significant inconvenience to most patients. Better identification of patients who might benefit from early therapy with such agents is needed. The data supporting combination therapy with insulin is sparse and, at the present time, in the absence of significant obesity/overeating and the presence of maintained insulin secretory capacity, unlikely to be of significant benefit in most patients on insulin. However, this is a rapidly evolving field and improved recognition of patients likely to benefit from such combination therapy may result in increased use in selected patients.

References

1. Hayden MR, Sowers JR. Isletopathy in type 2 diabetes mellitus: implications of islet RAS, islet fibrosis, islet amyloid, remodeling, and oxidative stress. *Antioxid Redox Signal.* **9**(7):891–910, 2007.
2. Florez JC, Jablonski KA, Bayley N, et al. TCF7L2 polymorphisms and progression to diabetes in the Diabetes Prevention Program. *N Engl J Med.* **355**(3):241–250, 2006.
3. Bock G, Dalla Man C, Campioni M, et al. Pathogenesis of pre-diabetes: mechanisms of fasting and postprandial hyperglycemia in people with impaired fasting glucose and/or impaired glucose tolerance. *Diabetes.* **55**(12):3536–3549, 2006.
4. Solomon DH, Cadarette SM, Choudhry NK, Canning C, Levin R, Sturmer T. A cohort study of thiazolidinediones and fractures in older adults with diabetes. *J Clin Endocrinol Metab.* **94**(8):2792–2798, 2009.
5. Rodbard HW, Jellinger PS, Davidson JA, et al. Statement by an American Association of Clinical Endocrinologists/American College of Endocrinology consensus panel on type 2 diabetes mellitus: an algorithm for glycemic control. *Endocr Pract.* **15**(6):540–559, 2009.
6. Dormuth CR, Carney G, Carleton B, Bassett K, Wright JM. Thiazolidinediones and fractures in men and women. *Arch Intern Med.* **169**(15):1395–1402, 2009.
7. Krentz AJ, Patel MB, Bailey CJ. New drugs for type 2 diabetes mellitus: what is their place in therapy? *Drugs.* **68**(15):2131–2162, 2008.
8. Drucker DJ, Nauck MA. The incretin system: glucagon-like peptide-1 receptor agonists and dipeptidyl peptidase-4 inhibitors in type 2 diabetes. *Lancet.* **368**(9548):1696–1705, 2006.
9. Amori RE, Lau J, Pittas AG. Efficacy and safety of incretin therapy in type 2 diabetes: systematic review and meta-analysis. *JAMA.* **298**(2):194–206, 2007.
10. Davidson JA. Advances in therapy for type 2 diabetes: GLP-1 receptor agonists and DPP-4 inhibitors. *Cleve Clin J Med.* **76**(Suppl 5):S28–S38, 2009.
11. Drucker DJ, Sherman SI, Gorelick FS, Bergenstal RM, Sherwin RS, Buse JB. Incretin-based therapies for the treatment of type 2 diabetes: evaluation of the risks and benefits. *Diabetes Care.* **33**(2):428–433, 2010.
12. Heine RJ, Van Gaal LF, Johns D, Mihm MJ, Widel MH, Brodows RG. Exenatide versus insulin glargine in patients with suboptimally controlled type 2 diabetes: a randomized trial. *Ann Intern Med.* **143**(8):559–569, 2005.
13. Charbonnel B, Karasik A, Liu J, Wu M, Meininger G. Efficacy and safety of the dipeptidyl peptidase-4 inhibitor sitagliptin added to ongoing metformin therapy in patients with type 2 diabetes inadequately controlled with metformin alone. *Diabetes Care.* **29**(12):2638–2643, 2006.
14. Garber AJ, Foley JE, Banerji MA, et al. Effects of vildagliptin on glucose control in patients with type 2 diabetes inadequately controlled with a sulphonylurea. *Diabetes Obes Metab.* **10**(11):1047–1056, 2008.
15. Bunck MC, Diamant M, Corner A, et al. One-year treatment with exenatide improves beta-cell function, compared with insulin glargine, in metformin-treated type 2 diabetic patients: a randomized, controlled trial. *Diabetes Care.* **32**(5):762–768, 2009.
16. Edelman S, Maier H, Wilhelm K. Pramlintide in the treatment of diabetes mellitus. *BioDrugs.* **22**(6):375–386, 2008.
17. Marrero DG, Crean J, Zhang B, et al. Effect of adjunctive pramlintide treatment on treatment satisfaction in patients with type 1 diabetes. *Diabetes Care.* **30**(2):210–216, 2007.
18. Whitehouse F, Kruger DF, Fineman M, et al. A randomized study and open-label extension evaluating the long-term efficacy of pramlintide as an adjunct to insulin therapy in type 1 diabetes. *Diabetes Care.* **25**(4):724–730, 2002.
19. Riddle M, Pencek R, Charenkavanich S, Lutz K, Wilhelm K, Porter L. Randomized comparison of pramlintide or mealtime insulin added to basal insulin treatment for patients with type 2 diabetes. *Diabetes Care.* **32**(9):1577–1582, 2009.
20. Sheffield CA, Kane MP, Busch RS, Bakst G, Abelseth JM, Hamilton RA. Safety and efficacy of exenatide in combination with insulin in patients with type 2 diabetes mellitus. *Endocr Pract.* **14**(3):285–292, 2008.
21. Yoon NM, Cavaghan MK, Brunelle RL, Roach P. Exenatide added to insulin therapy: a retrospective review of clinical practice over two years in an academic endocrinology outpatient setting. *Clin Ther.* **31**(7):1511–1523, 2009.

22. Viswanathan P, Chaudhuri A, Bhatia R, Al-Atrash F, Mohanty P, Dandona P. Exenatide therapy in obese patients with type 2 diabetes mellitus treated with insulin. *Endocr Pract.* **13**(5):444–450, 2007.

23. Vilsboll T, Rosenstock J, Yki-Jarvinen H, et al. Efficacy and safety of sitagliptin when added to insulin therapy in patients with type 2 diabetes. *Diabetes Obes Metab.* **12**(2):167–177, 2010.

11 HbA1c: Is it the most important therapeutic target in outpatient management of diabetes?

Steven A. Smith

Associate Professor of Medicine, Medical Director, Mayo Patient Education, Consultant in Endocrinology, Diabetes, Nutrition and Metabolism, Health Care Policy & Research, Mayo Clinic, Rochester, MN, USA

LEARNING POINTS

- HbA1c is the best clinical measure of glycemic exposure.
- HbA1c is only one of the several measures of glycemic control and does not accurately assess glycemic variation or hypoglycemia.
- HbA1c maybe valuable in predicting vacular complications and risk, independent of its association with measures of blood glucose and other measures of glycemic control.
- Similar to other laboratory tests, it is important to realize that there are limitations in the interpretation of HbA1c values.
- There are plausible biological and physiological explanations as well as evidence from observation/epidemiological studies, controlled trials, and meta-analysis that support the hypothesis that treatment of hyperglycemia will reduce microvascular complications of diabetes.
- There is an uncertain treatment effect for reducing macrovascular events.

In 1962, Huisman and Dozy reported a fast-moving electrophoretic band on hemoglobin electrophoresis in four patients taking tolbutamide for diabetes and attributed this to the medication's reaction with hemoglobin [1]. Six years later; Samuel Rahbar clarified the more specific association of this observation with diabetes, observing a two- to threefold increase in the red cells of diabetic patients [1]. Structurally, glycosylated hemoglobins are closely related to adult hemoglobin and are irreversibly formed from the nonenzymatic condensation of glucose or other reducing sugars with hemoglobin A. Cellulose acetate electrophoresis, high performance liquid, boronate affinity chromatography, as well as immunoassays have used charge and/or structure to separate the glycated forms of hemoglobin [2]. Because the concentration of glycated hemoglobin is determined by blood glucose, the life span of the red blood cell (RBC), and membrane permeability of glucose (or glycation gap), it has become the standard for assessing integrated glucose exposure and glycemic control.

For over 70 years, the relationship between the level of hyperglycemia and the development of long-term vascular complications has remained a primary hypothesis (Glucose Hypothesis) in the management of the complex metabolic disorders in diabetes. For this reason, clinical measures to assess an individual's degree of glucose exposure (fasting glucose, urinary glucose, glucose challenge tests, and glycosylated protein assays) and risk of diabetes complications have been the holy grail in the clinical management of people with diabetes.

As a clinical standard, the measure of glycosylated hemoglobin has served as the primary outcome for the Glucose Hypothesis and has been used to predict the impact of long-term glycemic control and risks for diabetes. Is it the most important therapeutic target in the management of diabetes? To address this question, we ask, is HbA1c the best measure of an individual's glycemic exposure, glucose control, and risk? Secondly, we examine the evidence for the importance of glucose control in managing the risks of diabetes.

Clinical Dilemmas in Diabetes, First Edition. Edited by Adrian Vella and Robert A. Rizza
© 2011 Blackwell Publishing Ltd. Published 2011 by Blackwell Publishing Ltd.

Is HbA1c the best measure for glycemic exposure, glucose control, and risk?

Prior to 1975, patients with both type 1 and type 2 diabetes monitored urine glucose and ketones to adjust medication to minimize glycosuria and symptoms. This was accompanied by the occasional blood glucose determination during visits with their physicians. Treating day-to-day symptoms required levels of glucose below renal threshold and was easily determined by the monitoring of urine sugars. Managing patients to lower target levels of glucose, as opposed to symptom relief, was made possible with the advent of home glucose monitoring (HBGM). This technology evolved rapidly as a standard of care such that by the time of the Diabetes Control and Complication trial (DCCT) [3], patients in the usual control group initially restricted to urine testing were allowed to monitor their own blood glucose levels.

HbA1c standardization

The DCCT, the United Kingdom Prospective Diabetes Study (UKPDS), and the Kumamoto Study were the first to provide evidence for the relationship between the control of glucose, HbA1c, and risk for diabetes complications [3–5]. From the DCCT trial it was recognized that there was a direct relationship between HbA1c and mean blood glucose over the preceding 8–12 weeks. Based largely on these findings, the National Glycohemoglobin Standardization Program (NGSP) in 1993 established a program for certification of clinical laboratories providing physicians and patients with measures of HbA1c, linked to the DCCT reference method [6]. By 2002, laboratories reporting to the NGSP had a coefficient of variation of less than 5% [6] and as of 2009, 97% of laboratories in the United States reported HbA1c that was NGSP certified. Despite this, systematic biases, drifts in analytic performance over time, and inter-method variability have been observed among NGSP-certified HbA1c methods. This variability has been a potential source of inaccuracy interpreting HbA1c results relative to clinical decision thresholds [7].

Relationship of HbA1c to average glucose

With the advent of continuous glucose monitoring systems (CGMS), it has become easier to estimate a patient's mean blood glucose with greater accuracy. A recent international study was completed to determine if HbA1c could serve as a reliable estimate of average glucose (eAG) for

TABLE 11.1 Relationship of HbA1c (%) and the estimate of average blood glucose (mgm/dl) (adapted from [8])

HbA1c (%)	Estimate of average blood glucose (mgm/dl)
5	97
6	126
7	154
8	183
9	212
10	240
11	269
12	298

individuals with and without diabetes [8]. A total of 587 patients (268 type 1, 159 type 2, and 80 without diabetes) used CGMS for 48 hours on 4 different occasions over a 3-month period, 8 point self glucose monitoring during CGMS days, 7 point self-glucose monitoring at least 3 days per week of the study, and monthly HbA1c assay that was DCCT referenced and performed in a central lab. Despite attempts to have a broad ethnic representation, the study participants were mainly non-Hispanic white (83%); Hispanic, Black and Asian American participants combined, accounted for 16% of the total group. In addition; as a first attempt in using CGMS to assess the association of HbA1c and eAG, the study included only patients with stable glycemic control and excluded children, pregnant women, and individuals with renal impairment. Despite these limitations, 90% of patients had average glucose values that were within +/− 15%; the predetermined minimal standard for data acceptability. Using the derived regression equation (eAG mgm% = $28.7 \times$ HgbA1c − 46.7) the authors report HgbA1c derived specific eAGs (Table 11.1).

While a specific eAG may seem to be more meaningful to patients and physicians; taking into account the confidence intervals, interpretation demonstrates a significant analytic and clinical imprecision. For example, a HbA1c of 7% could have an eAG of 123–185 mgm% which could have a HbA1c range of 6.7–9.2%. Despite the endorsement for the concept of eAG by major consensus groups (e.g., American Diabetes Association, International Diabetes Federation, and European Association for the Study of Diabetes), its impact in clinical care is still uncertain and its use has not been universally accepted [2, 9].

Other limitations for the measurement of HbA1c

HbA1c is not the complete expression of glycemic control, and is not a reliable measure of pre- and postprandial glycemic variation as well as hypoglycemia [10]. In addition, other clinical conditions where HbA1c may not accurately reflect glucose control are based on abnormalities in RBC production and half-life and include; hemolysis, hemoglobinopathies, severe anemias, and recent transfusion. It is often recognized that some patients have discrepant HbA1c values compared to their clinical presentation, HBGM, or other measures of glycated proteins (i.e., fructosamine). This has been hypothesized to be due to age, race, and other genetic factors determining differences in glycation rates, RBC life span, and membrane permeability [2].

Other considerations for the measurement of HbA1c

Somogyi was the first to report that for healthy individuals without diabetes, the ratio of serum to intracellular RBC glucose could range from 0.66 to 0.95 [11]. Since that time, there have been a number of reports that emphasize the potential implications regarding HbA1c as a measure of RBC intracellular glycation and differences in membrane permeability for circulating glucose. Consistent with this, from 4 to 12% of apparently healthy individuals have been found to have elevation in HbA1c without an association with glycemic control, glucose intolerance, caloric intake, or activity [12,13]. In addition, the fact that there could be substantial interindividual variation in RBC glucose exposure could help explain discordance in the measures of blood glucose and other glycated circulating protein such as albumin [14]. The observed association of HbA1c and tobacco use, aging, and atherosclerosis without other abnormalities in our traditional measures of glycemic control could suggest a unifying hypothesis for the contribution of intracellular hyperglycemia to risks for complications [12]. Consistent with these epidemiologic observations, expert panels have made recommendations that HbA1c be used for screening and diagnosis of glucose abnormalities and risk in individuals [15].

Why HbA1c is the best measure for glycemic exposure, glucose control, and risk?

1 At present, HbA1c is the best clinical measure of glycemic exposure.

2 HbA1c is only one of the several measures of glycemic control and does not accurately assess glycemic variation or hypoglycemia.
3 HbA1c may be valuable in predicting vascular complications and risk, independent of its association with measures of blood glucose and other measures of glycemic control.
4 Similar to other laboratory tests, it is important to realize that there are limitations in the interpretation of HbA1c values.

What is the evidence for glucose control in managing the risks of complications of diabetes?

In order to answer the question regarding the importance of HbA1c in the outpatient management of diabetes, we need to understand the importance of glycemia and the efficacy, effectiveness, and value of our current therapeutic options in glucose control for patient-important outcomes of morbidity, mortality, and quality of life.

Efficacy: What are the plausible arguments that glucose control can reduce risk?

Physiologic studies

Glucose reacts with many different proteins (circulating and tissue), which result in advanced glycation end products, increased protein kinase signaling, altered arterial structure/distensibility, plaque formation, and endothelial dysfunction [16–19]. It is proposed that these processes are cumulative and often result in subsequent atherosclerosis from decades of exposure to hyperglycemia.

Epidemiology and observational studies

From epidemiologic studies we know that diabetes is associated with high rates of complications related to microvascular (e.g., nephropathy, retinopathy, and neuropathy) and macrovascular (e.g., cardio- and cerebrovascular) disease [20], while observational studies demonstrate a strong association of chronic hyperglycemia with microvascular complications [21,22], cognitive impairment [23], and evidence that patients with microvascular disease such as retinopathy are also at increased risk for myocardial infarctions and cardiovascular morbidity and mortality [24]. In addition to the association of vascular events with glycemic control, it has long been recognized that associated metabolic abnormalities (e.g., hypertension, hyperlipidemia) are also important contributors to the risk of complications [25].

Randomized controlled trials

In randomized trials, improving glucose control significantly reduces the risk of microvascular disease in people with diabetes [3, 5, 26]. Alternatively; regarding macrovascular complications, clinical trials have historically depended on surrogate intermediate outcomes such as HbA1c because of being underpowered for hard cardiovascular outcomes, having insufficient follow-up to detect moderate cardiovascular risk reduction, and having insufficient follow-up to provide measurable feedback concerning the long-term success for interventions to improve glycemic control. While glycemic outcomes (e.g., HbA1c values) are important to providers and patients, Montori and others have emphasized that studies often lack other patient-important outcomes [27]. Recently three very large randomized trials have tried to address the value of interventions for glycemic control, the relationship of HbA1c, and important cardiovascular events [28–30]. While point estimates for hazard ratios for primary outcomes (nonfatal MI, nonfatal stroke, CVD death, and hospitalization for CHF revascularization) showed a favorable trend, these studies were collectively unable to show a significant association with aggressive glycemic control (Table 11.2).

In addition, the intensive glycemic control arm of the ACCORD trial was stopped early because of risk of death, hazard ratio (HR) (95% CI) 1.22 (1.01–1.46) [29].

Meta-analysis

Several meta-analyses, including observational studies, have suggested that chronic hyperglycemia as measured by HbA1c is associated with an increased risk for cardiovascular disease in people with diabetes [31]. Meta-analysis and pooled estimates for the recent large randomized trials suggest that intensive glucose control can reduce the risk for nonfatal myocardial infarction but not cardiovascular or all-cause mortality [32].

Effectiveness: What is the evidence that glucose control is effective in reducing risk and adds value?

What are the risks of glucose control (hypoglycemia)?

The risks of severe hypoglycemia during randomized trials have been reported to be up to 2–3 times greater for patients intensively treated for hyperglycemia [3, 4, 29, 30] but not found to be statistically different for patients in other studies [33, 34] where intensive treatment regimens were left up to the judgment of health care provider and patient. In addition to the immediate risks associated with hypoglycemia, an episode of severe hypoglycemia within 3 months has been reported to be the strongest predictor of a first primary outcome; HR 2.062 (1.132, 3.756) [30]. This time-dependent covariate raises the question of interaction with other significant predictors of first primary events, i.e., age HR 1.33 (1.191, 1.492) and duration of diabetes HR 1.019 (1.007, 1.030) and has lead to the hypothesis that the adverse risk of death in intensive intervention could be explained by the aggressiveness of treatment in an elderly population with longer duration of diabetes and established coronary disease. As compared to the ADVANCE trial where treatment goals (median A1c achieved of 6.4%) occurred over 12–18 months, most individuals in ACCORD achieved this target A1c within 6 months [29, 30]. To confirm or exclude the diagnosis of hypoglycemia, clinical trials will need to include more accurate measurement of the circulating glucose levels than HbA1c.

What are the risks of glucose control (weight gain)?

More individuals in the intensive arm of the ACCORD trial gained 10+ kg from baseline (29 vs. 14% $p < 0.001$) [29], while differences in weight at study end for ADVANCE were more favorable for standard intervention, attributed to ~1 kg weight loss compared to weight neutrality for the intensively treated group [30]. The large weight gain seen

TABLE 11.2 Effect of intensive glucose control and primary outcomes

	ACCORD	ADVANCE	VADT
Primary outcome	Nonfatal MI nonfatal stroke CVD death Hospitalization for CHF and revascularization	Nonfatal MI nonfatal stroke CVD death	Nonfatal MI nonfatal stroke CVD death
Hazard ratio 95% CI	0.87 0.73–1.04	0.90 0.78–1.04	0.94 0.84–1.06

in individuals in the ACCORD study has been attributed to the greater use of thiazolidinediones (TZD) in the intensive arm. No differences in weight gain were reported for the UKPDS follow-up or Steno 2 study [33, 34].

What are the benefits of glucose control (microvascular)?

In clinical practice, management of hyperglycemia in patients with diabetes is in concert with other management strategies for risk reduction (e.g., lipids, blood pressure). In the Steno 2 study, an example of a multifactorial intervention initiative, at the end of trial (7.8 years) and at the end of follow-up (13.3 years) there was a relative risk reduction (95% CI) of 0.44 (0.25, 0.77) for nephropathy, one patient in the intensive therapy group progressing to dialysis as compared to six patients in the conventional therapy group ($p < 0.04$). Relative risk for progression of retinopathy 0.57 (0.37, 0.88), laser treatment for proliferative retinopathy 0.45 (0.23, 0.86), and blindness 0.51 (0.17, 1.53) also favored the intensive intervention group [33].

What are the benefits of glucose control (macrovascular)?

Point estimates for hazard ratios for primary outcomes (nonfatal MI, nonfatal stroke, death from cardiovascular causes, and hospitalization for CHF revascularization) for the Action to Control Cardiovascular Risk in Diabetes (ACCORD), Action in Diabetes and Vascular Disease Preterax and Diamicron MR Controlled Evaluation (ADVANCE), and Veterans Administration Diabetes Trial (VADT) trials showed favorable trends (with significantly less events), but collectively were unable to show a significant association (Table 11.2). An observation that has been consistently observed in the Steno 2 and United Kingdom Prospective Diabetes Study (UKPDS) follow-up studies is the suggestion of a legacy effect of early management of hyperglycemia for macrovascular events. For example, the relative risk reduction for myocardial infarction for earlier glycemic control was 15% ($p = 0.014$), median 8.5 years posttrial follow-up in UKPDS [34], while the absolute risk reduction seen in Steno 2 was 29%, median follow-up 13.3 years [33].

What are glycemic treatment goals for hyperglycemia?

Guidelines for glycemic goals have used HbA1c values and are as a low of 6% in Latin America and up to 7.5% in the United Kingdom (see Figure 11.1).

Table 11.3 summarizes the median HbA1c values achieved in recent trials, intervention versus standard, as well as those seen in posttrial follow-up. Based on these studies to reduce cardiovascular events, a conservative HbA1c goal of <8% would seem appropriate as an accountability measure that could apply to all patients. Otherwise, it appears prudent to individualize treatment goals based on expected risks/benefits of treatment. For example, a goal of 7% to reduce the risks of microvascular

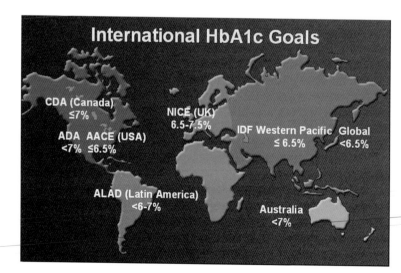

FIG 11.1 International HbA1c goals.

TABLE 11.3 Summary of intervention and follow-up studies for glycemic control

	Duration of follow-up (median/years)	Median A1c achieved	
		Intervention (%)	Standard (%)
ACCORD	3.5	6.4	7.5
ADVANCE	5	6.4	7.0
VADT	6	6.9	8.4
UKPDS follow-up	8.5	7.8	7.8
Steno 2 follow-up	13.33	7.8	7.8

complications should be balanced against the risks for occurrence of hypoglycemia.

What is the value of glucose control?

Diabetes is an expensive illness to manage, but it is more expensive not managed. In the United States, diabetes is reported to be associated with an annual direct medical expenditure of $91.8 billion, while the per capita cost totals $13,243 for individuals with diabetes compared to $2,560 for those without [35].

In the Steno 2 follow-up study, while a large part of the increased costs for care for people with diabetes was pharmacy and consultation, incremental costs for all complications and interventions were less for intensive compared to conservative treatment, despite the fact that patients lived longer (1.7 quality-adjusted life years) with intensive treatment. The incremental cost-effectiveness ratio was favorable; € 3927 ($6682 USA) per life year gained [35] and was likely related to a comprehensive approach to patient management and not solely glycemic control.

What is a patient's risk for micro- and macrovascular events?

In order to assess the value of glucose control it is necessary to assess an individual's risks. To do this, a clinician can turn to a number of statistical (e.g., UKPDS and Framingham) and simulation (e.g., Archimedes) models that have been validated against large clinical trials and other populations and are available to predict micro- and macrovascular complications for type 2 diabetes patients.

As an example, the patient described in Table 11.4 has a 10-year risk of myocardial infarction (MI) of 14%, 25%, and 14% for Archimedes, UKPDS, and Framingham respectively. With improvement in HbA1c to 7%, his risk drops by 13%, while there is a projected 50% or greater risk

reduction with improvement in LDL cholesterol to 100 mgm% or systolic blood pressure to 120. In contrast, he has a projected 21% risk of kidney failure in 30 years for which the models predict can be significantly reduced with glycemic control. In addition, and consistent with the importance of both bio and psychosocial measures, attention to other outcomes measures (e.g., weight loss, regular foot exams) can have a similar impact as glycemic control.

TABLE 11.4 Diabetes risk according to Archemedes PhD Simulation [37] Case: A 54-year-old Caucasian male with a family history of diabetes has had type 2 diabetes for 8 years. He is taking Metformin, Glimepiride, Aspirin, Simvastatin, and Lisinopril; has a blood pressure of 138/90, a BMI of 31 kg/m^2, and symptoms-signs of peripheral neuropathy. His HbA1c is 7.8%, cholesterol 235 mgm%, HDL 35 mgm%, and triglycerides are 280 mgm%.

Risk	10 year	30 year
Myocardial infarction		
HbA1c 7.8%[1,2]	14.3%	
HbA1c 7.0%	12.4%	
HbA1c 6.5%	11.0%	
Kidney failure		
HbA1c 7.8%[3]		21.0%
HbA1c 7.0%		6.0%
Foot problem		
HbA1c 7.8%[4]		20.0%
HbA1c 7.0%		13.0%

	10-year risk	30-year risk
[1]UKPDS [38]	25.2%	
Framingham [39]	14.0%	
[2]and LDL 100 mgm %	9.2%	
or Systolic blood pressure 120	9.5%	
or Weight loss		11.8%
[3]and Systolic blood pressure 120, LDL 100 mgm%		5.1%
[4]and regular foot exams		14.0%

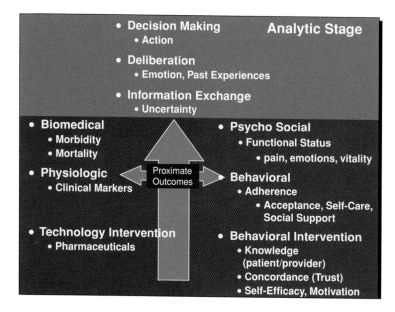

FIG 11.2 Process for decision making (from [36]).

What is the Evidence for Glucose Control in Managing the Risks of Complications of Diabetes?

1 There are plausible biological and physiological explanations as well as evidence from observation/epidemiological studies, controlled trials, and meta-analysis that support the hypothesis that treatment of hyperglycemia will reduce microvascular complications of diabetes.

2 There is an uncertain treatment effect for reducing macrovascular events. To reduce macrovascular events, the benefit of early treatment of hyperglycemia and/or conservative treatment regimens that minimize hypoglycemia seem prudent but require further study.

What can we conclude? Is HbA1c the most important therapeutic target in outpatient management of diabetes?

Summary

HbA1c, the current best measurement of glucose control, is one of the important therapeutic targets in the outpatient management of diabetes. Similar to the model of clinical decision making by Charles and Gaffini [36] (Figure 11.2), decision making in the management of diabetes is currently determined by guidelines and public policy that has uncertainty and, as a consequence, often there are strong emotions about the importance of glycemic control and HbA1c levels. Additional important therapeutic targets include lipid, hypertension, and behavioral outcomes.

Because it is unlikely that all "what if" questions will be effectively addressed by head-to-head comparisons in large well powered randomized trials, more effective modeling of outcomes with the inclusion of both biomedical (e.g., HbA1c) and psychosocial outcomes important to patients will be essential for comparative evaluation. Until that time, one can conclude that there is not a "most important" but many important outcomes in the care of people with diabetes.

References

1. Rahbar S. The discovery of glycated hemoglobin: a major event in the study of nonenzymatic chemistry in biological systems. *Ann N Y Acad Sci.* **1043**:9–19, 2005.
2. Little RR, Sacks DB. HbA1c: how do we measure it and what does it mean? *Curr Opin Endocrinol Diabetes Obes.* **16**(2):113–118, 2009.
3. Anonymous. The effect of intensive treatment of diabetes on the development and progression of long-term complications in insulin-dependent diabetes mellitus. The Diabetes Control and Complications Trial Research Group.[see comment]. *N Engl J Med.* **329**(14):977–986, 1993.

4. Anonymous. Effect of intensive blood-glucose control with metformin on complications in overweight patients with type 2 diabetes (UKPDS 34). UK Prospective Diabetes Study (UKPDS) Group. [see comment][erratum appears in Lancet 1998 Nov7;352(9139):1557]. *Lancet.* **352**(9131):854–865, 1998.

5. Shichiri M, Kishikawa H, Ohkubo Y, Wake N. Long-term results of the Kumamoto Study on optimal diabetes control in type 2 diabetic patients. *Diabetes Care.* **23**(Suppl 2):B21–B29, 2000.

6. Little RR. Glycated hemoglobin standardization–National Glycohemoglobin Standardization Program (NGSP) perspective. *Clin Chem Lab Med.* **41**(9):1191–1198, 2003.

7. Holmes EW, Ersahin C, Augustine GJ, et al. Analytic bias among certified methods for the measurement of hemoglobin A1c: a cause for concern? [see comment]. *Am J Clin Pathol.* **129**(4):540–547, 2008.

8. Nathan DM, Kuenen J, Borg R, et al. Translating the A1C assay into estimated average glucose values. [see comment]. *Diabetes Care.* **31**(8):1473–1478, 2008.

9. Brick JC, Derr RL, Saudek CD. A randomized comparison of the terms estimated average glucose versus hemoglobin A1C. *Diabetes Educ.* **35**(4):596–602, 2009.

10. Cox DJ, Gonder-Frederick L, Ritterband L, Clarke W, Kovatchev BP. Prediction of severe hypoglycemia. *Diabetes Care.* **30**(6):1370–1373, 2007.

11. Somogyi M. The distribution of sugar in blood. *J Biol Chem.* **78**(1):117–127, 1928.

12. Bloomgarden ZT. Cardiovascular disease, neuropathy, and retinopathy. *Diabetes Care.* **32**(6):e64–e68, 2009.

13. Selvin E, Zhu H, Brancati FL. Elevated A1C in adults without a history of diabetes in the U.S. *Diabetes Care.* **32**(5):828–833, 2009.

14. Khera PK, Joiner CH, Carruthers A, et al. Evidence for interindividual heterogeneity in the glucose gradient across the human red blood cell membrane and its relationship to hemoglobin glycation. *Diabetes.* **57**(9):2445–2452, 2008.

15. Fonseca V, Inzucchi SE, Ferrannini E. Redefining the diagnosis of diabetes using glycated hemoglobin. [comment]. *Diabetes Care.* **32**(7):1344–1345, 2009.

16. Feener EP, King GL. Vascular dysfunction in diabetes mellitus. *Lancet.* **350**(Suppl 1):SI9–SI13, 1997.

17. Schmidt AM, Yan SD, Wautier JL, Stern D. Activation of receptor for advanced glycation end products: a mechanism for chronic vascular dysfunction in diabetic vasculopathy and atherosclerosis. *Circ Res.* **84**(5):489–497, 1999.

18. Sheetz MJ, King GL. Molecular understanding of hyperglycemia's adverse effects for diabetic complications. [see comment]. *JAMA.* **288**(20):2579–2588, 2002.

19. Srivastava AK. High glucose-induced activation of protein kinase signaling pathways in vascular smooth muscle cells: a potential role in the pathogenesis of vascular dysfunction in diabetes (review). *Int J Mol Med.* **9**(1):85–89, 2002.

20. Harris MI. Diabetes in America: epidemiology and scope of the problem. [see comment]. *Diabetes Care.* **21**(Suppl 3):C11–C114, 1998.

21. Gaster B, Hirsch IB. The effects of improved glycemic control on complications in type 2 diabetes. *Arch Intern Med.* **158**(2):134–140, 1998.

22. Klein R, Klein BE, Moss SE. Relation of glycemic control to diabetic microvascular complications in diabetes mellitus. *Ann Intern Med.* **124**(1 Pt 2):90–96, 1996.

23. Cukierman-Yaffe T, Gerstein HC, Williamson JD, et al. Relationship between baseline glycemic control and cognitive function in individuals with type 2 diabetes and other cardiovascular risk factors: the action to control cardiovascular risk in diabetes-memory in diabetes (ACCORD-MIND) trial. *Diabetes Care.* **32**(2):221–226, 2009.

24. Reaven PD, Emanuele N, Moritz T, et al. Proliferative diabetic retinopathy in type 2 diabetes is related to coronary artery calcium in the Veterans Affairs Diabetes Trial (VADT). *Diabetes Care.* **31**(5):952–957, 2008.

25. Poulter NR. Blood pressure and glucose control in subjects with diabetes: new analyses from ADVANCE. *J Hypertens.* **27**(Suppl 1):S3–S8, 2009.

26. Anonymous. Intensive blood-glucose control with sulphonylureas or insulin compared with conventional treatment and risk of complications in patients with type 2 diabetes (UKPDS 33). UK Prospective Diabetes Study (UKPDS) Group.[see comment][erratum appears in Lancet 1999 Aug14;354(9178):602]. *Lancet.* **352**(9131):837–853, 1998.

27. Montori VM, Fernandez-Balsells M. Glycemic control in type 2 diabetes: time for an evidence-based about-face? *Ann Intern Med.* **150**(11):803–808, 2009.

28. Duckworth W, Abraira C, Moritz T, et al. Glucose control and vascular complications in veterans with type 2 diabetes.[see comment][erratum appears in N Engl J Med. 2009 Sep3;361(10):1024-5; PMID: 19726779]. *N Engl J Med.* **360**(2):129–139, 2009.

29. Action to Control Cardiovascular Risk in Diabetes Study G, Gerstein HC, Miller ME, et al. Effects of intensive glucose lowering in type 2 diabetes. [see comment]. *N Engl J Med.* **358**(24):2545–2559, 2008.

30. Group AC, Patel A, MacMahon S, et al. Intensive blood glucose control and vascular outcomes in patients with type 2 diabetes. [see comment]. *N Engl J Med.* **358**(24):2560–2572, 2008.

31. Selvin E, Marinopoulos S, Berkenblit G, et al. Meta-analysis: glycosylated hemoglobin and cardiovascular disease in diabetes mellitus. [see comment]. *Ann Intern Med.* **141**(6):421–431, 2004.

32. Kelly TN, Bazzano LA, Fonseca VA, Thethi TK, Reynolds K, He J. Systematic review: glucose control and cardiovascular disease in type 2 diabetes. *Ann Intern Med.* **151**(6):394–403, 2009.

33. Gaede P, Lund-Andersen H, Parving HH, Pedersen O. Effect of a multifactorial intervention on mortality in type 2 diabetes. [see comment]. *N Engl J Med.* **358**(6):580–591, 2008.

34. Holman RR, Paul SK, Bethel MA, Matthews DR, Neil HA. 10-year follow-up of intensive glucose control in type 2 diabetes. *N Engl J Med.* **359**:1577–1589, 2008.

35. Gaede P, Valentine WJ, Palmer AJ, et al. Cost-effectiveness of intensified versus conventional multifactorial intervention in type 2 diabetes: results and projections from the Steno-2 study. *Diabetes Care.* **31**(8):1510–1515, 2008.

36. Charles C, Whelan T, Gafni A. What do we mean by partnership in making decisions about treatment? *BMJ.* **319**(7212):780–782, 1999.

37. Association AD. Archimedes PhD; Available from: http://www.diabetes.org/diabetesphd/default.jsp, ed.

38. Oxford DU. UKPDS Risk Engine; Available from: http://www.dtu.ox.ac.uk/index.php?maindoc=/riskengine/download.php, ed.

39. Institute NHLB. Framingham Risk Calculator; Available from: http://hp2010.nhlbihin.net/atpiii/calculator.asp, ed.

PART III

Management of Associated Risk Factors and Disease

12 Primary therapy for obesity as the treatment of type 2 diabetes

Manpreet S. Mundi[1] and Michael D. Jensen[2]

[1] Senior Associate Consultant, Division of Endocrinology, Mayo Clinic, Rochester, MN, USA
[2] Tomas J. Watson, Jr. Professor in Honor of Dr. Robert L. Frye, Mayo Foundation, Rochester, MN, USA

LEARNING POINTS

- The treatment of obesity is an important part of the therapy of type 2 diabetes and may require oral agents as well as surgical intervention.
- Weight gain is a common side effect of the treatment of type 2 diabetes.
- Weight loss alone improves the metabolic status of patients with type 2 diabetes.

The obesity epidemic is escalating the incidence of diabetes in adults and children, requiring health care providers to reassess treatment options to best suit the obese patient. Obesity has long been recognized as the major risk factor for type 2 diabetes. Nearly 90% of type 2 diabetics in the United States are overweight or obese [1]. The association between obesity and the prevalence of diabetes in a population has been well documented. For example, data from the Nurses' Health Study (84,941 women followed for 20 years) indicated that body mass index (BMI) was the most important diabetes risk factor [2]. In that population the risk of diabetes was ~39 times greater in women with BMI of 35 kg/m^2 or greater, and ~20 times greater for women with BMI between 30.0 and 34.9 kg/m^2 compared to women with BMI of less than 23.0 kg/m^2. Similarly, the prevalence of diabetes was found to be 2.5 times greater in overweight men (BMI 25–29.9) and 3 times higher in overweight women compared to the normal weight group in the NHANES III study [3]. From these studies, it seems evident that the prevalence of diabetes increases as weight increases. This chapter will present cases highlighting the pharmacologic, dietary, and surgical options for treating the obese diabetic patient.

A 40-year-old male presents after routine preemployment blood tests revealed fasting plasma glucose of 132 mg/dL. He currently has no complaints and reports that he has not seen a physician for over 20 years. He is well appearing and has a BMI of 31.4 kg/m². His blood pressure is 154/87 with a heart rate of 94. Other than obesity, the physical examination is within normal limits. Repeat blood work reveals fasting blood glucose of 128 mg/dL and total cholesterol of 224 mg/dL with triglycerides of 314 mg/dL, HDL of 28 mg/dL, and LDL of 114 mg/dL.

This case highlights the fact that, in addition to the increased risk of diabetes, obesity complicates treatment by exacerbating metabolic complications such as hypertension and dyslipidemia [2–6]. Obesity itself may account for approximately 78% and 65% of essential hypertension in men and women respectively [7], with progressive increases in systolic blood pressure as BMI increases [8]. A similar relationship has also been noted between increasing obesity and hyperlipidemia. The NHANES III survey revealed approximately a 1.5 times higher prevalence of high cholesterol in obese men and women when compared to the normal weigh cohort [3].

The combination of diabetes and obesity, especially central obesity, is also strongly associated with insulin resistance and a pro-atherogenic lipid profile consisting of increased triglyceride and apolipoprotein B concentrations, an increased proportion of small dense LDL particles, and a low HDL cholesterol. This high-risk combination is often accompanied by a prothrombotic and a proinflammatory profile, which significantly worsens an individual's risk of cardiovascular disease and overall mortality [9]. Compared with normal-weight individuals with diabetes, mortality is 2.5 to 3.3 times higher in diabetics with body weights that are 20–30% greater than ideal weight and 5.2 to 7.9 times higher for those with body weights 40% above the ideal [10].

We suggest that this exponential increase in risk attributed to obesity indicates that weight management should be the first target for overweight/obese patients at presentation. Although many physicians seem pessimistic about the likelihood that lifestyle modification can result in long-term benefit, results of the Diabetes Prevention Program clearly show that this approach is feasible, given the proper support [11]. Furthermore, an effect on prevention of T2DM seems to be detectable as many as 10 years after beginning the intervention [12]. For physicians with a large number of obese patients with, or at risk for, T2DM, we believe that efforts to identify or develop successful lifestyle programs will improve practice outcomes.

Reduced energy diets, increased physical activity, and the accompanying weight loss have a positive effect on almost every risk factor associated with diabetes and obesity. Newly diagnosed type 2 diabetics in the UKPDS cohort who were treated successfully with dietary therapy experienced a substantial decrease in fasting blood glucose concentrations, from an average of 205 down to 146 mg/dL in the first 3 months [13]. This was accompanied by a decrease in fasting insulin concentrations [14], an increase in insulin sensitivity [15], and an improvement in beta-cell function [15]. Similar improvements were also noted in coexisting conditions such as hypertension and dyslipidemia. In the first few days of caloric restriction, VLDL and triglyceride concentrations decrease and LDL particle size increases [16]. With longer duration of therapy, a decrease in LDL concentration and an increase in HDL particle numbers occurs.

Although the improvements in metabolic characteristics are generally greater in patients who lose the most weight, modest weight loss can also produce significant benefit. The findings of a retrospective review of the medical records of 263 patients with type 2 diabetes treated at the Aberdeen Diabetic Clinic suggested that the lifestyle changes required for weight loss were associated with a three- to four-month prolonged survival for each 1 kg decrease in weight [17]. The investigators estimated that lifestyle changes required to maintain a 10-kg weight loss would eliminate 35% of the expected reduction in life expectancy seen with type 2 diabetes.

Despite the numerous benefits of weight loss in type 2 diabetes, it is often quite difficult for obese individuals to initially lose the desired weight and then maintain the weight loss. Even when patients achieve their goal of weight reduction with calorie restriction, they commonly regain most, if not all of the weight that was lost [18]. Long-term follow-up has shown that repeated episodes of weight loss and gain, also known as weight cycling, are common and can have more negative health impact than weight-stable obesity. Sub-analysis of the Framingham Heart Study Cohort examined the effects of weight fluctuations on total mortality, morbidity and mortality from coronary heart disease, and mortality from cancer [19]. Even after accounting for an individual's current weight and other confounding factors, weight variability was significantly positively associated with total and coronary heart disease mortality in both men and women. Because the relative risks attributable to fluctuations in weight were comparable in magnitude to the risks attributable to being overweight, we suggest that physicians place a high value on interventions that are more likely to result in permanent reductions in weight.

Although rapid weight loss due to severe calorie restriction can rapidly lower blood glucose in patients with type 2 diabetes, these diets can also have adverse metabolic consequences [20]. Very low calorie/liquid protein diets are associated with decreased thyroid hormone (T3) concentrations, elevated ketone bodies, and a rise in serum uric acid concentrations [21]. An average of 38% of rapid weight loss in the first 12 days of these diets consists of fluid [21]; loss of lean body mass accounts for only approximately 10% of the initial weight loss. Electrolyte imbalances and excess fluid losses may occur and may be problematic managing in patients with multiple underlying comorbidities.

We suggest that physicians emphasize a more modest goal for rates of weight loss that will carry less risk and encourage patients to develop long-term, healthy lifestyle patterns. Weight loss of about 0.4 to 0.6 kg/week, with an initial goal of 5–10% of body weight lost, appears to be safe and effective at improving metabolic control. The published literature suggests that this moderate caloric restriction in combination with mild exercise can result in an average weight loss of 4.4 ± 2.7 kg over 12 months (see Table 12.1). If the individual is able to achieve and maintain this loss, further weight reduction can then be attempted.

Diet changes should be focused on helping patients to reduce energy intake in a manner that is consistent with long-term adherence, rather than single-mindedly focusing

TABLE 12.1 Summary of selected clinical trials enrolling type 2 diabetic subjects

Treatment	Patients/characteristics	Trials (number of subjects)	Average duration of treatment (months)	Mean weight change (kg)	Mean change in HgbA1c (%)	Side effects
Lifestyle modifications (diet and exercise)	Newly diagnosed type 2 diabetics	22 (1870)	12.4 ± 17	-4.4 ± 4.2	0.25 ± 0.40	
Metformin alone	NIDDM	14 (8842)	14.6 ± 14	-2.35 ± 0.52	-0.87 ± 0.76	Common: nausea, vomiting, bloating, and diarrhea
Metformin plus diet/exercise	NIDDM	5 (624)	7.2 ± 2.7	-1.41 ± 2.51	-0.40 ± 1.07	Rarely can lead to lactic acidosis.
Metformin plus insulin	NIDDM	6 (1602)	13.9 ± 8.3	0.35 ± 1.03	-0.95 ± 0.51	Contraindicated in elderly and patients with renal insufficiency, liver
Secretagogues (sulfonylureas and meglinitides)						disease, and congestive heart failure
Metformin plus thiazolinedione	NIDDM	3 (952)	6.0 ± 0.0	1.68 ± 0.31	-0.78 ± 0.31	
Thiazolinediones	NIDDM	11 (3595)	12.1 ± 12.9	3.15 ± 1.62	-0.72 ± 0.51	Water retention and contraindicated in patients with decreased ventricular function
Sulfonylureas	NIDDM	7 (5425)	13.8 ± 15.8	1.68 ± 0.65	-1.00 ± 0.98	Hypoglycemia Contraindicated in pregnancy (teratogenic) and liver/kidney impairment
Exenatide plus sulfonylurea	NIDDM on sulfonylurea	2 (254)	7.5 ± 0.0	-1.30 ± 0.30	-0.70 ± 0.20	Nausea, vomiting, bloating, diarrhea, headache, and decreased appetite
Exenatide plus metformin	NIDDM on metformin	2 (223)	7.5 ± 0.0	-2.20 ± 0.60	-0.60 ± 0.20	Rarely can cause pancreatitis
Exenatide plus metformin/TZD	NIDDM on metformin/TZD	1 (121)	4	-1.8	-0.9	
Exenatide plus metfromin/sulfonylurea	NIDDM on metfromin/sulfonylurea	5 (1548)	13.9 ± 12.5	-3.13 ± 1.59	-0.92 ± 0.17	

(Continued)

TABLE 12.1 (Continued)

Treatment	Patients/ characteristics	Trials (number of subjects)	Average duration of treatment (months)	Mean weight change (kg)	Mean change in HgbA1c (%)	Side effects
DPP-4 inhibitors	NIDDM	10 (2779)	6.6 ± 1.9	-0.25 ± 0.51	-0.99 ± 0.25	Nasopharyngitis, diarrhea, contact dermatitis, and osteoarthritis
DPP-4 inhibitor plus TZD	NIDDM	3 (441)	6.0 ± 0.0	1.77 ± 0.35	-1.50 ± 0.53	Note that long term safety outcomes pending
DPP-4 inhibitor plus sulfonylurea	NIDDM on sulfonylurea	3 (445)	5.3 ± 1.2	0.72 ± 0.79	-0.53 ± 0.16	
DPP-4 inhibitor plus metformin	NIDDM on metformin	8 (2468)	6.9 ± 2.1	-0.92 ± 0.70	-0.87 ± 0.81	
Sibutramine	Obese NIDDM	8 (483)	7.3 ± 3.0	-6.00 ± 3.32	-0.47 ± 0.78	Insomnia, dry mouth, constipation, nausea, and elevation in blood pressure
Sibutramine plus sulfonylurea	NIDDM on sulfoyulurea	1 (44)	12	-4.1	0.6	
Orlistat	Obese NIDDM	10 (1048)	7.7 ± 2.8	-5.13 ± 1.37	-0.99 ± 1.00	Fecal urgency, oily stool, increased defecations, and fecal incontinence
Orlistat plus metformin	NIDDM on metformin	1 (250)	12	-4.7 ± 0.3	-0.75 ± 0.08	
Orlistat plus sulfonylurea	NIDDM on sulfonylurea	1 (139)	12	-6.2 ± 0.5	-0.28 ± 0.09	
Orlistat plus Metformin/sulfonylurea	NIDDM on metformin and sulfonylurea	2 (141)	8.0 ± 5.7	-4.28 ± 1.31	-1.23 ± 0.35	
Orlistat plus insulin	Type 2 diabetic on insulin	1 (274)	12	-4.0 ± 0.3	-0.62 ± 0.08	
Bariatric surgery (overall)	Obese diabetics	9 (452)	Variable	-40.55 ± 11.36	-2.13 ± 0.50	Initially associated with surgical risk, diarrhea, nausea, vomiting, and dumping syndrome
Gastric banding	Obese diabetics	3 (23)	Variable	-17.28 ± 9.36	-1.40 ± 1.00	Long-term associated with vitamin and mineral deficiencies
Gastric bypass	Obese diabetics	3 (161)	Variable	-42.65 ± 8.29	-2.18 ± 0.53	
Biliopancreatic Diversion/duodenal switc	Obese diabetics	3 (268)	Variable	-56.30 ± 10.11	N/A	

Data are presented as weighted means ± weighted standard deviations about the mean [39].

on a specific diet composition. Despite the plethora of diets and dieting guides available, head-to-head comparisons of the various diets have revealed that weight loss is similar between diets with varying macronutrient composition, provided that dietary adherence is comparable [22]. In one study comparing high carbohydrate, high monounsaturated fat, and high saturated fat diets, the participants lost an average of 6.6 kg in each of the three groups after 12 weeks. As expected, the participants in the high saturated fat group had the worst lipid profile. This supports the recommendation by the American Diabetes Association that saturated fats be limited to less than 7% of the total energy intake [23].

In summary, this patient with newly diagnosed T2DM deserves an aggressive trial of lifestyle modification if he is willing to attempt changes, with or without pharmacotherapy, as needed. Even though long-term success may not occur in the majority of patients, this approach is virtually risk-free. We suggest that not considering this approach will deprive the subset of patients who are "lifestyle responders" of a treatment that improves a host of metabolic abnormalities.

> *A 52-year-old asymptomatic female was diagnosed with diabetes 4 years ago and has been treated with glyburide and pioglitazone for the last two years. She is referred for consultation because of suboptimal glycemic control (HbA1c of 8.6%). Her BMI is 36 kg/m² and her blood pressure is 138/86 with a heart rate of 88.*

This patient would benefit from aggressive weight loss therapy, however, because she is on a sulfonylurea; this should be done with caution due to the increased risk for hypoglycemia while she is actively losing weight. Pharmacotherapy may need to be altered to avoid agents that cause hypoglycemia. Furthermore, agents that are associated with weight gain [insulin, sulfonylureas, and thiazolidinediones (TZDs)] (see Table 12.1) are counterproductive in this setting. Biguanides, of which metformin is the sole approved agent, are not associated with significant weight gain and are recommended as first-line pharmacotherapy by most treatment guidelines. Metformin enhances insulin sensitivity, thus inducing greater peripheral glucose uptake and decreasing hepatic glucose output [24]. The effect of metformin on body weight in large randomized controlled trials has been variable depending on the addition of other hypoglycemic agents [25].

The United Kingdom Prospective Diabetes Study (UKPDS) randomized 753 overweight newly diagnosed diabetics to conventional therapy (diet only) versus intensive glucose control with metformin, glibenclamide, or insulin. After a 10-year follow-up period, the change in bodyweight was similar in the metformin and conventional treatment groups with a ~1.5 and ~1.9 kg net weight gain. However, this was significantly less than the weight gain seen in the sulfonylurea or insulin-treated groups, who experienced ~3.7 and ~6.0 kg weight gains, respectively [26]. In addition to the lack of significant weight gain, metformin resulted in fewer hypoglycemic episodes than sulfonylurea or insulin therapy and achieved similar improvements in HbA1c. A Diabetes Outcome Progression Trial (ADOPT) showed significant weight loss associated with metformin treatment [27]. This 4-year, double-blind randomized control trial assigned 4,360 newly diagnosed type 2 diabetics to receive metformin, glyburide, or rosiglitazone. Over the duration of the trial, weight decreased in the metformin group by 2.9 ± 0.6 kg (see Table 12.1), while rosiglitazone was associated with a weight gain of 4.8 ± 0.5 kg. Glyburide was associated with a 1.6 ± 0.6 kg weight gain in the first year, with the weight remaining stable afterward. The weight gain noted with both glyburide and rosiglitazone was associated with an increase in the waist and hip circumferences. Metformin, however, resulted in a reduction in both hip and waist circumferences. These beneficial changes in fat distribution have been quantified in a randomized study comparing the effects of metformin and rosiglitazone monotherapy for 26 weeks [28]. They noted that metformin significantly decreased body weight by an average of 2.0 kg, while placebo and rosiglitazone groups remained weight stable. Metformin also resulted in a significant decrease in both abdominal subcutaneous (from 5.3 ± 0.6 to 4.9 ± 0.5 kg) and intra-abdominal fat masses (from 2.5 ± 0.3 to 2.2 ± 0.2 kg).

The weight benefits of metformin have also been found when it is used in combination with other antidiabetic agents (see Table 12.1). In patients with type 2 diabetes who were suboptimally controlled on a sulphonylurea, adding metformin improved HbA1c to the same extent as adding pioglitazone [29]. However, patients receiving the sulphonylurea-pioglitazone combination gained 2.8 kg in one year, whereas the sulphonylurea-metformin group lost an average of 1.0 kg. Although other studies noted less weight benefit, the addition of metformin to sulfony-lurea did significantly lessen weight gain when compared to the use of sulfonylureas alone (0.35 ± 0.94 vs. 1.68 ± 0.58, respectively). Similar results have been noted with the addition of metformin to TZDs or insulin [25].

Another class of medications, the "incretins," is reported to be weight neutral or display weight loss properties. These compounds are either glucagon-like peptide-1 (GLP-1) receptor agonists or prevent GLP-1 breakdown through inhibition of dipeptidyl peptidase-4 (DPP-4), the enzyme responsible for the rapid clearance of GLP-1 from the circulation. Numerous clinical trials have reported on the efficacy of exenatide as adjuvant therapy in type 2 diabetics who fail to achieve adequate glycemic control with standard oral hypoglycemic agents. With a maximum dose of 10 μg twice daily, exenatide allowed 32–62% of patients to achieve a HbA1c of 7% or less [30]. These trials also reported weight loss averaging 1.3 ± 0.3 kg after 30–52 weeks of treatment (see Table 12.1). Total weight loss of 5.3 ± 0.4 kg was found during an open label extension trial, with 46% of subjects achieving and maintaining a HbA1c of less than 7% with 3 years of treatment [31]. The caveat is that only responders stayed in the open label extension, so these results are likely not representative of "average" results.

Liraglutide, a long-acting GLP-1 analog, also produces significant weight reductions both as mono- and adjuvant-therapy. A 14-week trial comparing various dosages of liraglutide (0.65 mg, 1.25 mg, 1.90 mg daily) versus placebo noted a significant, average weight loss of 2.9 kg at the highest dose [32]. This weight loss was accompanied by a 1.5% reduction in HbA1c and 46% of patients achieved a HbA1c of less than 7% in the highest dose group. In a 5-week dose escalation study of 144 type 2 diabetics, the addition of liraglutide to metformin produced a 70 mg/dl reduction in fasting glucose, a 0.8% reduction in HbA1c and an additional 2.9 ± 0.7 kg weight loss [33].

Weight loss associated with the DDP-4 inhibitors (sitagliptin and vildagliptin) is not as remarkable and this class of drug is best characterized as weight neutral. Multiple studies utilizing sitagliptin and vildagliptin as both mono- and adjuvant therapeutic agents have revealed minimal to no significant weight loss or gain (see Table 12.1) [30]. Combination therapy with sulfonylureas and TZDs has been shown to result in small weight gain [30]. Overall, the incretin class of drugs is effective in reducing HbA1c and has not been shown to result in significant weight gain. For the obese patient with T2DM these agents offer a chance

to avoid the weight gain side effects of sulfonylureas and TZDs and should be utilized early on in patients such as those presented above.

> A 49-year-old female with T2DM is referred by her primary care physician after failing multiple attempts at weight loss. She has had T2DM for 5 years and has been successfully treated with metformin and glipizide; her current HbA1c is 7.2%. Over the last ten years she has tried numerous times to lose weight through diet and exercise but has been unsuccessful. She reports only minor success with dieting, but has usually rapidly regained the weight. Her BMI is 33 kg/m² and her blood pressure is 132/82 and heart rate is 78.

Diet and exercise, along with an adjustment in the hypoglycemic medications, may not be sufficient for a significant number of obese patients who may require additional weight loss therapy. For patients who have a BMI of 27 kg/m² or higher and have failed to achieve weight loss after at least 6 months of treatment with diet, exercise, and behavioral therapy, the use of obesity pharmacotherapy may be considered. Sibutramine, one of two currently approved drugs for long-term use, acts as an inhibitor of norepinephrine and serotonin reuptake in the CNS, resulting in a reduction in food intake through increased satiety. In a multicenter 12-month randomized double-blind trial, sibutramine produced significant weight loss with both 15 mg/day (5.5 ± 0.6 kg) and 20 mg/day (8.0 ± 0.9 kg) doses after 12 months of follow-up (see Table 12.1) [34]. Of note, weight loss of greater or equal to 10% was achieved by 14 and 27% of subjects receiving 15 and 20 mg, respectively, but by none given placebo. Subjects who experienced a weight loss of ≥10% also showed significant decreases in HbA1c (1.2 ± 0.4%) as well as fasting plasma glucose (32 mg/dl). The most common side effects reported with sibutramine use are insomnia, headache, dry mouth, constipation, and nausea. Cardiovascular side effects have also been reported. Treatment with 15 mg/d sibutramine raised diastolic blood pressure by ≥5 mmHg in 43% of subjects versus 25% in the placebo group [34]. Pulse rate increased by ≥10 bpm in 42% of treated patients versus 17% with placebo. Of note, an ongoing study, the Sibutramine Cardiovascular Outcome Trial (SCOUT), is currently being conducted to address the efficacy and safety of sibutramine in high-risk subjects with increased risk of cardiovascular events.

Orlistat, the remaining approved long-term weight loss compound, acts as an inhibitor of gastric and pancreatic lipases. The weight loss is believed to largely result from fat malabsorption and, as might be expected, the most common side effects are gastrointestinal symptoms such as fecal urgency, oily stool, increased defecation, and fecal incontinence [1]. Orlistat has also been more thoroughly studied than sibutramine with over 15 randomized placebo-controlled trials in obese subjects with type 2 diabetes (see Table 12.1) [35]. One such multicenter trial randomized 391 sulfonylurea-treated patients to either orlistat 120 mg tid or placebo in addition to a low calorie diet [36]. After 1 year of treatment the orlistat group lost $6.2 \pm 0.5\%$ of initial body weight versus $4.3 \pm 0.5\%$ in the placebo group and twice as many subjects receiving orlistat lost $\geq 5\%$ of their initial body weight (48.8 vs. 22.6%, $p = 0.001$). Orlistat treated patients also achieved greater improvements in glycemic control than placebo (HbA1c change of –0.28% vs. +0.18%, respectively) resulting in a significant decrease in sulfonylurea dosage (23% vs. 9%, respectively). Fasting glucose (–0.02 mmol/L vs. +0.54 mmol/L, respectively) as well as fasting insulin

(–5.2% vs. +4.3%, respectively) also improved significantly in the orlistat group versus placebo. Similar results were also noted in patients who were previously being treated with metformin [37] or insulin [1]. The plethora of data available as well as the lack of cardiovascular and systemic side effects makes orlistat a reasonable therapeutic option in obese type 2 diabetics such as the patient illustrated in the case above.

> A 51-year-old female with a long-standing history of diabetes is referred for consultation for diabetes management. She reports that she was diagnosed with diabetes in her mid-thirties, was initially treated with oral hypoglycemic agents, and then started on insulin therapy 2 years ago. She reports that over the last 10 years, she has gained over 100 lbs despite trying various diet and exercise programs. She is currently unable to exercise due to severe pain in both knees. On exam BMI is 42 kg/m² and her blood pressure is 152/88 and pulse is 94. She has acanthosis nigricans in her axillae and neck. Bilateral nonproliferative retinopathy is present and deep tendon reflexes in the ankles are absent.

Bariatric surgery may be another option in individuals who fail to have adequate weight loss with pharmacologic therapies and lifestyle changes and who have a BMI of > 40 or a BMI ≥ 35 kg/m² in the presence of multiple, severe medical complications such as the case described above. Numerous techniques fall under this category, ranging from gastric banding to the Roux-en-Y gastric bypass. The later procedure is more complex, involving the exclusion of the majority of the stomach and anastamosis of a small gastric remnant to an enteric limb carrying food. The remainder of the stomach, duodenum and jejunum (carrying the bilio-pancreatic secretions) are anastamosed to the nutrient-carrying portion of the intestine at variable distances from the ileocolonic junction to allow digestion and absorption of food. A review of studies published between 1990 and 2006 revealed a total weight loss of 38.5 kg or 56% of excess body weight in patients with an average presurgery BMI of 47.9 kg/m² [38]. For patients with diabetes the total weight loss with all procedures was 40.6 kg (64% of excess body weight). This weight loss appears to persist for at least 2 years as trials with follow-up of greater than 2 years note a weight loss of 42.9 kg (58% of excess body weight). Overall, 78% of patients had a complete resolution and 87% experienced an improvement or resolution of the clinical and laboratory manifestations of diabetes with a mean decline in HbA1c of 2.1%, a fall in fasting glucose of 79 mg/dl, and reduction in fasting insulin of 98 µU/mL. The resolution of diabetes was least following the gastric banding procedure (56.7%) and greatest with the Roux-en-Y gastric bypass—95%. Other studies have also revealed an improvement in both morbidity and mortality in type 2 diabetics after bariatric surgery [38]. Despite the impressive benefits associated with bariatric surgery, it is associated with significant long- and short-term complications such as malabsorption, vitamin deficiencies, and anemia, which have not been fully studied in long-term trials (> 10 years of follow-up). Therefore, candidates for bariatric surgery should be well informed of these risks and benefits and be chosen carefully to ensure adequate follow-up.

The treatment of type 2 diabetes is quite taxing for both the patient as well as health care workers and requires significant resources. Currently, the obesity epidemic has made this situation even more difficult both in terms of the prevalence of diabetes and a worsening of its prognosis. Thus, it is paramount for health care professionals caring for patients with type 2 diabetes to focus on treatment of obesity, as even moderate amounts of weight loss can produce significant benefits. An ideal approach can address this issue through many different methods focusing on patient education, diet, exercise, and a tailoring of hypoglycemic therapy toward weight loss. If these techniques are unsuccessful in producing the desired effects, focus can shift toward assessing other methods such as weight loss drugs or even surgery in the appropriate candidates. Due to the diversity of the disease and the factors that have created it, a multifaceted approach, armed with an equally diverse set of tools, can better yield a successful and sustainable weight loss, along with a reversal of the morbid complications of obesity.

References

1. Maggio CA, Pi-Sunyer FX. Obesity and type 2 diabetes. *Endocrinol Metab Clin North Am.* **32**(4):805–822, viii, 2003.

2. Hu FB, Manson JE, Stampfer MJ, et al. Diet, lifestyle, and the risk of type 2 diabetes mellitus in women. *N Engl J Med.* **345**(11):790–797, 2001.

3. Must A, Spadano J, Coakley EH, Field AE, Colditz G, Dietz WH. The disease burden associated with overweight and obesity. *JAMA.* **282**(16):1523–1529, 1999.

4. Allison DB, Fontaine KR, Manson JE, Stevens J, VanItallie TB. Annual deaths attributable to obesity in the United States. *JAMA.* **282**(16):1530–1538, 1999.

5. Despres JP, Fong BS, Julien P, Jimenez J, Angel A. Regional variation in HDL metabolism in human fat cells: effect of cell size. *Am J Physiol Endocrinol Metab.* **252**(5):E654–E659, 1987.

6. Kissebah AH, Alfarsi S, Adams PW, Wynn V. Role of insulin resistance in adipose tissue and liver in the pathogenesis of endogenous hypertriglyceridaemia in man. *Diabetologia.* **12**(6):563–571, 1976.

7. Kannel WB, Garrison RJ, Dannenberg AL. Secular blood pressure trends in normotensive persons: the Framingham Study. *Am Heart J.* **125**(4):1154–1158, 1993.

8. Kissebah AH, Krakower GR. Regional adiposity and morbidity. *Physiol Rev.* **74**(4):761–811, 1994.

9. Despres J, Lemieux I, Bergeron J, et al. Abdominal obesity and the metabolic syndrome: contribution to global cardiometabolic risk. *Arterioscler Thromb Vasc Biol.* **28**(6):1039–1049, 2008.

10. Blackburn GL, Read JL. Benefits of reducing–revisited. *Postgrad Med J.* **60**(Suppl 3):13–18, 1984.

11. Knowler WC, Barrett-Connor E, Fowler SE, et al. Reduction in the incidence of type 2 diabetes with lifestyle intervention or metformin. *N Engl J Med.* **346**(6):393–403, 2002.

12. Knowler WC, Fowler SE, Hamman RF, et al. 10-year follow-up of diabetes incidence and weight loss in the Diabetes Prevention Program Outcomes Study. *Lancet.* **374**(9702):1677–1686, 2009.

13. UK prospective diabetes study 7: Response of fasting plasma glucose to diet therapy in newly presenting type II diabetic patients. *Metabolism.* **39**(9):905–912, 1990.

14. Henry RR, Gumbiner B. Benefits and limitations of very-low-calorie diet therapy in obese NIDDM. *Diabetes Care.* **14**(9):802–823, 1991.

15. Henry RR, Wallace P, Olefsky JM. Effects of weight loss on mechanisms of hyperglycemia in obese non-insulin-dependent diabetes mellitus. *Diabetes.* **35**(9):990–998, 1986.

16. Markovic TP, Campbell LV, Balasubramanian S, et al. Beneficial effect on average lipid levels from energy restriction and fat loss in obese individuals with or without type 2 diabetes. *Diabetes Care.* **21**(5):695–700, 1998.

17. Lean ME, Powrie JK, Anderson AS, Garthwaite PH. Obesity, weight loss and prognosis in type 2 diabetes. *Diabet Med.* **7**(3):228–233, 1990.

18. Wadden TA, Foster GD, Letizia KA. One-year behavioral treatment of obesity: comparison of moderate and severe caloric restriction and the effects of weight maintenance therapy. *J Consult Clin Psychol.* **62**(1):165–171, 1994.

19. Lissner L, Odell PM, D'Agostino RB, et al. Variability of body weight and health outcomes in the Framingham population. *N Engl J Med.* **324**(26):1839–1844, 1991.

20. Isner JM, Sours HE, Paris AL, Ferrans VJ, Roberts WC. Sudden, unexpected death in avid dieters using the liquid-protein-modified-fast diet. Observations in 17 patients and the role of the prolonged QT interval. *Circulation.* **60**(6):1401–1412, 1979.

21. Henry RR, Wiest-Kent TA, Scheaffer L, Kolterman OG, Olefsky JM. Metabolic consequences of very-low-calorie diet therapy in obese non-insulin-dependent diabetic and non-diabetic subjects. *Diabetes.* **35**(2):155–164, 1986.

22. Heilbronn LK, Noakes M, Clifton PM. Effect of energy restriction, weight loss, and diet composition on plasma lipids and glucose in patients with type 2 diabetes. *Diabetes Care.* **22**(6):889–895, 1999.

23. Executive Summary: Standards of Medical Care in Diabetes–2009 [Internet]. Diabetes Care. 2009 Jan 1 [cited 2009 Apr 24]; Available from: http://care. diabetesjournals. org.

24. Cusi K, Consoli A, DeFronzo R. Metabolic effects of metformin on glucose and lactate metabolism in noninsulin-dependent diabetes mellitus. *J Clin Endocrinol Metab.* **81**(11):4059–4067, 1996.

25. Golay A. Metformin and body weight. *Int J Obes.* **32**(1):61–72, 2007.

26. UKPDS. Effect of intensive blood-glucose control with metformin on complications in overweight patients with type 2 diabetes (UKPDS 34). *Lancet.* **352**(9131):854–865, 1998.

27. Kahn SE, Haffner SM, Heise MA, et al. Glycemic durability of rosiglitazone, metformin, or glyburide monotherapy. *N Engl J Med*. 355(23):2427–2443, 2006.

28. Virtanen KA, Hallsten K, Parkkola R, et al. Differential effects of rosiglitazone and metformin on adipose tissue distribution and glucose uptake in type 2 diabetic subjects. *Diabetes*. 52(2):283–290, 2003.

29. Hanefeld M, Brunetti P, Schernthaner GH, Matthews DR, Charbonnel BH. One-year glycemic control with a sulfonylurea plus pioglitazone versus a sulfonylurea plus metformin in patients with type 2 diabetes. *Diabetes Care*. 27(1):141–147, 2004.

30. Chia CW, Egan JM. Incretin-based therapies in type 2 diabetes mellitus. *J Clin Endocrinol Metab*. 93(10):3703–3716, 2008.

31. Klonoff DC, Buse JB, Nielsen LL, et al. Exenatide effects on diabetes, obesity, cardiovascular risk factors and hepatic biomarkers in patients with type 2 diabetes treated for at least 3 years. *Curr Med Res Opin*. 24(1):275–286, 2008.

32. Vilsboll T, Zdravkovic M, Le-Thi T, et al. Liraglutide, a long-acting human glucagon-like peptide-1 analog, given as monotherapy significantly improves glycemic control and lowers body weight without risk of hypoglycemia in patients with type 2 diabetes. *Diabetes Care*. 30(6):1608–1610, 2007.

33. Nauck MA, Hompesch M, Filipczak R, Le TDT, Zdravkovic M, Gumprecht J. Five weeks of treatment with the GLP-1 analogue liraglutide improves glycaemic control and lowers body weight in subjects with type 2 diabetes. *Exp Clin Endocrinol Diabetes*. 114(8):417–423, 2006.

34. McNulty SJ, Ur E, Williams G. A randomized trial of sibutramine in the management of obese type 2 diabetic patients treated with metformin. *Diabetes Care*. 26(1):125–131, 2003.

35. Choussein S, Makri AA, Frangos CC, Petridou ET, Daskalopoulou SS. Effect of antiobesity medications in patients with type 2 diabetes mellitus. *Diabetes Obes Metab* [Internet]. 2009 Feb 18 [cited 2009 Apr 24]; Available from: http://www.ncbi.nlm.nih.gov/pubmed/19236442.

36. Hollander PA, Elbein SC, Hirsch IB, et al. Role of orlistat in the treatment of obese patients with type 2 diabetes. A 1-year randomized double-blind study. *Diabetes Care*. 21(8):1288–1294, 1998.

37. Miles JM, Leiter L, Hollander P, et al. Effect of orlistat in overweight and obese patients with type 2 diabetes treated with metformin. *Diabetes care*. 25(7):1123–1128, 2002.

38. Buchwald H, Estok R, Fahrbach K, et al. Weight and type 2 diabetes after bariatric surgery: systematic review and meta-analysis. *Am J Med*. 122(3):248–256.e5, 2009.

39. Bland JM, Kerry SM. Weighted comparison of means. *BMJ*. 316(7125):129, 1998.

13 Are statins the optimal therapy for cardiovascular risk in patients with diabetes? Are triglycerides an important independent risk factor for diabetes?

Michael O'Reilly[1] and Timothy O'Brien[2]

[1]Specialist Registrar in Endocrinology/Diabetes Mellitus, Department of Medicine and Endocrinology/Diabetes Mellitus, University College Hospital/National University of Ireland, Galway, Ireland
[2]Professor of Medicine, Consultant Endocrinologist/Director of REMEDI, Department of Medicine and Endocrinology/Diabetes Mellitus, University College Hospital/National University of Ireland Galway, Galway, Ireland

LEARNING POINTS

- Dyslipidemia is part of the adverse cardiovascular risk profile in type 2 diabetes mellitus.

- Syndrome X (the metabolic syndrome) refers to a constellation of abnormalities that frequently cluster together in type 2 diabetes.

- Therapy with statins is an important part of primary and secondary cardiovascular disease prevention in diabetes.

- Hypertriglyceridemia is an independent risk fact for cardiovascular disease in diabetes.

Dyslipidemia in type 2 diabetes

Type 2 diabetes mellitus (T2DM) is associated with a two- to fourfold increase in the risk of coronary heart disease compared to the nondiabetic population [1]. Dyslipidemia is the best-characterized risk factor for atherosclerosis in patients with T2DM. A number of features of dyslipidemia are characteristically associated with diabetes mellitus, increasing the predisposition to atherosclerosis. The most common derangement of lipid profile in diabetes mellitus is elevated triglycerides and decreased HDL cholesterol levels associated with increased circulating concentrations of remnant particles and a preponderance of dense LDL cholesterol particles [2].

Although LDL cholesterol levels in T2DM are not significantly different from the nondiabetic population, qualitative abnormalities of this lipid fraction exist [2]. For instance, patients with diabetes mellitus typically have smaller, denser LDL particles with likely increased atherogenicity, even if the total LDL concentration is not increased. In addition, studies have shown that the ratio of esterified to free cholesterol is increased in the LDL particle in diabetes mellitus [3]. This leads to increased oxidation of LDL particles, which increases the delivery of cholesterol to atherosclerotic plaques via macrophage uptake. Oxidized LDL is also known to be increased in T2DM [4]. Glycation of LDL is also believed to increase the atherogenicity of the particle by increasing the susceptibility to oxidation, and also increasing free radical production.

Levels of the cardioprotective lipid fraction, HDL cholesterol, are decreased in patients with diabetes mellitus. HDL particles are known to protect LDL from oxidation through paraoxonase activity. HDL composition is also altered in subjects with elevated plasma triglycerides [5].

Hypertriglyceridemia is the most common lipoprotein abnormality found in poorly controlled diabetes mellitus. The pathophysiology underlying hypertriglyceridaemia in T2DM is complex and is caused by disturbances in fatty acid metabolism. The key feature of diabetic dyslipidemia appears to be an increase in production of very low density lipoprotein (VLDL) by the liver in response to elevations

Clinical Dilemmas in Diabetes, First Edition. Edited by Adrian Vella and Robert A. Rizza
© 2011 Blackwell Publishing Ltd. Published 2011 by Blackwell Publishing Ltd.

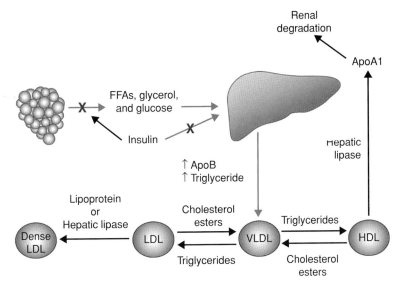

FIG 13.1 Insulin resistance and dyslipidemia. The suppression of lipoprotein lipase and very-low-density lipoprotein (VLDL) production by insulin is defective in insulin resistance leading to increased free fatty acid (FFA) flux to the liver and increased VLDL production, which results in increased circulating triglyceride concentrations. The triglycerides are transferred to low-density lipoprotein (LDL) and high-density liporotein (HDL), and the VLDL particle gains cholesterol esters by the action of the cholesterol ester transfer protein (CETP). This leads to increased catabolism of HDL particles by the liver and loss of apolipoprotein (Apo) A, resulting in low HDL concentrations. The triglyceride-rich LDL particle is stripped of the triglycerides, resulting in the accumulation of atherogenic small, dense LDL particles. (Copyright © 2008 by Saunders, an imprint of Elsevier Inc. All rights reserved)

in free fatty acids (FFAs). Insulin suppresses lipolysis, and mediates uptake of FFAs by striated muscle. Insulin resistance leads to derangements in this process, with increasing levels of FFAs available to the liver. This disorder is characterized by the accumulation of apo-B-containing lipoproteins, which are proatherogenic, in the plasma. In fact, fasting nonesterified free fatty acid (NEFA) levels are an independent predictor of insulin sensitivity [6], and elevations are the first lipid abnormality in impaired glucose tolerance. In addition, insulin-dependent lipoprotein lipase activity is defective in T2DM. This leads to an accumulation of triglyceride-rich lipoproteins in the plasma and a delay in the clearance of chylomicrons and VLDL with a consequent increase in remnant particles (Figure 13.1).

It is important to bear in mind, however, that as in non-diabetic individuals, lipids levels can be deranged independently of hyperglycemia or defective insulin action. Secondary causes of dyslipidemia such as renal disease, hypothyroidism, and genetically determined lipoprotein disorders (e.g., familial combined hyperlipidemia and familial hypertriglyceridemia) must be taken into consideration. Furthermore, alcohol, oestrogen, and antiretroviral agents may induce abnormalities of plasma lipids.

Syndrome X, or the metabolic syndrome, refers to a constellation of metabolic derangements frequently found in T2DM that are individually and continually associated with an increased risk of cardiovascular disease. These include low HDL cholesterol, elevated triglycerides, small, easily oxidized LDL molecules, and elevated serum uric acid concentration [7]. Central obesity and hypertension are usually clinically manifest. There is a strong association between the metabolic syndrome and incidence and mortality of cardiovascular disease. A Finnish Prospective cohort study showed the age-adjusted relative risk (RR) for coronary heart disease (CHD) mortality was 2.96 (95% CI 1.31–3.21) [8]. Hyperinsulinemia is likely the underlying link between hyperglycemia and CVD in these patients; several studies have shown elevated fasting insulin levels to be an independent predictor of CVD risk [9].

There are different sets of diagnostic criteria for the metabolic syndrome that have been published by the National Cholesterol Education Program (NCEP) Adult

Treatment Panel III (ATP III) (see Box 13.1), the World Health Organisation (WHO), and the International Diabetes Federation (IDF). It is important to remember that risk is conferred by the underlying risk factors and the definition of metabolic syndrome is an arbitrary aggregation of risk factors whose presence or absence is defined by discrete cut points. In practice, risk is conferred continuously.

Treatment of dyslipidemia in patients with diabetes mellitus

Evidence for treatment of dyslipidemia in T2DM for primary and secondary prevention of cardiovascular disease is well established (Figure 13.2). Hydroxymethylglutaryl coenzyme A reductase inhibitors (statins) have a particularly strong evidence base in several large trials in diabetic patients with and without CHD. In 1997, the Scandinavian Simvastatin Survival Study (4S) looked at 202 diabetic and 4242 nondiabetic subjects with known CHD treated with simvastatin or placebo for 5 years [10]. The RR of major CHD events (nonfatal myocardial infarction or revascularization) and mortality was 0.45 and 0.57, respectively. Subsequently in the Cholesterol and Recurrent Events (CARE) trial, pravastatin use in diabetes patients with established CHD had a significant 25% reduction in the incidence of CHD death, nonfatal myocardial infarction (MI), coronary artery bypass graft (CABG) surgery, and revascularization procedures [11]. Subgroup analysis of diabetes patients in the Long-term Intervention with Pravastatin in Ischemic Disease (LIPID) study showed a 19% reduction in major

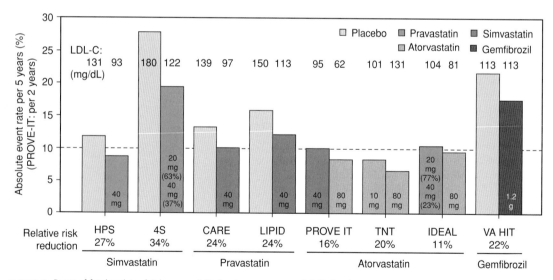

FIG 13.2 Rates of fatal and nonfatal myocardial infarction on recent major lipid-lowering trials conducted in patients with CHD or CHD-equivalent disorders. In all trials, lower LDL-C levels were associated with lower event rates. The relative risk reductions were 11% to 34%. Absolute event rates approached 10% per 5 years (2% per year) for all patients in all trials irrespective of treatment. In PROVE-IT (Pravastatin or Atorvastatin Evaluation and Infection Therapy), the only trial of patients with acute coronary syndrome, the 2-year event rate was 8.3% despite average on-treatment LDL-C = 1.61 mM/L(62 mg/dL). 4S, Scandinavian simvastatin survival study; CARE, cholesterol and recurrent events; IDEAL, incremental decrease in endpoints through aggressive lipid lowering; LIPID, long-term intervention with pravastatin in ischemic disease; TNT, treating to new targets; VA-HIT, Veterans Administration HDL intervention trial. (Copyright © 2008 by Saunders, an imprint of Elsevier Inc. All rights reserved)

CHD (fatal and nonfatal myocardial infarction) [12]. Haffer et al. studied simvastatin therapy across a range of glucose tolerance from normal to diabetes; treatment significantly reduced major adverse cardiovascular events and revascularization procedures in patients with diabetes mellitus. In the subgroup with impaired glucose tolerance, simvastatin treatment was also associated with a significant reduction in total and coronary mortality [13].

The Heart Protection Study (HPS) published in the *Lancet* in 2002 was a large, randomized placebo-controlled trial that examined the use of simvastatin 40 mg in 20,536 high-risk patients over 5 years [14]. Of this large number of study participants, 29% had T2DM. Treatment with simvastatin resulted in a significant reduction in major vascular events in patients with T2DM who had previous MI or other coronary artery disease (33.4% vs. 37.8% in simvastatin- and placebo-treated patients, respectively). This benefit extended to patients with T2DM who had no previous CHD (13.8% vs. 18.6%), and in both groups combined (20.2% vs. 25.1%). The HPS also demonstrated a significant 12% relative risk reduction in all-cause mortality, and an 18% relative risk reduction in coronary mortality in all patients in the simvastatin group. This study suggested that the benefit of statins was also seen in patients with "normal" LDL cholesterol, implying that all patients with diabetes mellitus should be treated with a statin regardless of LDL cholesterol levels.

The most recent large-scale intervention study for primary prevention in T2DM, the Collaborative Atorvastatin Diabetes Study (CARDS), demonstrated that 10 mg atorvastatin was beneficial [15]. This was a large ($n = 2838$) randomized, placebo-controlled trial that assessed the benefit of atorvastatin 10 mg od in the prevention of acute coronary heart disease events, coronary revascularization or stroke in patients with T2DM with no previous history of CVD and plasma LDL <160 mg/dL (<4.08 mmol/L). This study was terminated two years early after prespecified efficacy criteria were met. Patients treated with atorvastatin had a relative risk reduction of 37% of first cardiovascular events after a median of 3.9 years (95% CI −52, −17; $p = 0.001$) compared with placebo-treated patients. Acute coronary heart disease-related events were reduced by 36%, coronary revascularization by 31% and stroke by 48%. Benefit emerged within one year of initiating therapy.

The Treating to New Targets (TNT) study published in the Lancet in 2006 was an international, multicentre, double-blind trial that randomized 10,003 with clinically evident CHD who also met NCEP criteria for diagnosis of the metabolic syndrome to treatment with 10 mg or 80 mg of atorvastatin for a period of 4.9 years [16]. The study included 778 patients with T2DM (22% of study population). Treatment with 80 mg of atorvastatin was significantly more effective in reducing major cardiovascular events than the 10 mg dose (HR = 0.71, 95% CI 0.61–0.84, $p < 0.0001$). This is presumably due to the significantly greater reduction in LDL cholesterol in the aggressive treatment group. The relative risk of stroke alone in the 80 mg atorvastatin was 23% lower at the end of the study. There was also a 26% drop in risk of hospitalization for congestive cardiac failure in the aggressive treatment group. This was the first randomized trial to demonstrate the benefits of lowering LDL cholesterol below 2.6 mmol/L in patients with stable coronary artery disease. These benefits included a 22% reduced risk of cardiovascular events and a 25% reduction in the risk of stroke. Both of these benefits were achieved without additional significant safety risks in the high-dose group. When the percentage of patients with new CHD events was plotted against the average achieved LDL cholesterol in the TNT study compared with other major secondary prevention statin trials, the relationship remained linear, indicating that levelling of the effect of LDL cholesterol lowering did not occur in TNT. In other words, the LDL level below which vascular events ceased was not reached in this study.

Based on the literature at the time of writing, all patients with T2DM should be on statin therapy regardless of LDL cholesterol. As the TNT demonstrated, a lower LDL level below which vascular events no longer occur has not been reached. While target LDL cholesterol has traditionally been below 2.6 mmol/L, the TNT suggests that a target of ≤ 1.8 mmol/L may be reasonable. The ATP III guidelines have been updated to reflect this point, and suggest that the latter target may be very appropriate for those high-risk patients with T2DM and established CHD. However, aggressive pharmacotherapy with high-dose statins is not without side effects, and the likelihood of adverse events such as hepatotoxicity or myositis increases in a dose-dependent manner. Current ADA guidelines suggest an LDL cholesterol target of below 100 mg/dl (2.6 mmol/L) in patients both with and without CHD. Desirable HDL cholesterol levels are above 40 mg/dl (1.02 mmol/L). However, the lower the LDL cholesterol that can be achieved, the greater the reduction in vascular risk. This must be balanced against potential adverse effects of lipid-lowering therapy, and the clinician must thus target the lowest LDL possible with the maximum tolerated lipid-lowering agent.

The above literature refers almost exclusively to the management of dyslipidemia in patients with type 2 diabetes mellitus. Indeed, there is a paucity of evidence on the benefits of statin therapy in primary prevention in type 1 diabetes mellitus (T1DM). This group does have an increased incidence of CHD than nondiabetic patients, but diabetes is usually diagnosed at a young age when the absolute incidence of CHD is negligible. The benefit of statin therapy in T1DM has not been proven, given the very small numbers of these patients included in statin trials. A small number of patients with T1DM were included in HPS. Although they received a similar benefit to the diabetic group as a whole, this failed to reach statistical significance due to the small size of the group. It remains uncertain when to initiate statin therapy in people with T1DM; nevertheless, it seems reasonable to extrapolate the trial data from type 2 to type 1 diabetes.

While there is now a very large evidence base supporting the use of statins in T2DM, even in patients with "normal" LDL cholesterol levels, there still exists a significant increase in adverse outcomes related to coronary artery disease in statin-treated patients. This fact has been referred to as the *residual risk*. Attention is now focusing on how the residual risk may be further reduced in patients with diabetes mellitus and whether additional attention to CVD risk factors such as hypertriglyceridemia may be therapeutically beneficial.

Evidence linking hypertriglyceridemia to CHD risk in diabetes mellitus

Elevated LDL cholesterol is well established as a risk factor for cardiovascular disease in patients with normal and abnormal glucose metabolism. But what evidence do we have that elevated triglycerides, the most common lipid abnormality in T2DM, poses a cardiovascular risk independently of hyperglycaemia, elevated LDL, and low HDL? Is there evidence in the literature that lowering serum triglycerides reduces CHD risk and clinical outcomes? Growing evidence indicates that hypertriglyceridemia may be an independent risk factor for CAD in type 2 DM [17]. However, whether the atherogenicity is due to triglyceride particles per se, or to their metabolic consequences, is a matter of debate. In 1996, a Finnish group calculated that serum triglycerides were the major determinant of LDL size in both diabetic and nondiabetic subjects [18]. They con-

cluded that serum triglyceride levels should be kept as low as possible in subjects with T2DM to prevent atherogenic changes in LDL. Indeed there is growing epidemiological evidence to suggest that hypertriglyceridemia is a strong risk factor for CHD. The Paris Prospective Study in 1989 looked at 943 men with diabetes or impaired glucose tolerance and found that elevated triglycerides were a risk factor for CHD, but did not find that this risk was independent of cholesterol [19]. During a mean follow-up of 11 years, 26 of these 943 patients with abnormal glucose metabolism died from CHD. The distribution of plasma triglyceride level was clearly higher for the subjects who died from CHD compared to those who did not die from this cause or were alive at the end of follow-up.

More recently, the Hoorn study has shown hypertriglyceridemia to be an independent risk factor in patients with abnormal glucose metabolism [20]. In this population-based cohort study, which began in 1989, 869 men and 948 women had participated. The aim of the study was to investigate the association of triglyceride and non-HDL cholesterol concentration with cardiovascular disease in subjects with and without abnormal glucose metabolism. After 10 years, the age and sex-adjusted hazard ratios for cardiovascular disease were 1.35 (1.11–1.64) and 1.71 (1.40–2.08) for high triglycerides and high non-HDL cholesterol, respectively. After adjustment for abnormalities in glucose metabolism, the hazard ratios for non-HDL cholesterol were 1.71 (1.31–2.21) in normal glucose metabolism and 1.56 (1.12–2.18) in abnormal glucose metabolism. Triglycerides were not a risk factor for cardiovascular disease in subjects with normal glucose metabolism (HR 0.94; CI 0.73–1.22); however, in patients with abnormal glucose metabolism, the hazard ratio for cardiovascular disease was 1.54 (1.07–1.22). In subjects with abnormal glucose metabolism, the hazard ratio for the combined presence of high triglycerides and non-HDL cholesterol was 2.12 (1.35–3.34) (Table 13.1).

There is a large body of evidence that implicates hypertriglyceridemia as a risk factor for cardiovascular disease in both diabetic and nondiabetic patients [21, 22]. A large 1996 meta-analysis of 17 prospective trials with 57,000 patients also concluded that elevated triglycerides are a risk factor for CHD in nondiabetic subjects also [23]. There are several possible explanations for the discrepancy in contribution of hypertriglyceridemia to CHD risk in euglycemic and dysglycemic subjects. High fasting and, in particular, postprandial triglyceride levels in patients with abnormal glucose metabolism are due to defective insulin action in the liver

TABLE 13.1 Hazard ratios (95% CI) of cardiovascular disease (CVD) for medians of triglycerides (TG) and non-HDL-cholesterol, stratified for glucose metabolism (from [20]).

	Normal glucose metabolism			Abnormal glucose metabolism		
	n	Cases	CVD	n	Cases	CVD
Dichotomised						
Age- and sex-adjusted						
High TG[a]	547	112	1.10 (0.86–1.41)	314	111	1.67 (1.16–2.39)[d]
High non-HDL[b]	647	153	1.67 (1.30–2.15)	260	95	1.67 (1.20–2.33)
Mutually adjusted[c]						
High TG	547	112	0.94 (0.73–1.22)[d]	314	111	1.54 (1.07–2.22)[d]
High non-HDL	647	153	1.70 (1.31–2.21)[d]	260	95	1.56 (1.12–2.18)[d]
Multivariate model[e]						
High TG	529	105	0.70 (0.53–0.92)	303	106	1.48 (1.00–2.20)
High non-HDL	629	144	1.54 (1.17–2.03)	253	90	1.20 (0.84–1.71)
Combined categories						
Age- and sex-adjusted						
Low non-HDL, low TG	509	75	1	107	25	1
Low non-HDL, high TG	181	28	0.96 (0.62–1.48)	113	32	1.03 (0.55–1.93)
High non-HDL, low TG	281	69	1.71(1.23–2.37)	59	16	1.13 (0.67–1.91)
High non-HDL, high TG	366	84	1.60 (1.17–2.19)	201	79	2.12 (1.35–3.34)
Multivariate model[e]						
Low non-HDL, low TG	497	72	1	105	24	1
Low nonHDL, high TG	173	25	0.69 (0.44–1.10)	109	32	1.38 (0.79–2.41)
High non-HDL, low TG	273	64	1.54 (1.09–2.16)	59	16	1.09 (0.57–2.07)
High non-HDL, high TG	356	80	1.07 (0.77–1.50)	194	74	1.73 (1.06–2.81)

a Cut-off points for triglycerides are 1.4 mmol/l in men and 1.3 mmol/l in women (medians)

b Cut-off points for non-HDL-cholesterol are 5.2 mmol/l in men and 5.3 mmol/l in women (medians)

c Age- and sex-adjusted

d Interaction between triglyceride*non-HDL-cholesterol*glucose metabolism status $p = 0.14$

e Adjusted for age, sex, waist-to-hip ratio, hypertension, prevalent cardiovascular disease, smoking and alcohol consumption and peripheral tissues. This results in impaired suppression of hepatic VLDL production, reduced lipoprotein lipase activity and impaired clearance of triglyceride-rich particles due to competition for the same pathways. The net effect of this is the persistence of atherogenic triglyceride-rich particles in the circulation in patients with abnormal glucose metabolism. These particles last longer than in patients with normal glucose metabolism, and have increased atherogenicity.

Many epidemiological studies have reported on associations between high triglycerides and the risk of CHD. Sarwar et al. reported primary data on triglyceride concentrations from two prospective cohort studies in *Circulation* in 2007: the Rejkavik study and the European Prospective Investigation of Cancer (EPIC)–Norfolk study, which in total comprised 44,237 Western middle-aged men and women (predominantly Caucasian) and a total of 3582 incident cases of CHD (including 1089 female cases) [24]. In addition, previous meta-analyses were updated with a further 12 studies, providing information from a total of >10,000 CHD cases from 29 Western studies involving a total of 260,000 participants. After adjustment for baseline values of several established risk factors, odds ratio for CHD was 1.76 (95% CI, 1.39–2.21) in the Rejkavik study and 1.57 (95% CI, 1.10–2.24) in the EPIC-Norfolk study in a com-

parison of individuals in the top third with those in the bottom third of the usual log-triglyceride values. Similar overall findings (adjusted odds ratio, 1.72; 95% CI, 1.56–1.90) were observed in the updated meta-analysis involving a total of 10,158 cases of incident CHD from 262,525 participants in 29 studies (Figure 13.3). Although these data were not adjusted for normal and abnormal glucose metabolism, they indicate consistent, moderate, and highly significant associations between triglyceride and CHD risk.

Nordestgaard et al. examined the hypothesis that very high levels of nonfasting triglycerides were predictors of myocardial infarction, ischemic heart disease, and death [25]. This was a prospective cohort study of 7587 women and 6394 men from the general Danish population followed from 1976 to 2004. Baseline nonfasting triglycerides were stratified into categories of increasing severity of hypertriglyceridemia, and compared to triglyceride levels of less than 88.5 mg/dl (1 mmol/L). Nonfasting triglyceride levels of 5 mmol/L or more (≥442.5 mg/dl) were found to be predictive of CHD. This study also supported the concept that nonfasting triglyceride levels more strongly predict CHD risk than levels measured after a 12- to 14-hour fast. Postprandial lipoproteins are generally triglyceride-rich, and if an individual has a predisposition to small, dense LDL cholesterol or has insulin resistance, then clearance of these

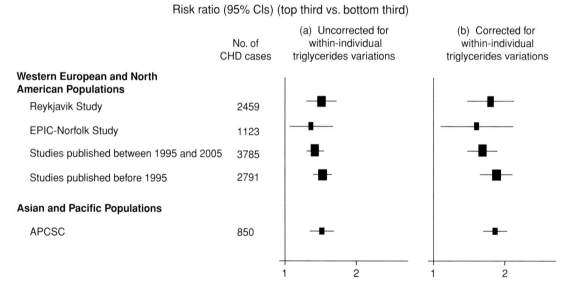

FIG 13.3 Available prospective studies of triglycerides and CHD in essentially general populations. APCSC indicates Asian and Pacific Cohort Studies Collaboration. *Includes three studies that were published before 1995 but were not included in the previous review from [24]).

lipoprotein particles can be delayed for up to 12 hours. The authors thus postulate that prolonged exposure of the endothelium to triglyceride-rich, atherogenic remnant particles, or the associated states in which atherogenic lipoprotein particles occur, such as obesity or the metabolic syndrome, may explain why nonfasting triglycerides are more predictive of CHD risk. Data from this study also suggested that women have greater risk associated with hypertriglyceridemia than men. The risk for atherosclerosis-related events is significantly increased when triglyceride levels are between 150 mg/dl and 1000 mg/dl (1.7–11.3 mmol/L), but whether this is the cause or effect remains unclear. Most previous studies on triglycerides have focused on fasting levels that exclude remnant lipoproteins. However, a previous Norwegian study found that nonfasting triglyceride levels of 3.5 mmol/L or more (≥309.7 mg/dl) versus less than 1.5 mmol/L (<132.7 mg/dl) was associated with a fivefold risk of death from coronary heart disease and a twofold risk of total death in women. Again it should be emphasized that these data were not adjusted for normal and abnormal glucose metabolism; however, studies to date indicate that if anything, the predictive value of triglycerides as a risk factor for CHD is even stronger in the setting of dysglycemia, as demonstrated in the Hoorn study.

There is strong epidemiological evidence to date that hypertriglyceridemia in an independent risk factor for CHD. Prospective randomized controlled trials examining this link are difficult, given the large number of patients with diabetes who are already on statin treatment (which modestly lower triglycerides) and the presence of other lipoprotein and metabolic derangements that may confound results. The data summarized above, however, suggest a consistent link between elevated plasma triglycerides and cardiovascular disease, and that this effect is more pronounced in patients with abnormal glucose tolerance.

Evidence that treating hypertriglyceridemia will reduce CV risk in DM

Pharmacological interventions for hypertriglyceridemia include fibrates, niacin (nicotinic acid), and omega-3 fish oils. The Fenofibrate Intervention and Event Lowering in Diabetes (FIELD) study assessed the effect of long-term fenofibrate therapy on cardiovascular events in patients with T2DM [26]. Patients were randomized to receive either micronized fenofibrate 200 mg qd (n = 4895) or placebo

(n = 4900). Marked hypertriglyceridemia (≥2.3 mmol/L) was associated with a higher CVD risk than merely meeting criteria for the metabolic syndrome, independent of HDL cholesterol. Multivariate modeling confirmed the independent contributions of HDL cholesterol, triglyceride levels, and blood pressure to CVD risk. This supports a continuous positive relationship between triglyceride concentrations and CVD. After 5 years of follow-up, coronary events were observed in 5.9% of placebo patients and 5.2% of fenofibrate-treated patients, but this difference was not statistically significant. However, fenofibrate treatment did significantly reduce total CVD events (HR 0.89, 95% CI 0.75–1.05, p = 0.035), coronary revascularization, progression of albuminuria, and the need for laser treatment of retinopathy. There was a significant 24% reduction in nonfatal MI, outcome of first MI, or CHD death. The secondary outcome of total cardiovascular disease events (the composite of cardiovascular disease death, myocardial infarction, stroke, and coronary and carotid revascularization) was significantly reduced by fenofibrate. It is possible that statistical significance was not reached for the primary end point due to the fact that, by the end of the study, 17% of the placebo patients were taking lipid-lowering agents (nonstudy drug, e.g., statins) compared with 8% in the fenofibrate group, thus masking the treatment effect. The effect of fibrates is to lower triglycerides by >25%. Individuals with elevated triglycerides thus appear to obtain the greatest benefits from fibrates in the study.

In the Bezafibrate Infarction Prevention (BIP), 3090 patients with a previous myocardial infarction or stable angina, total cholesterol of 180 to 250 mg/dl, HDL cholesterol <45 mg/dl, triglycerides <300 mg/dl, and LDL cholesterol <180 mg/dl were randomized to receive either 400 mg of bezafibrate daily or placebo, and followed for a mean of 6.2 years [27]. Bezafibrate reduced triglycerides by 21% and raised HDL cholesterol by 18%. No difference was apparent in the all-cause and cardiac mortality between the bezafibrate and placebo groups. However, on post hoc analysis, there was a significant reduction in the primary end point in 459 patients with high baseline triglycerides (≥200 mg/dl or 2.26 mmol/L). The reduction in the cumulative probability of the primary end point by bezafibrate was 39.5% (p = 0.02). Bezafibrate may thus have a prominent role in the management of dyslipidemia and CHD when targeted to a subgroup of patients with CHD. This supports the evidence from meta-analyses and epidemiological studies that triglycerides are indeed an independent risk factor for CHD in patients with both normal and abnormal glucose metabolism. The authors subsequently evaluated the effect of bezafibrate on the incidence of MI in patients enrolled in the BIP study who met the criteria for the metabolic syndrome [28]. The study sample for this post hoc subgroup analysis comprised 1470 patients aged 42 to 74 years who were randomly assigned to receive bezafibrate 400 mg daily (740 patients) or placebo (730 patients). The follow-up period was 6.2 years for events and 8.1 years for mortality data. New myocardial infarction was recorded in 82 patients from the bezafibrate group (11.1%) and 111 patients (15.2%) from the placebo group ($p = 0.02$). Bezafibrate was associated with a reduced risk of any MI and nonfatal MI with hazard ratios of 0.71 (95% CI, 0.54–0.95) and 0.67 (95% CI, 0.49–0.91) respectively. The cardiac mortality risk tended to be lower in patients taking bezafibrate (HR, 0.74; 95% CI, 0.54–1.03). However, post hoc analysis on the effect on MI risk of specifically lowering triglycerides within this group with metabolic syndrome was not performed. The primary prevention trial, the Helsinki Heart study, also showed that treatment with the fibric acid derivative gemfibrozil significantly reduced major cardiovascular events.

The Diabetes Atherosclerosis Intervention Study (DAIS) demonstrated that reduction of triglycerides with fibrates has coronary angiographic benefit [29]. This study was designed to assess the effects of correcting lipoprotein abnormalities with fenofibrate on coronary atherosclerosis in T2DM. DAIS took place in 11 clinical centres in Canada, Finland, France, and Sweden. In this study, 731 men and women with T2DM were screened by metabolic and angiographic criteria; of these, 418 were randomly assigned to receive fenofibrate 200 mg daily or placebo for at least 3 years. Half of the participants had a clinical history of coronary disease, making this a primary and secondary prevention trial. Total plasma cholesterol, HDL cholesterol, LDL cholesterol, and triglyceride concentrations all changed significantly more than baseline in the fenofibrate group ($n = 207$) than in the placebo group ($n = 211$). The fenofibrate group showed a significantly smaller increase in percentage diameter stenosis on coronary angiogram than the placebo group (mean 2.11 vs. 3.65, $p = 0.02$). Although the trial was not powered to examine clinical end points, there were fewer in the fenofibrate than placebo group (38 vs. 50). Although there was angiographic benefit in the setting of reduction of hypertriglyceridemia, as in most trials on triglycerides, it is difficult to deduce if this is a direct triglyceride-lowering effect or the result of correction of other lipoprotein abnormalities.

Other agents effective at lowering triglycerides include niacin (nicotinic acid) and fish oils. However, the evidence for these agents in T2DM is relatively sparse, and most trials focus on elevation of HDL cholesterol and cardiac end points rather than the effects of lower serum triglycerides. The Arterial Biology for the Investigation of the Treatment Effects of Reducing Cholesterol (ARBITER) was a randomized, double-blind study in which patients were assigned to receive extended-release niacin 500 mg titrated to 1000 mg qid ($n = 87$) or placebo ($n = 80$) on a background statin therapy [30]. The primary end point of the study was change in carotid intima media thickness (CIMT) after 1 year of niacin treatment. Despite a significant 21% increase in HDL cholesterol levels in patients receiving niacin, the overall difference in CIMT progression between the niacin- and placebo-treated groups only tended toward significance ($p = 0.08$). No studies on niacin have been conducted in diabetes due to concerns with regard to worsening of hyperglycemia. However, although niacin at a dose of <2.5 g/day increases fasting glucose by 4–5% and HbA1C by ~0.3%, these increases are modest, transient, and reversible, and typically amenable to adjustments in oral hypoglycemic regimens without discontinuing niacin. Two large trials on the addition of niacin to statin therapy that include patients with diabetes mellitus—AIM-HIGH and HPS2-THRIVE—are currently underway. These are primarily targeted at increasing HDL cholesterol in patients at target LDL but will provide useful information.

Discussion

Hypertriglyceridemia is associated with a constellation of metabolic abnormalities, most notably those that comprise the metabolic syndrome. While the metabolic syndrome and fasting hyperinsulinemia are recognized as independent risk factors for CHD, whether elevated triglycerides represent an independent marker of cardiovascular risk remains controversial. The approach to diabetic patients with LDL cholesterol at or below target but who have elevated plasma triglycerides and low HDL cholesterol is equally a matter of some debate. However, a mounting body of epidemiological evidence, including several meta-analyses over the past 20 years, as reviewed above, suggests that hypertriglyceridemia may confer additional risk, and that this risk may be greater in patients with abnormal glucose metabolism. Post hoc analysis of several large prospective trials mentioned above has also pointed toward an increased CHD risk with elevated plasma triglycerides. More recent interventional and intention-to-treat trials have shown varying degrees of clinical benefit in treating hypertriglyceridemia in diabetes mellitus. Such clinical outcomes range from improved CHD mortality and improved outcomes to angiographic benefit and coronary plaque regression. Ongoing studies such as ACCORD will provide additional information.

We suggest that all patients with T2DM should be on a statin to lower LDL cholesterol and thus reduce cardiovascular risk. The ADA currently recommends initiating a statin for primary prevention when LDL cholesterol is above 3.36 mmol/L (130 mg/dl), with the goal of reducing LDL to less than 2.57 mmol/L (100 mg/dl). Target LDL cholesterol on current guidelines is less than 2.6 mmol/L; we recommend the lowest possible LDL based on trial data from TNT. ATP III would suggest that a target of LDL cholesterol < 70 mg/dl (1.8 mmol/L) may be reasonable in patients with T2DM and CHD. This however must be taken in the context of increased risk of adverse events related to statin-lowering therapy on larger doses of these agents. Optimal HDL-cholesterol levels are >40 mg/dl (1.02 mmol/L) in men; a higher target may be more desirable in women (>50 mg/dl or 1.28 mmol/L) based on physiologically higher HDL levels in the female population. Raising HDL levels pharmacologically in patients with diabetes is very difficult, since the most effective agent increasing HDL is nicotinic acid, which is relatively contraindicated in diabetes mellitus.

The evidence is lacking in patients with T1DM but it is reasonable to extrapolate much of this data to this category of patient, in particular those with microalbuminuria. Patients with T1DM are typically younger, and therefore clinical experience and intuition is required in this group with regard to initiation of statin therapy. One approach is to commence patients with T1DM on statin therapy above the age of 30 years, or once micro- or macrovascular complications have developed.

We agree with current ADA guidelines that triglycerides are a recognized target for intervention in diabetes and that optimal triglyceride levels are <150 mg/dl (1.7 mmol/L). Initial therapeutic intervention for hypertriglyceridemia is behavioural modification with weight loss, increased physical activity, and moderation of alcohol consumption. Improving glycemic control will also lower triglycerides.

When LDL cholesterol is at or below target, but triglycerides are elevated and HDL cholesterol suboptimal (as in the introductory case to this chapter), the physician may consider adding a fibrate, niacin, or fish oil therapy. For more modest hypertriglyceridemia (1.7–3.0 mmol/L), fibrates such as fenofibrate, gemfibrozil, or bezafibrate can be considered as an adjunct to statin therapy. Nicotinic acid may also be used in combination with statins but must be used with caution in diabetes as the combination may worsen hyperglycemia, which would require adjustment of glycemic treatment. There are also issues surrounding tolerability due to facial flushing, although a new formulation is now available containing laropiprant, a novel flushing pathway inhibitor. High doses of niacin (>3 g/day) should generally be avoided in people with T2DM, although lower doses may effectively treat diabetic dyslipidemia without significantly worsening hyperglycemia.

References

1. Laasko M. Hyperglycemia and cardiovascular disease in type 2 diabetes. *Diabetes.* **48**:937–942, 1993.
2. Owens D, Maher V, Collins P, Johnson A, Tomkin GH. Cellular cholesterol regulation: a defect in the type 2 (non-insulin-dependent) patient diabetic patient in poor metabolic control. *Diabetologia.* **33**:93–99, 1990.
3. Bowie A, Owens D, Collins P, Johnson A, Tomkin GH. Glycosylated low-density lipoprotein is more sensitive to oxidation. Implications for the diabetic patient. *Atherosclerosis.* 102; 63–67, 1993.
4. Schaefer PG, Teerlink T, Heine RJ. Clinical significance of physiochemical properties in diabetes. *Diabetologia.* **48**:808–816, 2005.
5. Mastorikou M, Mackness M, Mackness B. Defective metabolism of oxidised phospholipids by HDL from people with type 2 diabetes. *Diabetes.* **55**:3099–3013, 2006.
6. Haber EP, Procopio J, Carvalho CR, Carpinelle AR, Newsholme P, Curi R. New insights into fatty acid modulation of pancreatic beta cell function. *Int Rev Cytol.* **248**; 1–41, 2006.
7. Kahn R, Buse J, Ferrannini E, et al. The metabolic syndrome: time for a critical appraisal: joint statement from the American Diabetes Association and the European Association for the Study of Diabetes. *Diabetes Care.* **28**(9): 2289–2304, 2005.
8. Lakka, H-M, Laaksonen DE, Lakka TA, et al. The metabolic syndrome and total cardiovascular disease mortality in middle-aged men. *JAMA.* **288**:2709–2716, 2002.
9. Howard G, O'Leary DH, Zaccaro D, et al. Insulin sensitivity and atherosclerosis. The Insulin Resistance Atherosclerosis Study (IRAS) Investigators. *Circulation.* **93**:1809–1817, 1996.

10. Pyorala K, Pedersen TR, Kjekshus J, Fraergeman O, Olsson AG, Thorgeirsson G. The Scandinavian Simvastatin Survival Study (4S) Group. Cholesterol-lowering with simvastatin improves prognosis of diabetic patients with heart disease. *Diabetes Care.* **20**:614–620, 1997.

11. Goldberg RB, Mellies MJ, Sacks FM, et al. Cardiovascular events and their reduction with pravastatin in diabetic and glucose-intolerant myocardial infarction survivors with average cholesterol levels: subgroup analyses in the cholesterol and recurrent events (CARE) trial. The Care Investigators. *Circulation.* **98**:2513–2519, 1998.

12. The Long-term Intervention with Pravastatin in Ischaemic Disease (LIPID) Study Group. Prevention of cardiovascular events and death in pravastatin patients with coronary heart disease and a broad range of initial cholesterol levels. *N Eng J Med.* **339**:1349–1357, 1998.

13. Haffner SM, Alexander CM, Cook TJ, et al. Reduced coronary events in simvastatin-treated patients with coronary heart disease and diabetes or impaired glucose levels. *Arch Intern Med.* **159**:2661–2667, 1999.

14. Heart Protection Study Collaborative Group. MRC/BHF Heart Protection Study of cholesterol-lowering with simvastatin in 20,536 high-risk individuals: a randomized, placebo-controlled study. *Lancet.* **360**:7–22, 2002.

15. Calhoun HM, Betteridge DJ, Durrington PN, et al. Primary prevention of cardiovascular disease with atorvastatin in type 2 diabetes in the Collaborative Atorvastatin Diabetes Study (CARDS): multi-centre randomised placebo-controlled trial. *Lancet.* **364**:685–696, 2004.

16. Deedwania P, Barter P, Carmena R, et al. Reduction of low-density lipoprotein cholesterol in patients with coronary heart disease and metabolic syndrome: analysis of the treating to new targets study. *Lancet.* **368**:919–928, 2006.

17. Assmann G, Schulte H, Funke H, von Eckardstein. The emergence of triglycerides as a significant independent risk factor in coronary artery disease. *Eur Heart J.* **19**(Suppl M): M8–M14, 1998.

18. Lahdenpera S, Syvanne M, Kahri J, et al. Regulation of low-density lipoprotein particle size distribution in NIDDM and coronary disease: importance of serum triglycerides. *Diabetologia.* **39**:453–446, 1996.

19. Fontbonne, Eschweg E, Cambien F, et al. Hypertriglyceridemia as a risk factor of coronary heart disease mortality in subjects with impaired glucose tolerance or diabetes. *Diabetologia.* **32**:300–304, 1989.

20. Bos G, Dekker JM, Nijpels G, et al. A combination of high concentrations of serum triglyceride and non-HDL cholesterol is a risk factor for cardiovascular disease in subjects with abnormal glucose metabolism: The Hoorn study. *Diabetologia.* **46**:910–916, 2003.

21. Ballantyne CM, Olsson AG, Cook TJ, Mercuri MF, Pedersen TR, Kjekshus J. Influence of low high-density lipoprotein cholesterol and elevated triglyceride on coronary heart disease events and response to simvastatin therapy in 4S. *Circulation.* **104**; 3046–3051, 2001.

22. Despres JP, Lemiieux I, Dagenais GR, Cantin B, Lamarche B. HDL-cholesterol as a marker of coronary heart disease risk: the Quebec cardiovascular study. *Atherosclerosis.* **153**; 263–272, 2000.

23. Hokanson JE, Austin MA. Plasma triglyceride level is a risk factor for cardiovascular disease independent of high-density lipoprotein cholesterol level: a meta-analysis of population-based prospective studies. *J Cardiovasc Risk.* **3**:213–219, 1996.

24. Sarwar N, Danesh J, Eiriksdottir G, et al. Triglycerides and the risk of coronary heart disease: 10,158 incident cases among 262,525 participants in 29 western prospective studies. *Circulation.* **115**; 450–458, 2007.

25. Nordestgaard BG, Benn M, Schnohr P, et al. Nonfasting triglycerides and risk of myocardial infarction, ischemic heart disease and death in men and women. *JAMA.* **298**(3): 299–308, 2007.

26. Scott R, O'Brien R, Fulcher G, et al. Effects of fenofibrate treatment on cardiovascular disease risk in 9,795 individuals with type 2 diabetes and various components of the metabolic syndrome. The Fenofibrate Intervention and Event Lowering in Diabetes (FIELD) study. *Diabetes Care.* **32**:493–498, 2009.

27. Secondary prevention by raising HDL cholesterol and reducing triglycerides in patients with coronary artery disease: the Bezafibrate Infarction Prevention (BIP) study. *Circulation.* **102**; 21–27, 2000.

28. Tenenbaum A, Motro M, Enrique Z, et al. Bezafibrate for the secondary prevention of myocardial infarction in patients with metabolic syndrome. *Arch Intern Med.* **165**; 1154–1160, 2005.

29. Effect of fenofibrate on progression of coronary-artery disease in type 2 diabetes: the Diabetes Atherosclerosis Intervention Study (DAIS), a randomised study. *Lancet.* **357**:905–910, 2001.

30. Taylor AJ, Sullenberger LE, Lee HJ, et al. Arterial Biology for the Investigation of the Treatment Effects of Reducing Cholesterol (ARBITER 2): a double-blind, placebo-controlled study of extended-release niacin on atherosclerosis progression in secondary prevention patients treated with statins. *Circulation.* **110**(23): 3512–3517, 2004. Erratum in *Circulation.* **110**(23): 3615, 2004. *Circulation.* **111**(24): e446, 2005.

14 The role of bariatric surgery in obese patients with diabetes: Primary or rescue therapy?

Praveena Gandikota[1] and Blandine Laferrère[2]

[1] Endocrine Fellow, Endocrine, Diabetes and Nutrition Division, Department of Medicine, St Luke's Roosevelt Hospital, New York, NY, USA

[2] Assistant Professor of Medicine, Division of Endocrinology, Diabetes and Nutrition Obesity Research Center Department of Medicine, St Luke's Roosevelt Hospital Center, Columbia University College of Physicians and Surgeons, New York, NY, USA

LEARNING POINTS

- Obesity and type 2 diabetes mellitus (T2DM) are major public health issues that are closely related. Lifestyle modifications (LSM) with diet and exercise leading to weight loss are cornerstones of T2DM management along with pharmacologic therapy. Limitations are cost, effectiveness, and short-term effect for LSM and compliance, cost and side effects for medications.

- Newer medications may help preserve beta-cell function over time.

- Bariatric surgery is increasingly becoming popular for management of morbid obesity and its related comorbidities including T2DM. Diabetes control improves for most patients after bariatric surgery, with full remission in over 50% of patients. The mechanisms of remission include, but are not limited to, caloric restriction with weight loss and changes of the incretins, particularly after gastric bypass (GBP).

- Although bariatric surgery is approved for diabetic patients with BMI $\geq$ 35 kg/m^2, the use of surgery to treat diabetes in less obese individuals is currently proposed. Limitations to this approach are lack of high quality data on short and long term complications of the surgery; and long-term data on diabetes remission and cost analysis.

- Emerging new endoscopic techniques may be an option in the future.

Introduction

The prevalence of type 2 diabetes mellitus (T2DM) and obesity is increasing worldwide and represents a considerable public health burden. Approximately half of patients with diabetes in the United States are obese. Medical therapy for patients with diabetes combines costly and often inefficient lifestyle modifications (LSM), with various medications, some of them inducing unwanted weight gain and/or hypoglycemia. However, in the last few years, management and prognosis of T2DM have changed considerably. Novel pharmacotherapies have emerged, with not only the capability to preserve beta-cell function, such as thiazolidinediones (TZDs) or incretin based therapies, but also to decrease body weight (incretins and amylin analogs). In addition, full remission of diabetes is achieved in 40–80 % of cases by various types of bariatric surgeries. T2DM, a chronic disease leading to progressive beta-cell death and vascular complications, is now a curable disease after weight loss surgery, and can go into remission [1, 2]. In view of the spectacular effect of bariatric surgery on T2DM, it is understandable that bariatric surgery be proposed as treatment of T2DM, independently of the beneficial weight loss effect, i.e., in patients with body mass index (BMI) < 35 kg/m^2. This could be a particularly attractive alternative in some ethnic groups, like Asians, who have a high risk of T2DM at lower BMI compared to Caucasians.

Clinical Dilemmas in Diabetes, First Edition. Edited by Adrian Vella and Robert A. Rizza
© 2011 Blackwell Publishing Ltd. Published 2011 by Blackwell Publishing Ltd.

The objective of this chapter is to discuss whether bariatric surgery should be offered as first-line therapy, or as rescue therapy, when medical options have failed to control diabetes. In addition, hypotheses on mechanisms of action of bariatric surgery on glucose homeostasis, the role of bariatric surgery in treatment of patients with T2DM with BMI < 35 kg/m^2, risks and benefits of different types of bariatric surgery, and future techniques will be discussed.

Possible mechanisms by which bariatric surgery improves T2DM

Effect of weight loss

T2DM is a very complex disorder with insulin resistance in the muscle and the liver, impaired beta- and alpha-cell function, impaired incretin effect, and alteration of glucose homeostasis in the kidney and the brain. A significant degree of beta-cell failure and vascular complications are often present at the time of diagnosis of T2DM. Reduced calorie intake and increased physical activity are essential for the management of T2DM.

Multiple studies have shown the effectiveness of LSM in preventing T2DM, with a risk reduction up to 58%. Similarly, weight loss and LSM in patients with established T2DM are beneficial [3]. A modest 10% weight loss is associated with significant improvement in diabetes and other obesity-related comorbidities such as hypertension and dyslipidemia. Contrary to LSM that result in weight loss of small magnitude and short duration [4] bariatric surgery results in weight loss of greater magnitude, 40–50% excess weight loss (EWL), sustained over time up to 14 years [1, 5]. Weight loss is a key factor in the improvement of T2DM after bariatric surgery.

Effect of incretins

Resolution of T2DM after bypass procedures has been described within days of the surgery, suggesting that factors other than weight loss could be responsible for the diabetes improvement. The change in incretins may explain part of diabetes remission after GBP. The two main incretins are glucagon like peptide 1 (GLP1) and glucose- dependent insulinotropic peptide (GIP), produced by the L and K cells, respectively. Together, they are responsible for the "incretin effect" or the greater insulin response after oral glucose compared to intravenous glucose. The incretins play a key role in postprandial glucose-mediated insulin secretion. In addition, GLP-1 decreases glucagon, induces weight loss

and, in animal models, decreased apoptosis and increased beta-cell mass. The incretin effect is blunted in T2DM. Both incretin levels and effect increase after GBP [6, 7], but not after diet [8] or purely restrictive procedures [9]. Levels of GLP-1 increase as early as 2 days [10] and persist up to 20 years [11]. The mechanisms of increased incretin levels after GBP are not fully understood. The rapid delivery of nutrients to the lower intestine after bypass surgeries or after vertical sleeve gastrectomy (VSG) [12] may increase the production of GLP-1 by direct nutrient exposure of the L cells. This hypothesis has been fueled by results of ileal transposition in rodents [13]. The foregut exclusion hypothesis emphasizes the role of exclusion of the proximal part of the gut from nutrients [14], suggesting the presence of a would-be anti-incretin factor secreted by the proximal small intestine. This hypothesis is the basis for the current trials with endoluminal sleeves (see below). It is possible that both mechanisms play a role in the changes of incretin release and glucose homeostasis after GBP.

Other possible mechanisms of successful weight loss and metabolic improvement after bariatric surgery include changes in ghrelin and PYY [9, 15], bile acids [16], changes in taste patterns, inflammatory markers, gastric emptying and intestinal transit time [7], and possibly in gut flora [17].

Role of bariatric surgery in T2DM: First-line therapy or rescue therapy when medical options fail?

Of the multiple pharmacological agents targeting physiopathological defects in diabetes, the insulin sensitizer thiazolidinediones (TZD) and incretin derived therapies have opened new perspectives for management of T2DM, as they both have the potential to preserve beta-cell function. Pharmacological agents used to treat T2DM [18] are not without risks and side effects. Weight gain, and/or the risk of hypoglycemia, especially with sulfonylureas and insulin, is a major hindrance in the management of the already obese patients. Additionally, challenges occur in patients with associated conditions like renal failure or heart failure. However, in spite of the various excellent pharmacological agents available in the United States, 43% of patients with T2DM fail medical therapy and do not achieve the HbA1C target of < 7% [19]. In a study by Holman et al, only 31.9–44.7% of patients achieved an HbA1c < 6.5% at 3 years with different insulin regimen [20]. None of the medical clinical trials report diabetes remission.

Nearly 30% of patients who undergo bariatric surgery have T2DM [1], although about a third of these patients are undiagnosed [21]. In the Buchwald meta-analysis [22], criteria used to define diabetes resolution was fasting blood glucose < 100 mg/dl and/or HbA1c < 6%, off diabetes medications. The percentage of diabetes remission varies according to surgery: 95% after BPD/duodenal switch, 80% after RYGBPP, 80% with gastroplasty and 57–73% after gastric banding (GB). The greater the malabsorption (BPD) and weight loss, the more likely the patient will achieve diabetes remission. Significant improvement in T2DM has also been shown in the Swedish Obesity Study (SOS), a long-term observational prospective study that compared surgical versus nonsurgical groups [5]. The surgical group fared better at both 2 years' and 10 years' follow-up with respect to decrease in glucose and insulin levels, incidence as well as recovery from T2DM. In a randomized controlled trial (RCT), Dixon et al. showed that GB resulted in a 73% diabetes remission rate at two years compared to conventional medical interventions (13%) [23]. The benefit of bariatric surgery include not only a ~40% weight loss, but the resolution and/or significant improvement of diabetes and most obesity-related comorbidities like hyperlipidemia (70%), hypertension (61.7%), and of obstructive sleep apnea (85.7%) [22]. Recent studies have shown a decreased mortality [24], particularly the mortality related to diabetes, after bariatric surgery.

Would patients failing medical treatment, who tend to be older, with longer duration of diabetes, with less optimal access to care, respond to bariatric surgery? Which bariatric surgery is more likely to help patients achieve their blood glucose target and/or go into remission? Should obese patients with BMI ≥ 35 kg/m^2 with T2DM be offered bariatric surgery as a first-line therapy? It is difficult to answer these questions as the data are scarce and the quality of surgical studies thus far is poor, with a high attrition rate. Available surgical studies on diabetes remission often do not report data on diabetes control and/or duration [25]. Diabetes duration, when provided, is short [23, 26] and few patients, 0.5% [23] to 39% [27], are insulin treated. The study by Schauer et al. [26] is the only one that provides outcome data analyzed according to preoperative diabetes status and duration. Patients with less severe disease had significantly better fasting plasma glucose and HbA1c post surgery compared with insulin-requiring patients with more severe disease. Additionally, the longer the duration of diabetes, the more likely patients were to remain on medications and/or insulin. However, the preoperative duration

of T2DM did not result in significant differences in postoperative glucose control among the groups [26]. Another issue in interpreting published data is the definition used for diabetes remission. As diabetes remission is indeed a novel concept [2], no uniform definition was used in previous surgical studies [22, 23]. The recent consensus statement proposed to define complete remission of T2DM as "normal glycemic measures (HbA1c in the normal range, fasting glucose < 100 mg/dl) for at least 1 year duration in the absence of active pharmacologic therapy or ongoing procedures" [2]. Whether this clinical definition of diabetes remission is accompanied by reversal of the pathophysiological defects seen with diabetes remains to be demonstrated.

According to the current guidelines, bariatric surgery is approved for patients with BMI ≥ 40 kg/m^2 or BMI ≥ 35 kg/m^2 in the presence of any comorbidity. Less than 3% of the patients who qualify for bariatric surgery undergo this treatment of their obesity and over 200,000 surgeries are performed yearly in the United States. As morbidly obese patients gain significant health and quality of life benefits from bariatric surgery, an effort to increase the number of surgeries on patients with higher BMI (> 45 kg/m^2) is a reasonable approach [28]. According to the latest ADA 2010 guidelines [18], bariatric surgery should be considered for adults with BMI ≥ 35 kg/m^2 and T2DM, especially if diabetes or other comorbidities are difficult to control with lifestyle and pharmacologic therapy. What defines "difficult to control" and for how long a patient has to be failing medical therapy prior to being offered bariatric surgery is unclear. Identifying preoperative predictors of diabetes resolution is critical not only for patient selection but also for determining which type of surgery would be the best. The amount of weight loss is clearly a major determinant. This is particularly true after GB when diabetes remission is directly proportional to the degree of weight loss [23]. The duration of diabetes and/or preoperative insulin use decreases the chances of diabetes remission [26, 27]. This implies that the less the deterioration of beta-cell function at the time of surgery, the higher the chances of diabetes remission. However, even if patients do not go into remission after bariatric surgery, most of them will experience significant improvement of their disease and achieve glucose control on less medications [26]. There are no data from RCT comparing aggressive medical treatment with bariatric surgery in morbidly obese persons. Even with the best medical scenario however, results of bariatric surgery will be likely hard to match, at least in the first 5–10 years after surgery.

Gastric banding or gastric bypass?

There are three main categories of bariatric surgery. Restrictive procedures, with or without gastrectomy, aim to reduce gastric volume in order to limit food intake and induce weight loss. These procedures include laparoscopic adjustable gastric banding (GB), vertical banded gastro-plasty (VBG), rarely performed now, and vertical sleeve gastrectomy (VSG). The Roux-en-Y gastric bypass (RYGBP) surgery, combines gastric restriction with some malabsorption and is the most commonly performed procedure in the United States. Finally, biliopancreatic diversion (BPD) is a procedure with significant malabsorption with (Figure 14.1) or without gastric restriction. Although

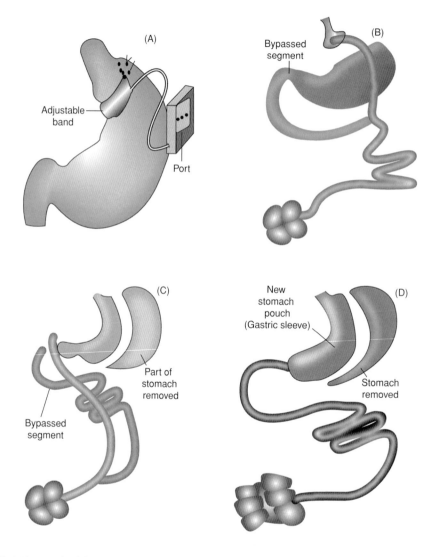

FIG 14.1 Bariatric surgeries. (A) Laparoscopic adjustable gastric banding (GB); (B) Roux-en-Y gastric bypass (RYGBP); (C) biliopancreatic diversion (BPD) with duodenal switch; (D) vertical sleeve gastrectomy (VSG). http://www.mayoclinic.org/bariatric-surgery/bariatric-procedures.html Figure used by permission of Mayo Foundation for Medical Education and Research. All rights reserved.

surgeons empirically tend to perform malabsorptive procedures in patients with BMI > 50 kg/m^2, rather than GB, there is no data and/or guidelines determining the best surgery for a particular patient. The choice of the type of surgery should not be based on surgeons' preference and/or on early 6–12 months weight loss outcome, but rather on short- and long-term data generated by RCT comparing various surgical procedures. Collecting long-term data is essential to learn about the effect of bariatric surgery on weight loss, resolution of comorbidities, as well as complications such as nutritional deficiencies. Data about nutritional deficiencies, weight regain, comorbidities resolution, and overall morbidity are essentially poorly known, as loss to follow-up is notably high for this patient population. In a recent review [29] only five studies were identified with data on nutritional deficiencies with at least 12 month follow-up and the data were suboptimal.

Morbid obesity is associated with an increased mortality. The mortality rate associated with bariatric surgery has been reported to be 0.1–1.1% [22]. In a recent prospective, multicenter observational study [28], the 30-day death rate was 0% after laparoscopic GB, 0.2% after laparoscopic RYGBP and 2.1% after open RYGBP. These rates are comparable to the 90-day mortality rate of 1% seen after cholecystectomy. Both prospective (e.g., SOS) [24] and retrospective studies [30] have shown decreased overall mortality after bariatric surgery. Specifically, cause-specific mortality in the RYGBP surgery group decreased by 92% for diabetes [30]. Bariatric surgery is associated with early postoperative complications such as thromboembolism, wound complications like infection/dehiscence, pulmonary complications like atelectasis, and late postoperative complications like anastomotic stricture, intestinal obstruction, incisional hernias, and gastrogastric fistula. In addition, dumping syndrome can be disabling. Long-term metabolic and nutritional complications related to altered micronutrient and vitamin absorption are frequently observed after malabsorptive surgeries [29] and need to be aggressively treated, often for a lifetime. Vitamin D deficiency may require weekly doses of ergocalciferol 50,000 units weekly or a few times a week and iron and B12 often are needed parenterally. Deficiencies need to be carefully monitored at least twice yearly, for a lifetime. At present, there are no established guidelines for mineral and vitamin supplementation after bariatric surgery.

Hyperinsulinemic hypoglycemia associated with histological appearances of nesidioblastosis in pancreatectomy specimen is rare. It usually occurs 2 years or more after RYGBP [31]. Patients present with severe postprandial neuroglycopenic symptoms in the presence of elevated endogenous hyperinsulinemia. Dietary management with or without glucosidase inhibitors, octreotide and other pharmacological treatment should always be tried first prior to performing partial pancreatectomy. The mechanism of nesidioblastosis is at present unknown.

Bariatric surgery is the treatment of choice for morbid obesity, with the additional benefit of diabetes improvement and/or remission in over 80% of cases. As all morbid obese individuals will greatly benefit from bariatric surgery, long duration and/or poor control of diabetes should not be contraindications to the surgery. Long-term high-quality data (>10 years) on weight loss, safety, and nutritional complications are essential. These long-term studies will help establish predictors of success, delineate the choice of surgery, and help implement guidelines for vitamin supplementation. As the number of bariatric surgeries increases, the number of patients in need of lifetime bariatric care will grow exponentially. Primary care physicians and/or endocrinologists need to be trained appropriately to optimize patient management both preoperatively and postoperatively.

Role of weight loss surgery in the treatment of patients with T2DM and BMI < 35 kg/m^2

There are currently few studies of bariatric surgery on patients with T2DM and BMI<35 kg/m^2. In the RCT by Dixon et al. [23], patients with well-controlled T2DM, of < 2 years duration, mean BMI of 37.1 kg/m^2 went into diabetes remission in 73% of cases after GB at 2 years (the dropout rate was low) versus 13% in the diet group [23]. The studies from De Paula et al. with complicated surgeries, including ileal transposition, report high remission rate, but a nonnegligible mortality, at least in the initial report [32]. A study reports remission of diabetes and improvement of insulin sensitivity 18 months after BPD in five patients with BMI< 35 kg/m^2 [33]. A recent nonrandomized study by Shah et al. in Asian Indians reported 100% remission rate in 15 patients 3 months after GBP surgery. Preoperatively, 80% of the patients were insulin treated, diabetes control was poor with HbA1C ~10%, and diabetes duration was 9 years [34]. The RCT by Dixon et al. provides the best evidence-based data to suggest the use of GB in patients with diabetes and lower BMI [23]. The diabetes remission was directly related to the amount of weight loss and the preoperative HbA1C levels. Participants had fairly mild diabetes. Whether these results can be achieved in a more severe diabetic population, different ethnic groups, and with a different health care system, is unknown. There is currently not enough evidence to suggest that bariatric surgery, particularly bypass, should be indicated for patients with BMI < 35 kg/m². As for more invasive surgeries (bypass ± ileal transposition), it is unclear whether the risk they represent is worth their use in clinical practice outside of very well controlled research RCT.

New techniques that can be an option in the future

Endoluminal duodenal sleeve either in lean diabetic rats [14] or in rats with diet-induced obesity [35] improves glucose metabolism and induces weight loss. The human trials of endoluminal treatments of obesity are limited to restrictive interventions such as intragastric balloons, transoral gastroplasty, and endoluminal vertical gastroplasty. More recently, the duodenojejunal bypass sleeve, the only endoluminal sleeve studied in humans, has been shown to promote weight loss and seems to improve glucose metabolism. This device aims to mimic the duodenal bypass effects of Roux-en-Y GBP without the need for intestinal anastomoses, and may offer novel outpatient therapeutic modalities for obese patients with T2DM. Early data in humans are encouraging, but long-term efficacy and safety data are lacking.

In conclusion, bariatric surgery should be the treatment of choice for patients with morbid obesity complicated by T2DM and with high metabolic and cardiovascular risks. The surgery has been proven to not only improve quality of life but also prolong life in these high-risk patients. In morbidly obese patients with T2DM, even with poor control, bariatric surgery can result in remission in about 50% of cases, an effect unmatched by medical treatment. There is not enough evidence to perform invasive bariatric surgeries and/or to experiment with new surgical procedures in patients with lower BMI and/or with milder diabetes, outside of well-controlled RCT. Optimizing chronic care after GB, a noninvasive procedure, to ensure proper weight loss and diabetes remission is important. Multidisciplinary teams including surgeons, endocrinologists, gastroenterologists, psychiatrists, nutritionists, and primary care are needed to follow up these patients. Bariatric surgery offers a

unique model to understand the complexity of T2DM and help develop new treatments for this chronic disease.

References

1. Pories WJ, Swanson MS, MacDonald KG, et al. Who would have thought it? An operation proves to be the most effective therapy for adult-onset diabetes mellitus. *Ann Surg.* **222**(3):339–350, 1995.
2. Buse JB, Caprio S, Cefalu WT, et al. How do we define cure of diabetes? *Diabetes Care.* **32**(11):2133–2135, 2009.
3. Pi-Sunyer X, Blackburn G, Brancati FL, et al. Reduction in weight and cardiovascular disease risk factors in individuals with type 2 diabetes: one-year results of the look AHEAD trial. *Diabetes Care.* **30**(6):1374–1383, 2007.
4. Wadden TA, Sternberg JA, Letizia KA, Stunkard AJ, Foster GD. Treatment of obesity by very low calorie diet, behavior therapy, and their combination: a five-year perspective. *Int J Obes.* **13**(Suppl 2):39–46, 1989.
5. Sjostrom L, Lindroos AK, Peltonen M, et al. Lifestyle, diabetes, and cardiovascular risk factors 10 years after bariatric surgery. *N Engl J Med.* **351**(26):2683–2693, 2004.
6. Laferrère B, Heshka S, Wang K, et al. Incretin levels and effect are markedly enhanced 1 month after Roux-en-Y gastric bypass surgery in obese patients with type 2 diabetes. *Diabetes Care.* **30**(7):1709–1716, 2007.
7. Morinigo R, Moize V, Musri M, et al. Glucagon-like peptide-1, peptide YY, hunger, and satiety after gastric bypass surgery in morbidly obese subjects. *J Clin Endocrinol Metab.* **91**(5):1735–1740, 2006.
8. Laferrère B, Teixeira J, McGinty J, et al. Effect of weight loss by gastric bypass surgery versus hypocaloric diet on glucose and incretin levels in patients with type 2 diabetes. *J Clin Endocrinol Metab.* **93**(7):2479–2485, 2008.
9. Bose M, Machineni S, Olivan B, et al. Superior appetite hormone profile after equivalent weight loss by gastric bypass compared to gastric banding. *Obesity (Silver Spring).* **18**(6):1085–1091, 2010.
10. le Roux CW, Welbourn R, Werling M, et al. Gut hormones as mediators of appetite and weight loss after Roux-en-Y gastric bypass. *Ann Surg.* **246**(5):780–785, 2007.
11. Naslund E, Gryback P, Hellstrom PM, et al. Gastrointestinal hormones and gastric emptying 20 years after jejunoileal bypass for massive obesity. *Int J Obes Relat Metab Disord.* **21**(5):387–392, 1997.
12. Vidal J, Ibarzabal A, Nicolau J, et al. Short-term effects of sleeve gastrectomy on type 2 diabetes mellitus in severely obese subjects. *Obes Surg.* **17**(8):1069–1074, 2007.
13. Strader AD, Vahl TP, Jandacek RJ, Woods SC, D'Alessio DA, Seeley RJ. Weight loss through ileal transposition is accompanied by increased ileal hormone secretion and synthesis

in rats. *Am J Physiol Endocrinol Metab.* **288**(2):E447–E453, 2005.

14. Rubino F, Forgione A, Cummings DE, et al. The mechanism of diabetes control after gastrointestinal bypass surgery reveals a role of the proximal small intestine in the pathophysiology of type 2 diabetes. *Ann Surg.* **244**(5):741–749, 2006.

15. Olivan B, Teixeira J, Bose M, et al. Effect of weight loss by diet or gastric bypass surgery on peptide YY3-36 levels. *Ann Surg.* **249**(6):948–953, 2009.

16. Patti ME, Houten SM, Bianco AC, et al. Serum bile acids are higher in humans with prior gastric bypass: potential contribution to improved glucose and lipid metabolism. *Obesity (Silver Spring).* **17**(9):1671–1677, 2009.

17. Zhang H, Dlbalse J, Zuccolo A, et al. Human gut microbiota in obesity and after gastric bypass. *PNAS.* **106**(7):2364–2370, 2009.

18. American Diabetes Association. *Diabetes Care.* **33**(Suppl 1):S1–S2, 2010.

19. Cheung BM, Ong KL, Cherny SS, Sham PC, Tso AW, Lam KS. Diabetes prevalence and therapeutic target achievement in the United States, 1999 to 2006. *Am J Med.* **122**(5):443–453, 2009.

20. Holman RR, Farmer AJ, Davies MJ, et al. Three-year efficacy of complex insulin regimens in type 2 diabetes. *N Engl J Med.* **361**(18):1736–1747, 2009.

21. Residori L, Garcia-Lorda P, Flancbaum L, Pi-Sunyer FX, Laferrère B. Prevalence of co-morbidities in obese patients before bariatric surgery: effect of race. *Obes Surg.* **13**(3):333–340, 2003.

22. Buchwald H, Avidor Y, Braunwald E, et al. Bariatric surgery: a systematic review and meta-analysis. *JAMA.* **292**(14):1724–1737, 2004.

23. Dixon JB, O'Brien PE, Playfair J, et al. Adjustable gastric banding and conventional therapy for type 2 diabetes: a randomized controlled trial. *JAMA.* **299**(3):316–323, 2008.

24. Sjostrom L, Narbro K, Sjostrom CD, et al. Effects of bariatric surgery on mortality in Swedish obese subjects. *N Engl J Med.* **357**(8):741–752, 2007.

25. Vetter ML, Cardillo S, Rickels MR, Iqbal N. Narrative review: effect of bariatric surgery on type 2 diabetes mellitus. *Ann Intern Med.* **150**(2):94–103, 2009.

26. Schauer PR, Burguera B, Ikramuddin S, et al. Effect of laparoscopic Roux-en Y gastric bypass on type 2 diabetes mellitus. *Ann Surg.* **238**(4):467–784, 2003.

27. Sugerman HJ, Wolfe LG, Sica DA, Clore JN. Diabetes and hypertension in severe obesity and effects of gastric bypass-induced weight loss. *Ann Surg.* **237**(6):751–756, 2003.

28. Purnell JQ, Flum DR. Bariatric surgery and diabetes: who should be offered the option of remission? *JAMA.* **301**(15):1593–1595, 2009.

29. Shah M, Simha V, Garg A. Review: long-term impact of bariatric surgery on body weight, comorbidities, and nutritional status. *J Clin Endocrinol Metab.* **91**(11):4223–4231, 2006.

30. Adams TD, Gress RE, Smith SC, et al. Long-term mortality after gastric bypass surgery. *N Engl J Med.* **357**(8):753–761, 2007.

31. Service GJ, Thompson GB, Service FJ, et al. Hyperinsulinemic hypoglycemia with nesidioblastosis after gastric-bypass surgery. *N Engl J Med.* **353**(3):249–254, 2005.

32. Depaula AL, Macedo AL, Mota BR, Schraibman V. Laparoscopic ileal interposition associated to a diverted sleeve gastrectomy is an effective operation for the treatment of type 2 diabetes mellitus patients with BMI 21-29. *Surg Endosc.* **23**(6):1313–1320, 2009.

33. Chiellini C, Rubino F, Castagneto M, Nanni G, Mingrone G. The effect of bilio-pancreatic diversion on type 2 diabetes in patients with BMI <35 kg/m2. *Diabetologia.* **52**(6):1027–1030, 2009.

34. Shah SS, Todkar JS, Shah PS, Cummings DE. Diabetes remission and reduced cardiovascular risk after gastric bypass in Asian Indians with body mass index <35 kg/m^2. *Surg Obes Relat Dis.* **6**(4):332–338, 2010.

35. Aguirre V, Stylopoulos N, Grinbaum R, Kaplan LM. An endoluminal sleeve induces substantial weight loss and normalizes glucose homeostasis in rats with diet-induced obesity. *Obesity (Silver Spring).* **16**(12):2585–2592, 2008.

15 Hyperglycemia should be avoided in critical illness and the postoperative period

Kalpana Muthusamy[1] and John M. Miles[2]

[1]Clinical Fellow, Division of Endocrinology, Mayo Clinic, Rochester, MN, USA
[2]Professor of Medicine, Endocrine Research Unit, Mayo Clinic, Rochester, MN, USA

LEARNING POINTS

- To discuss evidence for and against the use of insulin infusion to control hyperglycemia in the critically ill.

- To consider the role of hypoglycemia in the disparate results of large clinical trials investigating the use of intensive insulin therapy in the critically ill.

- To review the use of nutrition and its potential influence on insulin requirements and outcomes in the critically ill.

- To discuss mechanisms by which insulin infusion may modulate outcomes when used in critically ill patients.

Introduction

Hyperglycemia is a frequent finding in acute care hospitals, with a prevalence rate in excess of one-third of all inpatients [1, 2]. Among patients with hyperglycemia (admission glucose > 7 mmol/L or random glucose > 11.1 mmol/L), only two-thirds are known to have diabetes; the remainder either have newly diagnosed diabetes or temporary ("stress") hyperglycemia. Hyperglycemia has been identified as an independent predictor for higher infection rates [3, 4] and increased mortality [5, 6] in critically ill and postoperative patients. A number of large clinical trials have been conducted over the past 15 years to address the question of whether intravenous infusion of insulin could improve morbidity and mortality in the critically ill. One of these trials [7] led to a consensus conference convened in 2004 by the American College of Endocrinology and cosponsored by the American Diabetes Association, the American Heart Association, the American Society of Anesthesiologists, the

Endocrine Society, the Society of Critical Care Medicine, and the Society of Thoracic and Cardiovascular Surgeons [8]. The consensus conference concluded, again on the basis of a single clinical trial [7], that blood glucoses should be maintained < 6.1 mmol/L in critically ill patients, and that insulin infusion was the means to achieve that goal. The conference also recommended that a preprandial glucose target < 6.1 mmol/L in patients who are eating on general medical-surgical wards should be adopted. This latter recommendation, which in our view had and has very little evidence to support it, is not the subject of this chapter and will not be discussed further. Instead, we will address mechanisms of hyperglycemia-related morbidity and mortality in the critically ill and will undertake a detailed review of the evidence supporting the use of insulin infusion in the ICU, with emphasis on ten large clinical trials. We will also discuss the importance of hypoglycemia, nutritional support, and imprecision in blood glucose testing in interpreting the results of these trials. We conclude that there is strong evidence to support the use of insulin infusion to control hyperglycemia in the critically ill, but very little evidence to indicate what the blood glucose target should be.

Mechanisms mediating adverse effects of hyperglycemia during critical illness

During acute illness, hyperglycemia is exacerbated in people with diabetes as a consequence of the release of counterregulatory hormones and cytokines [9]. The same mechanisms, along with subtle defects in insulin secretion, contribute to stress, or temporary, hyperglycemia in some nondiabetic individuals. The exact mechanisms by which hyperglycemia mediates adverse outcomes such as infection and increased mortality are not fully understood, however, nor are the mechanisms responsible for improved outcomes resulting from correction of hyperglycemia. Several interesting hypotheses have been proposed involving both metabolic and non-metabolic pathways [10]. Hyperglycemia can cause direct cellular damage as well as indirect effects via increased generation of reactive oxygen species. Although the normal protective response of cells to hyperglycemia is to downregulate glucose transport, expression and localization of GLUT-1 and GLUT-3 in several cell types has been shown to be increased by elevated levels of cytokines, growth factors and hypoxia, which often occur together in the critically ill, potentially leading to cellular glucose overload [11]. Increased substrate availability for glycolysis results in excess superoxide formation that can overwhelm the normal detoxification process, leading to mitochondrial dysfunction [11]. Intensive insulin therapy has been shown to reverse or prevent hepatic mitochondrial abnormalities noted with critical illness [12]. There is also evidence showing improvement in the phagocytic and bactericidal activities of polymorphonuclear leukocytes with improved glycemic control in diabetic subjects, thus enhancing immunity [13]. Glucotoxicity can also impair β-cell secretory function, potentially initiating a vicious cycle of relative insulin insufficiency and further increases in glucose levels [14].

The pleiotrophic effects of insulin, independent of its glucose-lowering effect, have attracted considerable attention as a contributor to clinical benefits. Insulin has been shown to have anti-inflammatory properties, producing a decrease in concentration of acute phase reactants. Reduced mortality and organ failure in critically ill patients treated with insulin infusion is associated with decreased high sensitivity C-reactive protein levels, suggesting (but not proving) a role for reduced inflammation in improved outcomes [15]. Modulation of nitric oxide synthase expression, and activity by insulin therapy mitigates the increased nitric oxide levels seen during stress, thus protecting against endothelial damage [16]. Endothelial adhesion molecules such as ICAM-1 and E-selectin, despite being comparably elevated at admission are lower during intensive insulin therapy, indicating reduced endothelial activation [16]. These factors in combination likely help maintain the integrity of the microvasculature, leading to less organ damage and providing survival benefits.

There is also evidence that insulin therapy may favorably influence outcomes by improving altered lipid homeostasis. Plasma free fatty acids (FFA) are elevated in the critically ill, in spite of hyperinsulinemia due to resistance to insulin's antilipolytic effects in adipocytes [17]. This is of potential importance because elevated FFA contribute to acute endothelial dysfunction [18], have pressor effects [19], and can contribute to the dyslipidemia of critical illness by driving hepatic VLDL production [20]. Mesotten et al., in a post hoc analysis of a large clinical trial, found that intensive insulin therapy in the critically ill produced substantially lower triglyceride levels [21]. There was a four- to fivefold increase in mortality over a range of triglyceride levels, although in a multivariate analysis HDL cholesterol had the strongest association with mortality. The mechanism for increased morbidity and mortality related to dyslipidemia is not known, but could involve impairment of reticuloendothelial function, as discussed elsewhere [22]. Other proposed mechanisms of benefit are insulin-induced increase in expression of adiponectin [23] and a potential role in enhancing innate immunity [24]. Collectively, the evidence supports a role for nonglycemic effects of insulin therapy in improving outcomes in critical illness, although the relative contribution of these factors is an important area for future research.

Large intervention studies

Background

As recently as a decade ago, at a time when hyperglycemia was recognized as a predictor of adverse outcomes, elevated blood glucose in the critically ill was often ignored. However, since that time the results of large clinical trials have forced a reconsideration of this attitude of indifference. These results have produced wide swings in the pendulum of expert opinion. Initially, the changes were subtle, proposed glucose targets were quite liberal and, in fact, were based more on associations than on harder evidence; blood glucose levels of < 12.2 mmol/L were considered by some to be optimal, as they were associated with improved postoperative infection rates [25].

In 2004, an expert committee declared that a glucose target of < 6.1 mmol/L was appropriate for most critically ill patients [8]. As recently as January, 2009, the ADA stated in a position paper that "Critically ill surgical patients' blood glucose levels should be kept as close to 110 mg/dl (6.1 mmol/L) as possible . . ." [26]. Four months later, in a joint statement with the American Association of Clinical Endocrinologists, the ADA declared that "a glucose range of 140 to 180 mg/dl (7.8 to 10.0 mmol/L) is recommended for the majority of critically ill patients." [27]. What is the explanation for these wide shifts in prevailing views?

In 2001, Van den Berghe and colleagues published a landmark study (hereafter referred to as "Leuven 1") of more than 1500 patients in a surgical ICU. In this study, they aimed for (and achieved) a target blood glucose of 4.4–6.1 mmol/L in an intensive control group and 10–11.1 mmol/L in a conventional treatment group [7]. The in-hospital mortality was significantly lower in the intensive group at 7.2% compared to 10.9% in the conventional arm. They also reported a reduction in mortality during intensive care from 8% in the conventional group to 4.6% in the intensive group (42% relative reduction). Most of these benefits were observed in the patients who stayed in the intensive care unit (ICU) longer than 5 days. There was significant improvement in morbidity related to fewer days on mechanical ventilation, shorter ICU stay, reduced infection, acute renal failure, critical-illness polyneuropathy, and fewer blood transfusions. These overwhelmingly positive results were the sole basis for the target recommended in the 2004 consensus statement and obviously the driving force behind the January, 2009 ADA recommendation. A recently published survey revealed that the majority of intensivists prefer a target blood glucose of 6.1 mmol/L [28]. Although there was little published disagreement with the guidelines, it is not clear that they penetrated to the local level; a 2008–2009 informal poll of over 30 medium-sized hospitals in the United States, most of which did not have a critical care service, revealed that whereas there was a general recognition of the value of insulin infusion in the critically ill, virtually none were strictly adhering to the 6.1 mmol/L benchmark (*JMM*, unpublished observations).

In March 2009 the results of the NICE-SUGAR trial were published, demonstrating that excessively tight control (target 6.0 mmol/L, average glucose 6.4 mmol/L) might actually be harmful compared to a less stringent target (10 mmol/L, average glucose 8.0 mmol/L) [29]. The odds ratio for death in the intensive arm of this study was 1.14 ($p = 0.02$). The ADA-AACE consensus statement relaxing the guidelines was published less than two months later.

Where does this leave us? The results of meta-analyses [30, 31] conclude that intensive insulin therapy does not reduce mortality in critically ill patients and increases the risk of hypoglycemia, although one report [31] acknowledges it might benefit surgical patients. Taken at face value, it could be argued that these studies provide a rationale

for abandoning intensive treatment with insulin infusion altogether. The fact that the authors of the ADA-AACE consensus statement still endorse intensive treatment, albeit in a less aggressive form [26], indicates that they must see merit in the several studies that have reported benefit from this treatment. For this chapter, we will review in detail the results of ten large clinical trials that have produced disparate, difficult-to-reconcile results [7, 29, 32–39]. We included all trials of >500 patients in which glycemic targets were part of the study design, but we excluded studies in which glucose infusion was employed in one group but not the other for the purpose of allowing infusion of insulin at higher rates than would otherwise be necessary to control hyperglycemia [40]. Our purpose is to attempt to identify features of the studies that might explain divergent findings leading to conflicting conclusions and recommendations. Specifically, we hoped to determine whether variables such as acuity of illness in the study population, hypoglycemia, blood glucose testing methodology, and nutritional support might explain differences among studies.

General findings (Tables 15.1 and 15.2)

Table 15.1 shows the ten studies in chronological order and provides details on trial design and study populations, together with glucose targets and levels achieved. Eight of the studies were randomized, controlled trials; two used historical controls. Diabetes mellitus was an entry criterion for two of the studies; in the other eight, the majority of patients did not have diabetes. Patients were receiving nutritional support in eight of the studies but did not receive artificial nutrition in two [32, 33]. Table 15.2 provides information on severity of illness (APACHE II scores) and mortality.

We believe that the first five studies should be considered to indicate benefit from intensive insulin therapy, whereas the second five studies should be considered negative. Certainly, this interpretation could be questioned. The DIGAMI study was likely underpowered, and showed benefit in the whole cohort only with long-term follow-up. However, in-hospital mortality was significantly improved with intensive therapy in the diabetic patients who were lower risk and not previously treated with insulin [32]. The Portland and Stamford studies utilized historical controls, an inherently weaker design, but both had the strength of a large sample size. The Leuven 2 study has been interpreted as unequivocally negative by some authors because there was no difference in the primary end point, i.e., mortality in the aggregate cohort [35]. However, in the subset of individuals who were in the ICU for ≥3 days, mortality

TABLE 15.1 Trial design, patient characteristics

Study	Type of study	Patient population	Number of patients	Diabetes (%)	Mean blood glucose target (mmol/L)		Mean blood glucose achieved (mmol/L)	
					intensive	conventional	intensive	conventional
DIGAMI, 1997 [32]	RCT, multicenter	Coronary care unit	620	100	7.0–10.9	Usual care	9.6	11.7
Leuven-1, 2001 [7]	RCT, single-center	Surgical ICU	1548	13	4.4–6.1	10–11.1	5.7	8.5
Furnary, 2003 [33]	Historical controls, single-center	CABG	3554	100	variable	<11.1	9.8	11.9
Krinsley, 2004 [34]	Historical controls, single-center	Medical-surgical ICU	1600	17	<7.8	Usual care	7.3	8.4
Leuven-2, 2006 [35]	RCT, single-center	Medical-surgical ICU	1200	17	4.4–6.1	10–11.1	5.8	8.6
De La Rosa, 2008 [36]	RCT, single-center	Medical-surgical ICU	504	29–32	4.4–6.1	10–11.1	6.5	8.2
VISEP, 2008 [37]	RCT, multicenter	Medical-surgical ICU	537	30	4.4–6.1	10–11.1	6.2	8.4
Arabi, 2008 [38]	RCT, single-center	Medical-surgical ICU	523	32–48	4.4–6.1	10–11.1	6.4	9.5
NICE-SUGAR, 2009 [29]	RCT, multicenter	Medical-surgical ICU	6104	20	4.5–6.1	<10	6.4	8.0
Glucontrol, 2009 [39]	RCT, multicenter	Medical-surgical ICU	1078	16–21	4.4–6.1	7.8–10	6.5	8.0

TABLE 15.2 APACHE scores and mortality data

Study	APACHE score	Mortality (%) Intensive	Conventional	Relative reduction in mortality (%)	Basis for difference in mortality v controls
DIGAMI, 1997 [32]	NR	19 (at 1 year followup)	26	30	NR
Leuven-1, 2001 [7]	9 (median)	7.2 (in-hospital)	10.9	34	↓sepsis, MOF
Furnary, 2003 [33]	NR	2.5 (in-hospital)	5.3	47	Cardiac related
Krinsley, 2004 [34]	15 (median)	14.8	20.9	20.9	↓in subpopulation with septic shock, neurological or surgical diagnosis
Leuven-2, 2006 [35]	23 (mean)	37.3 (43 for >3 ICU days (in-hospital)	40 (52.5 for >3 ICU days)	NS (18,P<0.05*)	Multiple
De La Rosa 2008 [36]	16 (mean)	36.6 (in-hospital)	32.4	NS	–
VISEP, 2008 [37]	20 (mean)	39.7 (90 day)	35.4	NS	–
Arabi, 2008 [38]	23 (mean)	13.5	17.1	NS	–
NICE-SUGAR, 2009 [29]	21 (mean)	27.5	24.9	Increased by 14	Increases in cardiovascular death
Glucontrol, 2009 [39]	15 (mean)	15.3	17.2	NS	–

NR = Not reported; NS = Not significant; MOF = multiple organ failure; *long-stayers (>3 ICU days) only.

was significantly reduced with intensive therapy. This delay in apparent benefit was also observed to a lesser extent in the surgical ICU study from the same investigators [7]. The benefit in the long-stayers in ICU in Leuven 2 was least apparent in patients in the highest quartile of APACHE II scores [35]. The mortality data in Table 15.2 clearly indicate the Leuven 2 patients to be the sickest of those in any of the ten studies. It has been pointed out that a failure of benefit with short-term therapy could dilute to insignificance an effect in patients with longer ICU stays [41].

The last five of the studies found no benefit of intensive insulin therapy, and the NICE-SUGAR study actually reported higher mortality in intensively treated patients [29]. Three of the five studies were smaller and perhaps underpowered. Furthermore, in two of the five studies the glucose target range in the control group was lower than the Leuven trials. The threshold for initiating insulin infusion (a higher value than the actual target range in many studies) in the control group was lower than in the Leuven studies in two of the trials [29, 37] and not stated in two others [38, 39]. It is therefore not surprising that the average glucose in the control group of four of the five negative studies was lower or equal to the average glucose in the control group of all of the positive studies. Mesotten and van den Berghe suggest that this is due to the strong influence of the

positive studies on the design of the subsequent negative studies, and could have minimized differences in mortality between groups [42].

Role of hypoglycemia in interpretation of study results (Table 15.3)

Hypoglycemia (defined as a blood glucose ≤2.2 mmol/L, or <40 mg/dl) was reported in the landmark van den Berghe study of surgical patients as more common in patients receiving intensive treatment than in the control group, but not leading to hemodynamic deterioration or convulsions. It was not discussed further. The frequency of hypoglycemia was remarkably low in the Krinsley study of medical ICU patients, especially considering that a more liberal definition of hypoglycemia (<3.3 mmol/L) was employed. The Leuven 2 study was the first of the trials to indicate that hypoglycemia might be responsible for mortality in some patients. In three of the five subsequent negative studies there was an association between hypoglycemia and mortality [37–39]. An association between hypoglycemia and mortality was confirmed in the NICE-SUGAR study, and the authors speculated that hypoglycemia could be partly responsible for adverse effects observed with intensive therapy [29]. Thus, there is substantial evidence that hypoglycemia could have material harmful effects on

TABLE 15.3 Hypoglycemia data

Study	Definition of hypoglycemia (mmol/L)	Incidence of hypoglycemia (%)		Association between hypoglycemia and mortality?
		Intensive	Conventional	
DIGAMI, 1997 [32]	<3.0	15.0	0.0	NR
Leuven-1, 2001 [7]	≤2.2	5.1	0.8	No
Furnary, 2003 [33]	NR	NR	NR	NR
Krinsley, 2004 [34]	<3.3	1.4	0.9	No
Leuven-2, 2006 [35]	≤2.2	18.7	3.1	Yes
De La Rosa, 2008 [36]	≤2.2	8.3	0.8	NR
VISEP, 2008 [37]	≤2.2	12.1	2.1	Yes
Arabi, 2008 [38]	≤2.2	28.6	3.1	Yes
NICE-SUGAR, 2009 [29]	≤2.2	6.8	0.5	No
Glucontrol, 2009 [39]	≤2.2	8.7	2.7	Yes

outcomes in patients receiving intensive treatment with insulin infusion.

It is noteworthy that hypoglycemia is conventionally defined in the critical care literature as a value ≤2.2 mmol/L [7, 29, 35–39]. It appears that this definition is used because of a prevailing view that less severe hypoglycemia is not clinically important. In fact, a recent survey of adult intensivists showed that over 40% thought hyperglycemia was more dangerous than hypoglycemia, and a majority preferred a target of 6.1 mmol/L [28]. Ironically, in the same survey the median value for blood glucose that was considered to be the hypoglycemic threshold was 3.33 mmol/L. In fact, severe symptoms of hypoglycemia can occur at glucose concentrations much higher than 2.2 mmol/L, and the counterregulatory response, including sympathoadrenal activation, routinely occurs as glucose levels descend through the 3.6–3.8 mmol/L range [43]. Moreover, defective counterregulation [41] and lack of clinical cues of hypoglycemia may make hypoglycemia more difficult to identify, but not necessarily less threatening. For this reason, hypoglycemia experts have argued that the threshold for clinical important hypoglycemia lies in the 3.5 mmol/L [44] to 3.9 mmol/L [45] range. It is therefore simply not reasonable to dismiss glucose levels of 2.3–3.8 mmol/L as clinically unimportant in patients who are intubated [7], receiving propofol or other sedatives [36, 38], or both. Most of the studies reviewed here are encumbered by the limitation that clinically important hypoglycemia may have been excluded from consideration by an inappropriately narrow definition of hypoglycemia. A rather high incidence of hypoglycemia (15%) was reported in the intensive arm of the DIGAMI

study [32], but this is likely because a liberal definition (<3.0 mmol/L) of hypoglycemia was used. The incidence of "severe" (<2.2 mmol/L) hypoglycemia in the DIGAMI study is not known.

In summary, it is clear that hypoglycemia is a potentially serious limitation to the pursuit of near-euglycemia with intensive insulin therapy in the critically ill. It is possible, even likely, that hypoglycemia mitigated beneficial effects of intensive insulin therapy in negative [29, 35–39] and equivocal [35] studies. Failure to consider less severe (2.3–3.8 mmol/L) hypoglycemia is a serious limitation of these studies. A recent retrospective analysis of hypoglycemia in 1109 patients from two Australian ICUs demonstrated a stepwise and significant increase in mortality associated with increasingly severe hypoglycemia, including patients with glucose values of 4.0–4.5 mmol/L [46]. This indicates that even very mild hypoglycemia may have significant effects on survival in the critically ill.

Methodology for glucose testing

The observation that glucose values (4.0–4.5 mmol/L) not considered to be in the hypoglycemic range by even the most liberal definition of hypoglycemia could be associated with increased mortality is difficult to understand. In people with diabetes, there may be a shift upward in the glycemic threshold for the sympathoadrenal response [47]. Another possible explanation would apply to nondiabetic as well as diabetic patients, and relates to the methods used to measure glucose in the critically ill. Point-of care (POC) blood glucose testing was used in a number of the studies, and it has been shown to be very inaccurate and imprecise, especially during hypoglycemia. CLIA defines inaccuracy with POC glucose devices as values >20% different from the laboratory value except in the case of hypoglycemia, where values >0.83 mmol/L different are considered inaccurate. Thus, a true glucose level of 4.0 mmol/L could be reported as 3.2 mmol/L, or a true level of 2.8 could be reported as 3.6 mmol/L, and both values would be considered to be accurate. Critchell et al. reported that POC devices, when used by trained laboratory technicians, were inaccurate in 19% of samples [48]. Kanji et al. found the agreement of POC measurements with a central laboratory to be 56%, and only 26% in hypoglycemia samples [49]. The potential for error when POC devices are used is thus readily apparent. POC devices may also systematically overestimate true glucose [48]. Among the large clinical trials reviewed here, a bedside meter was used exclusively in two of the negative studies [36, 38]. NICE-SUGAR used both a blood gas machine, which has excellent precision and accuracy [50], and a POC device. When a POC device was used in NICE-SUGAR, laboratory confirmation was obtained only 60% of the time. Even when hypoglycemic values were confirmed, it should be recognized that the antecedent glucose level was unconfirmed and thus could have dictated an inappropriate decision about insulin infusion rate that led to the subsequent hypoglycemic episode. The Leuven 1 study used a blood gas instrument, and Leuven 2 used the Hemocue, a POC device that is designed for clinical use, not for self-monitoring. The VISEP study utilized both a blood gas device and the Hemocue [37]. Thus, the techniques used for blood glucose measurement in several of the studies may have contributed to hypoglycemia, failed to identify hypoglycemia, and even overcalled hypoglycemia.

The role of nutritional support in results of trials

A physician, so the story goes, once gave 1 mg of thyroxine daily to an elderly, frail woman who complained of fatigue. When the patient developed acute atrial fibrillation and died, the physician concluded that death was to be expected from thyroxine administration, and that it should never be used again. This kind of reasoning has been attributed to the "Chagrin Factor," which derives from aversion to a course of action that has produced an unexpected poor outcome [51].

Nutrition support is often used in the care of the critically ill, affecting glucose levels and insulin requirements. In two of the ten large trials [32, 33], nutrition was given

to very few patients [22]. Enteral nutrition was used almost exclusively in the study of Krinsley (J Krinsley, personal communication to *JMM*). Enteral nutrition was used primarily in four studies [29, 36, 38, 39], whereas enteral and parenteral nutrition were used equally in the VISEP study [37]. In the two Leuven studies, the majority of nutritional support was parenteral, at least for the first 7 days in the ICU. This has an impact on interpretation of the data from the Leuven 1 study, since parenteral nutrition is known to increase infection rates [52], and differences in infection, especially sepsis, accounted for most of the differences in mortality between the intensive and control groups in Leuven 1 [22, 53]. Enteral feeding does not appear to confer the same risk of infection [53], although control data on this issue are not available. In contrast, the differences in mortality in the NICE-SUGAR study were based primarily on cardiovascular outcomes, which may be influenced adversely by hypoglycemia [54].

In addition to the route of nutrition, the amount of nutrition given may influence the results of studies of glycemic control in the critically ill. We calculated energy supply in the Leuven 1 trial in relation to estimated basal energy expenditure, and thus basal energy requirements, using the Harris-Benedict equation [22]. This can be done for any study in which the calories given are reported and height and weight are provided. In the absence of height and weight data, the calculation can be made from body mass index and estimated height [22]. We therefore calculated energy given in relation to energy requirements in five of the reports where adequate information was available [7, 29, 35–37], using data on the intensively treated arm of the studies. Height was estimated from online information (e.g., http://forums.interbasket.net/f10/average-male-height-by-country-updated-9287/ and http://en.wikipedia.org/wiki/Human_height). Including protein in the energy calculation (estimated to be 1.0 g/kg per day when not provided), the values used for daily feeding rate were 27 kcal/kg for Leuven 1 [22], 25 kcal/kg for Leuven 2 [35], 25.5 kcal/kg for De La Rosa [36], 1236 kcal/day for VISEP [37] [from online appendix], and 1624 kcal for NICE-SUGAR [29] [from online appendix]. In several of the studies [7, 29, 37] the average energy intake on days 3–5 was used. Energy intake in the Arabi study was provided only as an average given over the first 7 days, and was much lower than expected based on the method for feeding described by the authors—using the Harris-Benedict equation and adjusting for stress factors

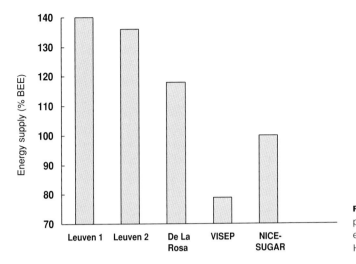

FIG 15.1 Energy supply expressed as a percentage of estimated basal energy expenditure (BEE, calculated from the Harris-Benedict equation) in five studies.

[38]; for this reason, we excluded the Arabi study from the analysis. Energy intake expressed as a percentage of estimated basal energy requirements is shown in Figure 15.1. The feeding rates among the various studies are surprisingly different. The amount of nutrition given in the Leuven studies, although within published guidelines, is greater than probable energy requirements in the critically ill [55] and may account for the rather high insulin requirements in the intensively treated groups in those studies, especially noteworthy considering that very few of the participants had diabetes. In contrast, studies that relied primarily on enteral feedings such as the

NICE-SUGAR study provided energy more in line with probably energy requirements [55]. This may be in part because tube feeding intolerance tends to limit infusion rate of enteral formulae. The relationship between amount of feeding and insulin infusion rate for the intensive groups of five studies is shown in Figure 15.2. As can be seen, there was a strong correlation between feeding rate and insulin requirement, particularly impressive since the modes of feeding were heterogenous among the studies, and when energy supply is controlled for, insulin requirements related to intravenous feeding are greater than requirements during enteral feeding [56]. The data

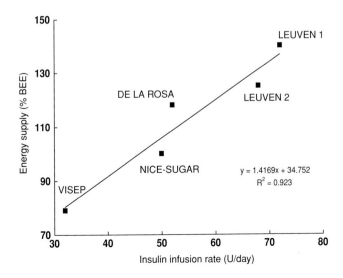

FIG 15.2 Energy supply versus insulin infusion rate in five studies.

shown in the figures are admittedly estimates, but do serve to illustrate how variable approaches to nutrition support can impact insulin requirements in the critically ill. This is an important point, as it is common to invoke "stress" as the cause of temporary hyperglycemia in critically ill nondiabetic patients, without sufficient attention to the role of overfeeding [55].

A recently published meta-analysis concluded that there is no evidence to support the use of intensive insulin therapy in general medical-surgical patients who are fed according to current guidelines [57]. The study was unusual in that it attempted to assess the role of nutritional support in the outcomes of some of the same clinical trials reviewed here. It found that there was a high incidence of hypoglycemia and increased risk of death in patients on intensive insulin therapy not receiving parenteral nutrition [29, 36, 38, 39]. Unfortunately, the authors did not consider the impact of how hypoglycemia is defined or the methodology used for blood glucose testing on frequency of hypoglycemia, and did not consider the possibility that (1) hypoglycemia could be avoided, that (2) selection of more reasonable glucose targets and use of better glucose testing techniques could facilitate avoidance of hypoglycemia, and (like the physician who gave up on thyroxine rather than consider a different dose) that (3) successful avoidance of hypoglycemia might completely change study outcomes and conclusions.

Conclusions

Available data concerning intensive therapy of hyperglycemia in the critically ill is inconsistent and confusing. However, much of the contradictory data is likely related to differences in experimental design that result in different frequency and severity of hypoglycemia. In most of the studies reviewed here, hypoglycemia was poorly defined and insufficiently respected. It should be emphasized that hypoglycemia may exert adverse effects of its own, masking beneficial effects of glycemic control. Problems with the accuracy and precision of available blood glucose testing methodology impose considerable limitations on interpretation of data and contribute to safety concerns. Nutritional support may also confound the interpretation of large clinical trials, although avoidance of overfeeding [55] should minimize concerns in that regard. Based on available data, we believe that intensive insulin therapy has a role in the management of the critically ill, although it is unclear what the optimal target range should be. Pending further research and in the interest of minimizing hypo-

glycemia, we believe that the current ADA/AACE guidelines for treatment of hyperglycemia on the critically ill, which recommend insulin infusion with a blood glucose target of 7.8–10 mmol/L, are appropriate. Robust and carefully standardized methods for blood glucose testing should be used, staff should be well trained, and hypoglycemia should be appropriately defined and assiduously avoided.

Acknowledgments

This work was supported in part by the USPHS (HL67933) and the Mayo Foundation. We thank P. E. Cryer for helpful comments on the manuscript.

References

1. Umpierrez GE, Isaacs SD, Bazargan N, You X, Thaler LM, Kitabchi AE. Hyperglycemia: an independent marker of in-hospital mortality in patients with undiagnosed diabetes. *J Clin Endocrinol Metab* **87**:978–982, 2002.

2. Cook CB, Kongable GL, Potter DJ, Abad VJ, Leija DE, Anderson M. Inpatient glucose control: a glycemic survey of 126 U.S. hospitals. *J Hosp Med.* **4**:E7–E14, 2009.

3. Golden SH, Peart-Vigilance C, Kao WH, Brancati FL. Perioperative glycemic control and the risk of infectious complications in a cohort of adults with diabetes. *Diabetes Care* **22**:1408–1414, 1999.

4. Zerr KJ, Furnary AP, Grunkemeier GL, Bookin S, Kanhere V, Starr A. Glucose control lowers the risk of wound infection in diabetics after open heart operations. *Ann Thorac Surg* **63**:356–361, 1997.

5. Weir CJ, Murray GD, Dyker AG, Lees KR. Is hyperglycaemia an independent predictor of poor outcome after acute stroke? Results of a long-term follow up study. *BMJ.* **314**:1303–1306, 1997.

6. Krinsley JS. Association between hyperglycemia and increased hospital mortality in a heterogeneous population of critically ill patients. *Mayo Clin Proc.* **78**:1471–1478, 2003.

7. van den Berghe G, Wouters P, Weekers F, et al. Intensive insulin therapy in critically ill patients. *N Engl J Med.* **345**:1359–1367, 2001.

8. Garber AJ, Moghissi ES, Bransome ED, Jr., et al. ACE position statement. *Endocr Pract* **10**:5–9, 2004.

9. McCowen KC, Malhotra A, Bistrian BR. Stress-induced hyperglycemia. *Crit Care Clin.* **17**:107–124, 2001.

10. Andreelli F, Jacquier D, Troy S. Molecular aspects of insulin therapy in critically ill patients. *Curr Opin Clin Nutr Metab Care.* **9**:124–130, 2006.

11. van den Berghe G. How does blood glucose control with insulin save lives in intensive care? *J Clin Invest.* **114**:1187–1195, 2004.

12. Vanhorebeek I, De Vos R, Mesotten D, Wouters PJ, De Wolf-Peeters C, Van Den Berghe G. Protection of hepatocyte mitochondrial ultrastructure and function by strict blood glucose control with insulin in critically ill patients. *Lancet.* **365**:53–59, 2005.

13. Bagdade JD, Stewart M, Walters E. Impaired granulocyte adherence. A reversible defect in host defense in patients with poorly controlled diabetes. *Diabetes.* **27**:677–681, 1978.

14. Poitout V, Robertson RP. Glucolipotoxicity: fuel excess and beta-cell dysfunction. *Endocrine Rev.* **29**:351–366, 2008.

15. Hansen TK, Thiel S, Wouters PJ, Christiansen JS, Van den Berghe G. Intensive insulin therapy exerts antiinflammatory effects in critically ill patients and counteracts the adverse effect of low mannose-binding lectin levels. *J Clin Endocrinol Metab.* **88**:1082–1088, 2003.

16. Langouche L, Vanhorebeek I, Vlasselaers D, et al. Intensive insulin therapy protects the endothelium of critically ill patients. *J Clin Invest.* **115**:2277–2286, 2005.

17. Stoner HB, Little RA, Frayn KN, Elebute AE, Tresadern J, Gross E. The effect of sepsis on the oxidation of carbohydrate and fat. *Br J Surg.* **70**:32–35, 1983.

18. Steinberg HO, Tarshoby M, Monestel R, et al. Elevated circulating free fatty acid levels impair endothelium-dependent vasodilation. *J Clin Invest.* **100**:1230–1239, 1997.

19. Stojiljkovic MP, Zhang D, Lopes HF, Lee CG, Goodfriend TL, Egan BM. Hemodynamic effects of lipids in humans. *Am J Physiol.* **280**:R1674–R1679, 2001.

20. Lewis GF, Uffelman KD, Szeto LW, Weller B, Steiner G. Interaction between free fatty acids and insulin in the acute control of very low density lipoprotein production in humans. *J Clin Invest.* **95**:158–166, 1995.

21. Mesotten D, Swinnen JV, Vanderhoydonc F, Wouters PJ, Van Den Berghe G. Contribution of circulating lipids to the improved outcome of critical illness by glycemic control with intensive insulin therapy. *J Clin Endocrinol Metab.* **89**:219–226, 2004.

22. Miles JM, McMagon MM, Isley WL. For debate: no, the glycemic target in the critically ill should not be <6.1 mmol/L. *Diabetologia.* **51**:916–920, 2008.

23. Langouche L, Vander Perre S, Wouters PJ, D'Hoore A, Hansen TK, Van Den Berghe G. Effect of intensive insulin therapy on insulin sensitivity in the critically ill. *J Clin Endocrinol Metab.* **92**:3890–3897, 2007.

24. Weekers F, Van Herck E, Coopmans W, et al. A novel in vivo rabbit model of hypercatabolic critical illness reveals a biphasic neuroendocrine stress response. *Endocrinology.* **143**:764–774, 2002.

25. Pomposelli JJ, Baxter JK, 3rd, Babineau TJ, et al. Early postoperative glucose control predicts nosocomial infection rate in diabetic patients. *JPEN: J Parenter Enteral Nutr.* **22**:77–81, 1998.

26. ADA: Standards of Medical Care in Diabetes—2009. *Diabetes Care* **32**:S41, 2009.

27. Moghissi ES, Korytkowski MT, DiNardo M, et al. American Association of Clinical Endocrinologists and American Diabetes Association consensus statement on inpatient glycemic control. *Diabetes Care.* **32**:1119–1131, 2009.

28. Hirshberg E, Lacroix J, Sward K, Willson D, Morris AH. Blood glucose control in critically ill adults and children: a survey on stated practice. *Chest* **133**:1328–1335, 2008.

29. Investigators N-SS, Finfer S, Chittock DR, et al. Intensive versus conventional glucose control in critically ill patients. *N Engl J Med.* **360**:1283–1297, 2009.

30. Wiener RS, Wiener DC, Larson RJ. Benefits and risks of tight glucose control in critically ill adults: a meta-analysis. [Erratum appeared in *JAMA.* 2009 Mar4;301(9):936]. *JAMA.* **300**:933–944, 2008.

31. Griesdale DEG, de Souza RJ, van Dam RM, et al. Intensive insulin therapy and mortality among critically ill patients: a meta-analysis including NICE-SUGAR study data. *CMAJ.* **180**:821–827, 2009.

32. Malmberg K. Prospective randomised study of intensive insulin treatment on long term survival after acute myocardial infarction in patients with diabetes mellitus. DIGAMI (Diabetes Mellitus, Insulin Glucose Infusion in Acute Myocardial Infarction) Study Group. *BMJ.* **314**:1512–1515, 1997.

33. Furnary AP, Gao G, Grunkemeier GL, et al. Continuous insulin infusion reduces mortality in patients with diabetes undergoing coronary artery bypass grafting. *J Thorac Cardiovasc Surg.* **125**:1007–1021, 2003.

34. Krinsley JS. Effect of an intensive glucose management protocol on the mortality of critically ill adult patients. *Mayo Clin Proc.* **79**:992–1000, 2004.

35. Van den Berghe G, Wilmer A, Hermans G, et al. Intensive insulin therapy in the medical ICU. *N Engl J Med.* **354**:449–461, 2006.

36. De La Rosa GDC, Donado JH, Restrepo AH, et al. Strict glycaemic control in patients hospitalised in a mixed medical and surgical intensive care unit: a randomised clinical trial. *Crit Care (London, England).* **12**:R120, 2008.

37. Brunkhorst FM, Engel C, Bloos F, et al. Intensive insulin therapy and pentastarch resuscitation in severe sepsis. *N Engl J Med.* **358**:125–139, 2008.

38. Arabi YM, Dabbagh OC, Tamim HM, et al. Intensive versus conventional insulin therapy: a randomized controlled trial in medical and surgical critically ill patients. *Crit Care Med.* **36**:3190–3197, 2008.

39. Preiser J-C, Devos P, Ruiz-Santana S, et al. A prospective randomised multi-centre controlled trial on tight glucose control by intensive insulin therapy in adult intensive care units: the Glucontrol study. *Intensive Care Med.* **35**:1738–1748, 2009.

40. Gray CS, Hildreth AJ, Sandercock PA, et al. Glucose-potassium-insulin infusions in the management of post-stroke hyperglycaemia: the UK Glucose Insulin in Stroke Trial (GIST-UK). *Lancet Neurol.* **6**:397–406, 2007.

41. Cryer PE. Hypoglycaemia: the limiting factor in the glycaemic management of the critically ill? *Diabetologia.* **49**:1722–1725, 2006.

42. Mesotten D, Van den Berghe G. Clinical benefits of tight glycaemic control: focus on the intensive care unit. *Best Practice & Research Clinical Anaesthesiology.* **23**:421–429, 2009.

43. Cryer PE. Hierarchy of physiological responses to hypoglycemia: relevance to clinical hypoglycemia in type I (insulin dependent) diabetes mellitus. *Horm Metab Res.* **29**:92–96, 1997.

44. Frier BM. Defining hypoglycaemia: what level has clinical relevance? *Diabetologia.* **52**:31–34, 2009.

45. Cryer PE. Preventing hypoglycaemia: what is the appropriate glucose alert value? *Diabetologia.* **52**:35–37, 2009.

46. Egi M, Bellomo R, Stachowski E, et al. Hypoglycemia and outcome in critically ill patients. *Mayo Clin Proc.* **85**:217–224.

47. Boyle PJ, Schwartz NS, Shah SD, Clutter WE, Cryer PE. Plasma glucose concentrations at the onset of hypoglycemic symptoms in patients with poorly controlled diabetes and in nondiabetics. *N Engl J Med.* **318**:1487–1492, 1988.

48. Critchell CD, Savarese V, Callahan A, Aboud C, Jabbour S, Marik P. Accuracy of bedside capillary blood glucose measurements in critically ill patients. *Intens Care Med.* **33**:2079–2084, 2007.

49. Kanji S, Buffie J, Hutton B, et al. Reliability of point-of-care testing for glucose measurement in critically ill adults. *Crit Care Med.* **33**:2778–2785, 2005.

50. Beneteau-Burnat B, Bocque M-C, Lorin A, Martin C, Vaubourdolle M. Evaluation of the blood gas analyzer Gem PREMIER 3000. *Clin Chem Lab Med.* **42**:96–101, 2004.

51. Feinstein AR. The 'chagrin factor' and quantitative decision analysis. *Arch Int Med.* **145**:1257–1259, 1985.

52. Perioperative total parenteral nutrition in surgical patients. The Veterans Affairs Total Parenteral Nutrition Cooperative Study Group. *N Engl J Med.* **325**:525–532, 1991.

53. Braunschweig CL, Levy P, Sheean PM, Wang X. Enteral compared with parenteral nutrition: a meta-analysis. *Am J Clin Nutr.* **74**:534–542, 2001.

54. Adler GK, Bonyhay I, Failing H, Waring E, Dotson S, Freeman R. Antecedent hypoglycemia impairs autonomic cardiovascular function: implications for rigorous glycemic control. *Diabetes.* **58**:360–366, 2009.

55. Miles JM. Energy expenditure in hospitalized patients: implications for nutritional support. *Mayo Clin Proc.* **81**:809–816, 2006.

56. van den Berghe G, Wouters PJ, Bouillon R, et al. Outcome benefit of intensive insulin therapy in the critically ill: Insulin dose versus glycemic control. *Crit Care Med.* **31**:359–366, 2003.

57. Marik PE, Preiser J-C. Toward understanding tight glycemic control in the ICU: a systematic review and metaanalysis. *Chest.* **137**:544–551, 2010.

16 Is there an optimal revascularization strategy in diabetic patients with ischemic heart disease?

Stephen H. McKellar[1], Morgan L. Brown[2], and Robert L. Frye[3]

[1] Resident, Division of Cardiovascular Surgery, Mayo Clinic, Rochester, MN, USA
[2] Resident, University of Alberta, Edmonton, AB, Canada
[3] Professor of Medicine, Division of Cardiovascular Diseases, Mayo Clinic, Rochester, MN, USA

LEARNING POINTS

- Coronary artery disease is a leading cause of death among patients with diabetes.

- Outcomes after coronary events/interventions are worse among patients with DM compared to those without DM.

- Patients with no or mild stable symptoms may have extensive multivessel CAD.

- Risk stratification is essential.

- Control of symptoms and reduction in risk of death and MI are reasons for invasive intervention.

- Choice of CABG or PCI depends on individual patient characteristics with CABG preferred for those with the most extensive disease.

Introduction

Coronary heart disease (CHD) is the leading cause of death among adults with diabetes mellitus [1]. While a major decline in CHD mortality has been observed since the 1960s in the general population, those with DM, particularly women, have not experienced the same decline [2]. Moreover, there are striking health disparities in the burden of disease and poor outcomes among specific minority, ethnic, and disadvantaged populations [3]. Also of concern is the rising obesity and type 2 DM epidemic and its likely impact on cardiovascular disease. Recent data suggest a leveling off of the reduction of CHD mortality in younger patients as a result of the metabolic consequences of obesity and DM [4]. These findings call for a careful assessment of how we manage CHD in the setting of DM.

Advances in understanding the basic pathophysiologic mechanisms that account for the more aggressive vascular disease in DM are important when considering the optimal strategy for coronary revascularization [5]. While percutaneous coronary intervention (PCI) has the advantage of being less invasive, the hostile metabolic milieu of DM may alter the response to injury of the arterial wall inherent in such interventions [6] and fails to anticipate new disease that may develop in untreated segments [7]. Coronary artery bypass grafting (CABG) has the inherent risks of major surgery with a more prolonged recovery time but provides more complete revascularization. To help clinicians decide which revascularization strategy is best for diabetic patients, this chapter will focus on: (1) the indications for coronary revascularization (2) selection of PCI or CABG if revascularization is needed and (3) the importance of aggressive medical management regardless of the specific revascularization procedure. Screening for CHD in patients with diabetes is discussed in Chapter 4.

Coronary revascularization

The optimal revascularization strategy for patients with diabetes depends on the following:

- clinical characteristics of the individual patient;
- severity, extent, and location of anatomic coronary artery disease (CAD);

Clinical Dilemmas in Diabetes, First Edition. Edited by Adrian Vella and Robert A. Rizza
© 2011 Blackwell Publishing Ltd. Published 2011 by Blackwell Publishing Ltd.

TABLE 16.1 Class I indications for CABG

- For asymptomatic patients with left main disease (or left main equivalent) and triple-vessel disease
- For patients with stable angina with left main disease (or left main equivalent), triple-vessel disease, two-vessel disease with LVEF < 50%, two-vessel disease (without proximal left main disease) if large territory is at risk, and for refractory, disabling angina
- For patients with unstable angina/NSTEMI with left main (or left main equivalent) disease, and ongoing, refractory ischemia
- For patients with STEMI who have failed PCI or unsuitable PCI anatomy, mechanical complications of myocardial infarction (MI), cardiogenic shock, and life-threatening arrhythmias with left main or triple-vessel disease
- For patients with left ventricular dysfunction with left main (or left main equivalent) disease and multivessel disease

---

- physiologic consequences of the CAD, (documentation of ischemia), and
- patient comorbidities and preferences.

The ACC/AHA [8–10] and European Society of Cardiology [11] Guidelines are essential references for a detailed set of recommendations for coronary revascularization. The latter provides extensive data for the broad management of cardiovascular disease. The Class 1 recommendations for all patients are listed in Table 16.1 (CABG) and Table 16.2 (PCI) from the ACC/AHA document. The recommendations that are specific for the patient with DM and CAD

TABLE 16.2 Class I recommendations for PCI

- For patients with unstable angina/NSTEMI with at least one of the following high-risk features: refractory ischemic or heart failure symptoms, elevated biochemical markers of ischemia, new ST-segment depression, LV dysfunction with or without hemodynamic instability, prior PCI or CABG
- For patients with STEMI with new MI or left bundle branch block*
- For patients with STEMI who develop shock within 36 hours of acute MI**
- For patients with STEMI with severe heart failure and/or pulmonary edema*
- (* must be performed within 12 hours of symptom onset. ** must be within 36 hours of symptom onset)

TABLE 16.3 Diabetes and coronary revascularization (Euroepan Society of Cardiology and European Association for the Study of Diabetes)

Recommendation	Class[a]	Level[b]
Treatment decisions regarding revascularization in patients with diabetes should favor coronary artery bypass surgery over percutaneous intervention	IIa	A
Glycoprotein IIb/IIIa inhibitors are indicated in elective PCI in a diabetic patient	I	B
When PCI with stent implantation is performed in a diabetic patient, drug-eluting stents (DES) should be used	IIIa	B
Mechanical reperfusion by means of primary PCI is the revascularization mode of choice in a diabetic patient with acute MI	I	A

[a]Class of recommendation
[b]Level of evidence
(from *European Heart Journal* 2007;28:88–136).

are included in the European Society Guidelines Table 16.3. Our goal is to provide a clinical overview on the approach to individual patients based on existing guidelines for (1) selecting patients who need coronary revascularization and (2) selection of the specific procedure for an individual patient, while emphasizing the importance of careful medical management for all patients regardless of the invasive procedure.

There are two basic reasons to consider an invasive coronary revascularization procedure (PCI or CABG) in a patient with CHD regardless of the presence of DM: (1) for control of symptoms due to myocardial ischemia in spite of optimal medical therapy, and (2) to reduce morality and subsequent nonfatal myocardial infarction in high-risk patients regardless of symptoms. These are not mutually exclusive, as highly symptomatic patients may also have clear survival and survival-free-of-MI benefits from revascularization. It is now clear from recent trials that patients with less severe but definite anatomic CAD may usually be managed first with medical therapy and with revascularization later, if the disease progresses. We will review the rationale and justification for recommending invasive coronary revascularization in each setting, noting specific findings in patients with DM when available, as most of the trials included a majority of patients without DM.

Control of symptoms in spite of optimal medical therapy (stable patients)

Rationale

The placebo effect for any intervention to control symptoms, such as angina, is well recognized and calls for carefully controlled studies [12]. Considerable skepticism regarding surgery for CHD developed in the era of ligation of the internal thoracic artery (ITA), for angina, and later implantation of the ITA in the myocardium after sham procedures demonstrated no therapeutic effectiveness of such procedures [13]. However, it is now clear from multiple studies in patients with and without diabetes that coronary revascularization improves symptoms and quality of life compared to medical therapy alone, both with CABG and PCI. [14,15] An advantage of CABG compared to PCI in duration of benefit in relief of angina without need for a repeat procedure has been shown by multiple studies.

A practical challenge for practitioners is in assessing the nature of symptoms that may be disabling and raise the necessity of coronary revascularization This includes dealing with the possibility that patients with DM may not perceive the classic symptoms of myocardial ischemia; dyspnea is a frequent angina equivalent. Moreover, because of the widespread use of noninvasive CT coronary angiography, many patients are found to have evidence of anatomic coronary artery disease and it may be difficult to determine if the symptoms truly relate to the physiologic consequences of the anatomic findings. Such a dilemma is evident also with invasive angiography and the finding of borderline lesions in terms of luminal diameter narrowing.

It is quite clear from studies of CABG [16] and PCI that pre-intervention [17] documentation of ischemia increases the probability of symptom relief after either intervention. The final resolution of the significance of flow limitation in borderline lesions (50–75% narrowing) calls for fractional flow measurement and/or intracoronary ultrasound imaging at the time of the diagnostic study. Unless the free flow ratio (FFR) is less than 0.75 across lesions with moderate narrowing, the likelihood of symptomatic improvement is reduced [17]. Gould has emphasized the need for careful consideration of physiologic factors in coronary flow dynamics and avoiding fixation on angiographic findings.

Selecting PCI or CABG patients with DM for symptom control

Having determined the presence of ischemia producing poorly controlled symptoms and coronary anatomy suitable for PCI or CABG, what is the basis for choosing one procedure over the other with the primary goal of reducing symptoms? In patients with single-vessel disease, PCI is the preferred strategy unless there is an anatomic reason to consider CABG regardless of the presence of DM. Some have erroneously concluded from the original BARI (Bypass Angioplasty Revascularization Investigation) trial that PCI is inappropriate for any patient with DM. This is a serious error in generalizing results of a randomized clinical trial, as there were no patients with single-vessel disease in BARI-l. Thus, it is quite appropriate for PCI to be the first choice for revascularization in a patient with DM and single-vessel disease with angina not responding to medical therapy, presuming the anatomy is suitable for PCI. In DM patients and single-vessel disease not suitable for PCI, CABG with an arterial graft is an alternative. In such a setting it is important to ensure medical therapy is intense, as it is best to defer CABG if possible until there is multivessel involvement. The bottom line for patients with severe multivessel disease is clearly articulated by the SYNTAX (Synergy between PCI with Taxus and Cardiac Surgery) investigators: "CABG remains the standard of care for patients with three-vessel or left main coronary artery disease, since the use of CABG, as compared with PCI, resulted in lower rates of the combined end point of major adverse cardiac or cerebrovascular events at 1 year" [18].

For less extensive multivessel disease PCI may have a role, particularly if comorbidities call for the less invasive strategy. In the original BARI Registry where decisions were made by choosing the presumed optimal procedure, it was demonstrated that physicians could select the patients with DM and multivessel disease who would likely do well with PTCA [19]. This was based on selecting those for PTCA with less extensive disease. In the BARI 2D trial, which included only patients with type 2 DM and in whom PCI or CABG was chosen, most patients with single-vessel disease were selected for PCI, and those with more extensive disease, for CABG [20]. Thus, one may intervene in patients with less severe disease to control symptoms without affecting survival.

Acute coronary syndromes

Acute coronary syndromes include unstable angina, non-ST-segment elevation myocardial infarction (NTEMI) and ST elevation myocardial infarction (STEMI). Prompt PCI is the preferred treatment for patients with STEMI regardless of the presence or absence of DM. Emphasis on reducing/eliminating delays to the cath lab for prompt treatment of the infarct-related artery provides real benefit. In patients with the most extensive anatomic disease, CABG is the preferred invasive revascularization strategy. The Global Registry of Acute Coronary Events has documented that one in four patients presenting to a participating hospital with ACS have DM [21] and are at increased risk for heart failure, renal failure, cardiogenic shock, and death, compared to those without DM. Also noted were differences between those with and without DM in terms of use of PCI and specific drugs such as beta-blockers and aspirin. Of particular importance was a much greater delay in seeking care in the setting of ACS among those with DM. This is a particular issue for primary providers in counseling patients to present promptly to an emergency room with symptoms suggesting ACS. It was noted in this observational experience that more patients with DM and STEMI went to CABG than those without DM, reflecting more extensive disease. However, it is clear that patients with DM benefit from early revascularization in the setting of STEMI combined with aggressive medical management.

For patients with unstable angina and NSTEMI, there is also evidence that early coronary revascularization is of benefit in reducing death and MI. The advantage of prompt coronary revascularization is well established by several prospective randomized trials and extends to patients with DM based upon post hoc analysis of the DM subgroup(s). The Framingham and Fast Revascularization During Instability in Coronary Artery Disease (FRISC) II trial has also focused on experience with diabetic patients in the setting of unstable CAD [22]. The benefit in long-term outcomes (death, MI) among those with DM randomized to early invasive therapy was actually greater than among patients without DM; the number needed to treat to reduce death and MI was 11 for those with DM as opposed to 32 for those without DM [11].

Coronary revascularization for prolonging life and preventing subsequent MI in stable patients

Clinical trials—Coronary artery revascularization

Studies demonstrating a survival benefit from coronary revascularization began with trials comparing coronary artery bypass grafting (CABG) to best medical therapy in the 1970s and 1980s [24–27]. These trials showed the most benefit was derived from revascularization in patients with the greatest disease burden (multivessel disease) as well as specific anatomic lesions such as left main or proximal left anterior descending with two-vessel disease and in

patients with decreased left ventricular function [28–30]. These findings have been also been noted in observational studies and meta-analyses. In contrast, no trial has shown a survival benefit for stable mildly symptomatic patients for coronary revascularization via PCI compared to medical therapy. Though unproven in randomized trials, the presence of a critical proximal LAD lesion amenable to PCI is thought to be of enough risk to justify invasive treatment, regardless of the presence of DM. Pooling of data from the original CABG trials was the basis of a careful meta-analysis by Yusuf confirming a survival benefit with CABG overall but also demonstrating the importance of risk stratification. Those at high risk noted improved survival, those at low risk did not benefit in terms of survival (or may have been harmed). A significant limitation in the early CABG trials relates to the absence of modern medical therapy. The studies, however, clearly demonstrated the gradient of risk in relation to the extent of disease and LV function. Recent observational data have demonstrated improved survival with CABG in stable asymptomatic patients with DM who were identified as being at high risk by nuclear stress imaging.

Several more trials are of interest in considering the reduction of risk for subsequent cardiac events. The Randomized Intervention Treatment of Angina (RITA) 2 trial randomized stable patients to PTCA or medical therapy and demonstrated an advantage of PTCA in reducing symptoms, but there was more frequent MI in the PTCA group [15]. The Angioplasty Compared to Medical Therapy (ACME) trial also demonstrated better symptom control but no effect on event rates. Two other trials, the Medicine Angioplasty of Surgery Study (MASS) and Trial of Invasive versus Medical Therapy in Elderly Patients with Chronic Symptomatic Coronary-Artery Disease (TIME), failed to demonstrate improved survival. The TIME trial, which included highly symptomatic patients, showed reduced cardiac event rates and improved symptoms in the revascularization group. The most currently relevant trial in the general population is the Clinical Outcomes Utilizing Revascularization and Aggressive Drug Evaluation (COURAGE) trial, which recently reported with no advantage of early revascularization for stable angina. About a third of the patients had DM. Based on these data, the indications for coronary revascularization to reduce risk of death or subsequent MI regardless of the presence of DM have been established. In stable patients with high-risk anatomy, a survival benefit for coronary revascularization has been demonstrated. Less severe disease can usually be managed medically regardless of the presence or absence of DM (Table 16.1 and 16.2). Class I indications exist for both PCI and CABG and are shown in the table. In all of these trials it must be emphasized that strict long-term treatment comparisons were not possible. Thus, patients randomized to an initial strategy of medical therapy might "cross over" to have revascularization. Thus the medical therapy groups undoubtedly benefitted from subsequent revascularization if they became unstable.

It is important to note, however, that these guidelines and Class I indications were derived from studies of patient cohorts where the majority of patients did not have diabetes. It is thus important to look at subgroups of patients with DM and also the few trials comprised only of patients with type 2 DM.

Diabetes subgroup analysis

The BARI trial was the first to observe a survival benefit, at 5 years, for patients with treated diabetes undergoing CABG with at least one internal thoracic artery (ITA) as a conduit compared to patients treated with PTCA. This observation in patients with treated diabetes was not a predefined end point but had been selected by the study's data safety and monitoring board to monitor for safety. Subsequent reports from the BARI trial with longer follow-up confirm the initial observation of improved survival among patients revascularized with CABG vs. PCI (76% vs. 56% at 7 years). This difference is due, in part, to poorer outcomes among diabetic patients randomized to PTCA with a subsequent Q-wave MI resulting in a tenfold higher 30-day mortality compared to patients experiencing Q-wave MI subsequent to CABG. A recent meta-analysis of 7812 patients based upon pooled data from ten clinical trials found improved survival for patients with diabetes undergoing CABG ($n = 615$) compared to PCI ($n = 618$) (HR 0.7 95% CI 0.56–0.87) but no difference in survival among nondiabetics. Comparable conclusions were reached in the New York State Registry [23]. Although drug eluting stents have reduced restenosis rates, they remain higher in those with DM than those without DM and furthermore it seems unlikely that mortality is linked to restenosis.

Is coronary artery disease different in patients with diabetes?

It is estimated CAD accounts for nearly 3 times as many deaths among diabetic compared to nondiabetic patients [1]. Are diabetic patients adequately represented in randomized clinical trials and large registry data? In Hlatky's meta-analysis of 7812 patients, patients with diabetes comprised only 16% of the total patient sample (range 6–28%). The impact of diabetes remained even after adjustment for other risk factors and excluding patients from the BARI trial. Since diabetic patients have been under-represented in earlier clinical trials, conclusions about patients with diabetes have been drawn from subgroup analyses with all its inherent biases. Fortunately, the BARI-2D trial has studied coronary revascularization in an exclusively diabetic population.

BARI 2D trial

BARI 2D was designed to test treatment strategies in patients with type 2 DM and angiographically documented CAD to determine if, in mildly symptomatic patients not requiring revascularization to control symptoms or instability, prompt revascularization would reduce mortality or subsequent MI compared to an initial strategy of optimal medical therapy with delayed or no revascularization. An insulin-sensitizing strategy was also compared to an insulin-providing strategy to achieve target glycemia control levels. The randomization was stratified by the procedure determined to be optimal for the individual patients, i.e., PCI or CABG. No difference in mortality/MI/stroke was observed for either treatment strategy. However, when analyzed by prespecified strata there was a significant reduction in the combined end point of death, MI and stroke for patients having prompt CABG. Furthermore, there was some evidence that insulin-sensitizing therapy may enhance the benefit of CABG. About 40% of the patients randomized to initial medical therapy alone had subsequent revascularization. The benefit of CABG was observed only in the patients with the most extensive disease (high myocardial jeopardy scores).

Therefore, for asymptomatic or mildly symptomatic patients with type 2 DM with less extensive disease, no advantage was seen with prompt revascularization and waiting until symptoms develop is a safe and reasonable option. In contrast, among patients with extensive disease with high myocardial jeopardy scores, a reduction in death/MI/stroke (compared to medical therapy) was shown with revascularization using CABG. Since the majority of patients presented with mild or no symptoms, identifying those with high-risk anatomy in the clinical practice of managing patients with type 2 DM remains a challenge.

Why is CAD different in patients with diabetes? Brown-lee et al. have suggested that damage to vascular endothelial cells in diabetes is predominantly caused by oxidative stress secondary to intracellular hyperglycemia. Vascular endothelial cells cannot reduce glucose transport into the cell, rendering them unable to regulate intracellular hyperglycemia. This, in turn, leads to overproduction of oxidative species from a dysfunctioning mitochondrial electron transport chain. Excessive oxidative species leads to cellular damage through modification of intracellular proteins involved in gene transcription and regulation, cell signaling dysfunction, and increased production of inflammatory cytokines [5]. Predictably, patients with diabetes often present with a more diffuse pattern of coronary disease rather than isolated culprit lesions, given the damaging intracellular milieu found throughout all vascular endothelial cells. Such a pattern of disease is best suited for a revascularization strategy using CABG, as available data shows improved outcomes compared to PCI. This is likely due to the ability of CABG to offer more complete revascularization instead of revascularization of a single culprit lesion.

Long-term studies demonstrate a survival advantage when arterial conduits are used for surgical revascularization. The BARI study demonstrated survival benefit only for diabetic patients in whom the ITA was used as conduit to revascularize the LAD. Since then, long-term survival has also been demonstrated in large surgical series using ITA to LAD revascularization. Moreover, data from the Cleveland Clinic at 10- and 20-year follow-up suggest a survival advantage with revascularization using bilateral ITA conduits compared to one ITA conduit, despite an increased risk of deep sternal wound infections. It is important to note that the majority of these patients (nearly 70%) had advanced two- or three-vessel disease. More recent observational studies from that group also demonstrate that use of the contralateral ITA, as a second conduit, is beneficial regardless of whether it is used to revascularize the right coronary or circumflex coronary artery.

Risk factor modification

Secondary prevention of ischemic events is critical following coronary revascularization and is a critical part of deciding on optimal revascularization. The benefits of any invasive procedure may be compromised by continued smoking and lack of attention to all the details of medical management. The combined efforts of the European Society of Cardiology and the European Association for Diabetes Guidelines provide in-depth review of all aspects of medical management in patients with CAD and diabetes. Lifestyle modification, such as complete smoking cessation, exercise, and weight management, coupled with controlling metabolic risk factors, can reduce mortality. Clinical trials have demonstrated the benefits of reducing hypertension and hyperlipidemia. Additionally, antiplatelet therapy is also beneficial following revascularization. For patients treated with PCI and if drug-eluting stents were used, clopidogrel is mandatory to prevent in-stent thrombosis in the postprocedure setting and often becomes lifelong in an attempt to prevent in-stent restenosis or thrombosis. Lifelong aspirin therapy, however, is sufficient in most patients following CABG. Angiotensin converting enzyme (ACE) inhibitor and beta-blockade therapies are recommended for most patients following revascularization. Starting an ACE inhibitor early for patients following MI is important and should be continued indefinitely for patients with LV dysfunction to prevent adverse ventricular remodeling. Similarly, beta-blockade should be initiated in high-risk patients following infarction and, likewise, is usually continued indefinitely. In addition to their lipid-lowering effects, HMG-CoA reductase inhibitors, or statins, have also been shown to strengthen atherosclerotic plaques and reduce myocardial events and should be part of the program for each patient unless there is lack of tolerance because of side effects. Glycemic control is essential and more complicated, given the results of the Action to Control Cardiovascular Risk in Diabetes (ACCORD) study. Current ADA guidelines should be observed.

Intensive insulin therapy in patients following cardiac surgery is controversial and may lead to worse outcomes. Van den Berghe reported the results of a randomized controlled trial in patients mechanically ventilated in a surgical ICU. They observed a survival benefit among patients with receiving intensive insulin control who stayed in ICU for 5 or more days and those with sepsis. Furnary has been a strong proponent of continuous insulin infusions during the perioperative period of CABG. However, in randomized studies of cardiac surgery patients, intensive insulin therapy showed no benefit and potential harm. It should also be noted that glycemic control at the time of PCI may influence outcomes, though there is evidence to the contrary.

Regardless of the impact of perioperative glycemic control on mortality, a growing body of evidence shows improved outcomes with aggressive, long-term multifactorial interventions among patients with diabetes. The Steno-2 trial has shown a nearly 50% reduction in cardiovascular and microvascular events as well as a reduction in all-cause and cardiovascular-related mortality by implementing a multifactorial approach to risk factor modification in patients with diabetes. This prospective, randomized observational study randomized patients to receive conventional risk factor modification compared to multifactorial intervention consisting of treatments aimed at diabetic and concomitant risk factor management reduction similar to published guidelines by the American Diabetic Association. Patients were treated for nearly 8 years then followed for another 5 years. The hazard ratio for death was 0.54 (95% CI 0.32, 0.89; $p = 0.02$) and cardiovascular-related mortality was 0.41 (0.25, 0.67; $p < 0.001$) demonstrating significant reduction in death from all causes with intensive, multifactorial interventions.

Conclusions

Coronary revascularization can be highly beneficial in selected patients with DM and CAD. While many patients with mild symptoms and documented CAD that is not severe may be managed without invasive intervention for many years, it must be recognized that there are high-risk patients with extensive CAD who present with mild symptoms, and risk stratification is important as BARI 2D has demonstrated selected patients with extensive CAD may benefit from early CABG. Patient preferences are frequently strong and must be considered, though with a frank discussion of potential adverse outcomes. In general, CABG is the preferred procedure in the diabetic patient with the most extensive disease. However, many patients with less extensive disease but severe symptoms may benefit from PCI, but there is no evidence in those patients that survival or survival free of MI is enhanced. The critical role of aggressive medical management of all aspects of the patient's risk factors and metabolic consequences of DM cannot be overemphasized. Insulin sensitization needs further study in reducing event rates after coronary revascularization. Regardless of PCI or CABG, aggressive and continued medical management is critical.

References

1. Diabetes in American (2nd edition); Available from: http://diabetes.niddk.nih.gov/dm/pubs/America/pdf, p. 221, 233.

2. Gregg EW, Gu O, Cheng YI, Narayan KMV, Cowie CC. Mortality trends in men and women with diabetes, 1971 to 2000. *Ann Intern Med.* **147**(3):149–155, 2007.

3. Ford ES, Capewell S. Coronary heart disease mortality among young adults in the U.S. from 1980 through 2002: concealed leveling of mortality rates. *J Am Coll Cardiol.* **50**:2128–2132, 2007.

4. Brownlee M. The pathobiology of diabetic complications: a unifying mechanism. *Diabetes.* **54**(6):1615–1625, 2005.

5. Cutlip DE, Chhabra AG, Baim DS, et al. Beyond restenosis: five-year clinical outcomes from second-generation coronary stent trials. *Circulation.* **110**:1226–1230, 2004.

6. Eagle KA, et al. ACC/AHA 2004 guideline update for coronary artery bypass graft surgery: a report of the American College of Cardiology/American Heart Association Task Force on Practice Guidelines (committee to update the 1999 guidelines for coronary artery bypass graft surgery). *Circulation.* **110**(14):e340–e437, 2004.

7. Eagle KA, et al. ACC/AHA guidelines for coronary artery bypass graft surgery: a report of the American College of Cardiology/American Heart Association Task Force on practice guidelines (committee to revise the 1991 guidelines for coronary artery bypass graft surgery). American College of Cardiology/American Heart Association. *J Am Coll Cardiol.* **34**(4):1262–1347, 1999.

8. Smith SC, Jr., et al. ACC/AHA/SCAI 2005 guideline update for percutaneous coronary intervention – summary article: a report of the American College of Cardiology/American Heart Association Task Force on practice guidelines (ACC/AHA/SCAI writing committee to update the 2001 guidelines for percutaneous coronary intervention) *Circulation.* **113**(1):156–175, 2006.

9. Ryden L, Standl E, et al. Guidelines on diabetes, pre-diabetes, and cardiovascular disease: executive summary. *Eur Heart J.* **28**:88–136, 2007.

10. Cobb LA, et al. An evaluation of internal mammary ligation by a double blind technic. *NEJM.* **260**:1115–1118, 1959.

11. CASS PRINCIPAL INVESTIGATORS AND THEIR ASSOCIATES. Coronary Artery Surgery Study (CASS): A randomized trial of coronary artery bypass surgery Quality of life in patients randomly assigned to treatment groups. *Circulation.* **68**:951–960, 1983.

12. Jones RH. Floyd RD. Austin EH. Sabiston DC, Jr. The role of radionuclide angiocardiography in the preoperative prediction of pain relief and prolonged survival following coronary artery bypass grafting. *Ann Surg.* **197**(6):743–754, 1983.

13. Bech GIW, De Bruyne B, Pijls NHJ, et al. Fractional flow reserve to determine the appropriateness of angioplasty in moderate coronary stenosis. A randomized trial. *Circulation.* **103**:2928–2934, 2001.

14. Serruys PW, et al. Percutaneous coronary intervention versus coronary-artery bypass grafting for severe coronary artery disease. *N Engl J Med.* **360**(10):961–972, 2009.

15. Feit F, et al. Coronary revascularization in diabetic patients: a comparison of the randomized and observational components of the Bypass Angioplasty Revascularization Investigation (BARI). **99**(5):633–640, 1999.

16. Lagervist B, Husted S, Kontny F, et al. A long-term perspective on the protective effects of an early invasive strategy in unstable coronary artery disease & the FRISC II Investigator two-year follow-up of the FRISC-II invasive study. *J Am Coll Cardiol.* **43**:585–591, 2004, doi:10.1016/j.jacc.2003.08.05.

17. Yusuf S, et al. Effect of coronary artery bypass graft surgery on survival: overview of 10-year results from randomised trials by the Coronary Artery Bypass Graft Surgery Trialists Collaboration. *Lancet.* **344**(8922):563–570, 1994.

18. Sorajja P, Chareonthaitawee P, Rajagopalan P, et al. Improved survival in asymptomatic diabetic patients with high-risk Spect imaging treated with coronary artery bypass grafting. *Circulation.* **112**(9 Suppl):I311–I316, 2005.

19. Trial of invasive versus medical therapy in elderly patients with chronic symptomatic coronary-artery disease (TIME): a randomised trial. *Lancet.* **358**(9286):951–957, 2001.

20. Boden WE, O'Rourke RA, Teo KK, et al. Optimal medical therapy with or without PCI for stable coronary artery disease. *NEJM* **356**:1503–1516, 2007.

21. Influence of diabetes on 5-year mortality and morbidity in a randomized trial comparing CABG and PTCA in patients with multivessel disease: the Bypass Angioplasty Revascularization Investigation (BARI). *Circulation.* **96**(6):1761–1769, 1997.

22. Hlatky MA, et al. Coronary artery bypass surgery compared with percutaneous coronary interventions for multivessel disease: a collaborative analysis of individual patient data from ten randomised trials. *Lancet.* **373**(9670):1190–1197, 2009.

23. Hannan EL, Racz MJ, Walford, et al. Long-term outcomes of coronary-artery bypass grafting versus stent implantation. *NEJM.* **352**:2174, 2005.

24. BARI 2D investigators. A randomized trial of therapies for type 2 diabetes and coronary artery disease. *N Engl J Med.* **360**(24):2503–2015, 2009.

25. Sabik JF, 3rd, et al. Does location of the second internal thoracic artery graft influence outcome of coronary artery bypass grafting? *Circulation.* **118**(14):S210–S215, 2008.

26. Accord 53 van den Berghe G, et al. Intensive insulin therapy in the critically ill patients. *N Engl J Med.* **345**(19):1359–1367, 2001.

27. Furnay 55 Gandhi GY, et al. Intensive intraoperative insulin therapy versus conventional glucose management during cardiac surgery: a randomized trial. *Ann Intern Med.* **146**(4):233–243, 2007.

28. Corpus RA, George PB, et al. Optimal glycemic control is associated with a lower rate of target vessel revascularization in treated type II diabetic patients undergoing elective percutaneous coronary intervention. *J Am Coll Cardiol.* **43**:8–14, 2004.

29. Gaede P. et al. Multifactorial intervention and cardiovascular disease in patients with type 2 diabetes. *N Engl J Med.* **348**(5):383–393, 2003.

30. American Diabetes Association. Standards of medical care in diabetes–2007. *Diabetes Care.* **30**(1):S4–S41, 2007.

Index